"Cancer is one of the leading causes of death in the U.S. and most conventional treatments are tragically ineffective and counterproductive. Defeat Cancer is a highly useful resource that provides insights from some of the leading natural medicine cancer experts. If you or a loved one are challenged with cancer, this book will provide you with a valuable perspective that you will likely not hear from your oncologists."

—Dr. Joseph M. Mercola, DO
Founder, Mercola.com
World's Most Visited Natural Health Site

"I have practiced medicine for 53 years, and a world without cancer is possible NOW. This book is a must-read and belongs in the hands of anyone who is affected by cancer."

—Garry F. Gordon, MD, DO, MD(H)
Coordinator of the Kobayashi Cancer Study
GordonResearch.com

"Defeat Cancer is a superb compilation of rarely discussed approaches to treating cancer using integrative therapies. If I were diagnosed with cancer, Defeat Cancer would be a must-have resource. I'd read every chapter until I found the doctor that resonated with me the most strongly. Then, I'd make an appointment and start my journey back to better health the very next day."

—Scott Forsgren
Founder & Editor
BetterHealthGuy.com

"I wish this book had been available to me twelve years ago when I was first diagnosed with cancer. Without exception, due to their passion, dedication, intelligence and courage, the doctors portrayed in this book are all true healers. I consider them to be intrepid fellow explorers, who are seeking to find help and comfort for their patients."

—Richard M. Linchitz, MD, Glen Cove, NY
Founder and Medical Director, Linchitz Medical Wellness
Glen Cove, NY

"Here are well-experienced physicians you can 'interview' by reading their philosophy and approach. Cancer does not have to be a death sentence, even late stage. Please read and study the information in this book. You do have many wonderful and often effective alternatives to conventional 'slash, burn and poison' cancer therapy."

—Robert Jay Rowen, MD
Editor-in-Chief
Second Opinion Newsletter, SecondOpinionNewsletter.com
(707) 578-7787

Defeat Cancer

15 Doctors of Integrative & Naturopathic Medicine Tell You How

Defeat Cancer

15 Doctors of Integrative & Naturopathic Medicine Tell You How

Written By
Connie Strasheim

Forewords By
Richard Linchitz, MD
Robert Rowen, MD

Edited by Robin McCully

BioMed Publishing Group
www.CancerBookSource.com

BioMed Publishing Group
P.O. Box 550531
South Lake Tahoe, CA 96155
www.BioMedPublishers.com

Copyright 2011 by Connie Strasheim.
ISBN 13: 978-0-9825138-2-8

Disclaimer

This book is not intended as medical advice. It is also not intended to prevent, diagnose, treat or cure disease. Instead, the book is intended only to share the research and opinions of the included interviewees, as well as that of author Connie Strasheim. The book is provided for informational and educational purposes only, not as treatment instructions for any disease. Much of the book is a statement of opinion in areas where the facts are controversial or do not exist. The information in this book should not be considered any more valid than any other type of informal opinion.

The physicians and health care providers who appear in this book were interviewed under informal circumstances and their statements herein do not necessarily represent their professional opinions.

The book was not written to replace the advice or care of a qualified health care professional. Be sure to check with your own qualified health care provider before beginning any protocols or procedures discussed in this book, or before stopping or altering any diet, lifestyle, or other therapies previously recommended to you by your health care provider.

Cancer treatment is a complex topic and this book should not be regarded as the final word on cancer care. The book should be viewed only as an unsubstantiated piece of literary work. The statements in this book have not been evaluated by the FDA.

Acknowledgements

To my publisher, Bryan: Thank you for being so patient with me during the long and grueling process of writing this book, and for being my best cheerleader and encouraging me with your brilliant ideas and optimism.

To Scott Forsgren and Robin McCully: Thank you for providing thoughtful and wise editing suggestions.

To the doctors of this book: Thank you for investing so much time and energy into interviewing and editing your chapters. I know you are busy, and I am grateful that you squeezed this project into your already heinous schedules. I believe that the priceless information you provided will help thousands. May the blessing come back to you tenfold.

To my friends and family: Thank you for always supporting me in my work, with words of wisdom and encouragement. May God reward you richly for the honor and love you have shown me.

And to my best friend, mentor and Savior, Jesus Christ: Thank you for providing me with wisdom and discernment during this project. For redeeming my life from the grave after nearly a decade of chronic illness, and for joy and peace, in this world and in the hereafter.

Dedication

To all the brave cancer doctors who daily put it all on the line to help their patients. Your selfless actions are truly embodied by the Hippocratic Oath:

"Whatever houses I may visit, I will come for the benefit of the sick, remaining free of all intentional injustices ..."

Also by Connie Strasheim

The Lyme Disease Survival Guide: Physical, Lifestyle,
and Emotional Strategies for Healing

Insights Into Lyme Disease Treatment: 13 Lyme-Literate Health Care
Practitioners Share Their Healing Strategies

*Available from **www.BioMedPublishers.com**
and **www.LymeInsights.com***

Healing Chronic Illness: By His Spirit, Through His Resources

*Available from **www.HealingChronicIllness.org***

Table of Contents

CHAPTER 6: Elio Martin Rivera Celaya, MD, with Steven Hines

CHAPTER 8: Robert Eslinger, DO, HMD 223

CHAPTER 10: Julian Kenyon, MD, MB, ChB 271

CHAPTER 11: Constantine A. Kotsanis, MD 293

CHAPTER 12: Joe Brown, NMD 311

Foreword by Richard Linchitz, MD

I wish this book had been available to me twelve years ago when I was first diagnosed with cancer. I am a medical doctor, and at that time, I was the director of a busy multi-specialty pain management program in Long Island, New York. I was also athletic, and had competed in many triathlons, swim events, and cycling/running races. Although I had never smoked in my life, I was diagnosed with an aggressive form of lung cancer. My cancer specialist told me that the five-year survival rate for this type of cancer was 55 percent, but I subsequently found out that it was more like 25 percent. To say I was shocked was an understatement! I wondered how this could happen to me. I thought I was the healthiest person in the world and immune to this kind of problem. It was a rude awakening, but it sent me on a fervent quest to find a cure.

I spent days and nights on the Internet, searching for the latest and best treatments for my condition. I visited all of the so-called "experts," but they all offered the same solution: chemotherapy. However, my research suggested that chemotherapy might only prolong my life for a month or two, and would leave me with a poor quality of life from the moment I began treatment. I felt there had to be a better way. I was determined to keep an open mind when I started looking at so-called "alternative" treatments, which we now more properly know as integrative medicine.

I was trained in traditional medicine at Cornell University Medical College, which is affiliated with the famous Memorial Sloan-Kettering Cancer Center. While Memorial Sloan-Kettering is known as a world-class cancer center, the doctors there could only offer me the same unsatisfactory treatments as everyone else. So I decided to look beyond mainstream medical research. After searching extensively, I began to realize that there was widespread information on effective cancer treatments in alternative, complementary and integrative medicine, but this information isn't usually published in the mainstream medical or specialty journals that we (doctors) are all expected to read.

We must go beyond these journals and the handouts that we receive from pharmaceutical company sales representatives, but it requires real effort. We must look at small, independent studies and apply logic in evaluating them, to help us understand how these findings might help our patients. We must look for the causes of disease and deal with those, rather than focus solely on symptom management, an unfortunate reality of pharmaceutically-based medicine. We must be willing to try new approaches, as long as we believe that what we do will not harm the patient, which is the first principle of medicine. It is this quest that led me to found Linchitz Medical Wellness, in Glen Cove, New York. The doctors who work at my center treat all types of medical conditions; however, my portion of the practice is devoted exclusively to cancer patients.

As I read *Defeat Cancer* I was struck by the fact that all of the doctors demonstrated incredible courage to face disapproval, and sometimes, outright attacks from mainstream medicine. In this regard, Stanislaw Burzynski, MD, is almost in a class by himself. He has probably been the most persecuted and prosecuted doctor in the modern history of "alternative" medicine. He faced fourteen years of attacks by the FDA and conventional doctors, and spent millions of dollars before he finally prevailed. The FDA is now finally cooperating with him in his study of antineoplastons, but still prohibits him from using them as he sees fit, outside of clinical trials. Many of the doctors featured in the book still face ridicule and condemnation by conventional doctors. Try to imagine what could motivate an intelligent, well-trained doctor, who could have easily succeeded in a conventional practice, to step outside of mainstream medicine and face criticism, and even sanctions on his work, in order to pursue a different path. What motivated him and the other doctors in this book is a passion for truth!

Mainstream medicine concentrates on what is often called "evidence-based" medicine. This term suggests that all of what is done in mainstream medicine is based upon rigorous studies. In evidence-based medicine, the "gold standard" for testing the effectiveness of different treatments is the double-blind, placebo-controlled trial, which involves the participation of hundreds or thousands of patients. After a rigorous mathematical analysis of the results of a trial, researchers look for "statistically significant" evidence, which can be defined as evidence that is different from what may be expected as a result of pure chance. Thus, even small benefits that patients experience as a result of different treatments are noted as statistically significant. Therefore, those treatments become valid options for use in clinical practice, but they may not, in fact, be all that effective, as you will see in the next few paragraphs.

There are several problems with this so-called "evidence-based" medicine:

- The first problem is that pharmaceutical companies control the publication of these studies, which is a well-documented reality. These companies can sponsor, or pay for, a dozen studies, in exchange for having the last word on whether these studies ever get published. In this way, a study that shows favorable results for a particular drug will never be overshadowed by another eleven studies which have negative outcomes, because the negative studies never get published.

- The next problem is that conventional medicine and peer-reviewed medical journals only seem to respect and focus on the large, expensive, pharmaceutically-sponsored trials. The careful and thoughtful observations of dedicated practitioners and their clinical outcomes with patients are dismissed as "anecdotal evidence." Yet it is just such anecdotal evidence that led to Louis Pasteur, MD's, discovery of the rabies vaccine, or James Lind,

MD's, discovery of the fact that citrus fruit can cure scurvy. Dr. Lind did an experiment on twelve people with scurvy and found that cures only occurred in those to whom he gave citrus fruit. Unfortunately, his recommendations weren't implemented for decades, during which time thousands of people died from scurvy. This private practitioner could have never afforded to do a large scale, double-blind, placebo-controlled trial. Only large pharmaceutical companies can afford to pay for this gold standard type of testing. What's more, pharmaceutical companies would never pay for studies on treatments such as herbs and supplements, because herbs and supplements can't be patented; therefore, no profits can be generated from them.

- Another problem with this evidence-based approach is that it focuses on large groups, rather than individuals. It seeks to find the common denominator among people, while ignoring their unique biochemical differences. For example, suppose a treatment works 100 percent of the time, but only on one or two people in a thousand within a particular study. Usually, with such results, the treatment would be completely dismissed as a statistical aberration; meaning, the results would be assumed to be due to chance, rather than an important finding that applies only to a certain segment of the population. On the other hand, in the clinical environment, some dedicated practitioners who decide to use the treatment might note positive results in their patients, and so would continue to offer it to those who met specific criteria, even though the therapy had been disproven by the gold standard. All of the doctors featured in this book focus on the individual patient and eschew the one-size-fits-all approach.

- The last, and perhaps most unfortunate, result of the so-called evidence based approach is its attempt to factor out the influence of the practitioner when determining the effectiveness of certain treatments. In double-blind studies, both the patient and practitioner are "blind" to whether or not the patients, or the study subjects, are getting placebo (fake) or real treatments. The reason studies are conducted this way is to try to eliminate the effects that patients' and practitioners' expectations and beliefs might have on the outcome of the study. However, over the centuries, the greatest healers have been great healers precisely *because* of their ability to influence their patients' expectations and beliefs. To eliminate this factor from consideration during studies is to ignore a potentially powerful healing force.

Without exception, due to their passion, dedication, intelligence and courage, the doctors portrayed in this book are all healers. I know some of them personally through our mutual membership in professional organizations and attendance at meetings, as well as through patient discussions. Others I've read about over the years in my quest to find a better way to treat my patients, as well as myself (during my own cancer ordeal). Still others were first introduced to me through the pages of this book. I consider them all to be intrepid fellow explorers, who are seeking to find help and comfort for their patients. Their patients are also fellow explorers, displaying even greater courage, through their willingness to look for and find better, more humane ways to deal with the cruel disease that we call cancer.

Richard M. Linchitz, MD, Glen Cove, NY

- *Founder and Medical Director, Linchitz Medical Wellness, Glen Cove, NY*
- *Chairman, Integrative Medicine Consortium*
- *Board of Directors, American College for Advancement in Medicine*
- *Board of Directors and Secretary, International College of Integrative Medicine*
- *Board of Directors and Scientific Advisory Board, International Association of IPT Physicians*
- *Certified Trainer for IPT*
- *Board of Directors, Best Answer for Cancer Foundation*
- *Board Certified, American Board of Psychiatry and Neurology, American Board of Integrative Holistic Medicine, American Academy Anti-Aging Medicine, American Academy of Medical Acupuncture, Certified Chelation Practitioner*

Foreword by Robert Jay Rowen, MD

Nothing strikes fear into a person more than sitting in front of the doctor and hearing the word "cancer." All of a sudden, everything goes blank and your mortality stares you in the face. And immediately, you are hustled in to one, two, or all of three "therapies" (slash, burn and poison) seemingly at the speed of light, with dire warnings to act quickly or face death. Sadly, most Americans submit, due to abject fear.

Look at the persons to your right, or left. Statistically, one of them will be struck with cancer. The treatment is an industry, and its politics are gruesome. In California, for example, it is a crime to treat cancer with anything other than the aforementioned "therapies" to "protect" you, the consumer. Yet there is a Catch-22. A cure has never been reported for these gruesome treatments for stage 4 cancer, except for a few limited tumors like testicular or some blood dyscrasias. At best, they extend life by a few weeks or months but at a horrific cost to your bank account and worse to your quality of life.

The pundits will scream, "Early detection saves lives," but by the time a cancer is detectable, almost 100 percent of people have circulating cancer cells in their bloodstream. Hence, it's really a joke to cut the tumor out, and an absolute lie for the surgeon to say "We got it all." (Johnson and Johnson is developing a blood test which detects cancer cells in the bloodstream as this book is printed). Cut it out? What happens when you cut a section of mold off a piece of cheese? In a few days three more mold spots appear. Cancer behaves no differently. It's usually just a matter of time before micro metastases or circulating cancer cells manifest into new tumors. Interestingly, about twenty percent of many cancers are destined to go nowhere even if not treated at all. Could the apparent "cures" of these early excisions be nothing more than a reflection of tumors that were destined to be contained by a functioning immune system? I personally think so!

The only answer to cancer is prevention. But, that, too, is difficult. We are so awash in a sea of poisons that even unborn babies are marinating in up to 200 different man made toxic chemicals. Our foods are sprayed with them. Monsanto is condemning us to GMO Frankenfood with the blessing and protection of our own government. Our soils are depleted of minerals and the Standard American Diet (SAD) makes all but a few of us dangerously nutritionally depleted. Most all of us are at risk of eventually hearing the "C" word.

A Canadian survey of oncologists found that few oncologists, if any, would take their own potions. In my 22 years in Alaska, I knew of one oncologist who clandestinely flew to Mexico for treatment rather than submit to chemo. You don't need to go to Mexico. There are brave American physicians who are thinking outside of the box and, in some cases, risking their necks to bring you less toxic or even non-toxic treatments. A century ago, doctors were injecting pancreatic enzymes and inducing remissions. In my 22 years in Alaska, I met several people "cured" by the pioneering work of Dr. William Donald Kelley (a dentist no less!) who simply changed their diets, provided them with enzymes orally, and detoxified them. You'll read about that treatment, among others, in this book.

Successful cancer treatment doesn't have to be expensive, either. Decades ago, Max Gerson, MD, documented scores of cures with diet and juicing alone. I've had several patients go into remission with just diet, supplements and detox strategies. But cancer is a lifelong treatment. It represents a failure of the immune system. Once a cancer patient, always a cancer patient. Two such women with stage four breast cancer who went into total remission felt that they had beat the disease and jumped off the diet wagon a few years later. Shortly afterward, their cancers returned with a vengeance.

The cancers of today are not the same as just two generations ago, in Gerson's day. We are far more toxic and nutritionally depleted. Our stresses are far higher. All these impair the ultimate killer of cancer—your immune system. While some patients might respond to simple measures, others may require more intensive treatment to reduce their tumor burden while supporting the immune system. The questions become "what therapies to do?" and "who to go to?"

This book may provide you the answer. Here are well-experienced physicians you can "interview" by reading their philosophy and approach. There is no "one size fits all" as there seemingly is in orthodox medicine. I like it when patients come to me having done a lot of personal research and "homework," prepared with lots of questions about approaches, whether they have cancer or other challenges. Your choices are not limited to just the handful of therapists in this book. Quite possibly there are integrative physicians near you who employ methods you'll read about shortly.

Cancer, even late stage, does not have to be a death sentence. I recently saw a 76-year-old Indian swami with cancer encircling his cecum (colon) with huge metastases (11 and 9 cm) in his liver. He looked terminal when he barely could cross the threshold into my office on his own power. Within three months, his tumors had shrunk 75 percent, his liver function returned to normal, and he was back at work full time in his spiritual duties. No toxic therapies were applied, only immune support (oral and IV). Though still bearing a tumor, he is still alive and functioning normally fifteen months after first coming to my office.

Please read and study the information in this book. You do have many wonderful and often effective alternatives to "slash, burn and poison."

Robert Jay Rowen, MD
Editor-in-Chief, Second Opinion Newsletter
www.secondopinionnewsletter.com
Phone: (707) 578-7787

Preface by Connie Strasheim

Cancer is an elusive, complex, and difficult disease to treat. Unfortunately, medical politics and pharmaceutical interests have added to this complexity by heavily influencing the kinds of treatments available to people with cancer. Conventional treatments, such as chemotherapy, radiation, and surgery, are usually the only options offered to cancer patients, but they aren't always effective.

Fortunately, integrative, naturopathic, and other types of "alternative" medicine frequently offer more effective solutions, which have been proven in clinical outcomes studies and in doctors' experiences with their patients. I put the word alternative in quotes because I believe that labeling non-conventional treatments as such is to assign them an undeserved inferior status.

In this book, a wide variety of treatments are described, all of which have effectively helped many cancer patients live long, productive lives. The physicians in this book practice integrative medicine, which takes the best of conventional, naturopathic, and other medical disciplines such as Traditional Chinese Medicine (TCM) and homeopathy, to formulate protocols that treat the underlying cause of disease, rather than just its symptoms. These doctors share the goal of treating their patients with whatever works, regardless of medical politics or other non-beneficial influences.

While conventional medicine has proven to be useful for treating a handful of cancers, for most types of cancer, its track record has been dismal. Dr. Robert Eslinger, DO, one of the doctors who participated in this book states that, "From 1990-2004, over 150,000 people with all types of cancer were studied, and it was found that only 2.1 percent of them were still alive after five years. All had done full dose chemotherapy." (Journal of Clinical Oncology, 2004) Eslinger adds that more than 250 billion dollars have been spent on cancer research over the past 60 years, and yet, the cure rate for cancer hasn't improved much since 1950.

In my interviews with the fifteen physicians in this book, I learned that conventional treatments for cancer have their place, but are useful only for certain types of cancer, are often inappropriately prescribed, and are inadequate in the absence of a holistic approach that includes botanicals, dietary modifications, and other therapies which augment the effects of anti-neoplastic (anti-cancer) therapies.

The physician participants in this book have discovered better, and in some cases, incredibly effective ways to heal the body from cancer, without weakening the immune system and producing the same side effects as most conventional treatments. Research studies have proven their success, as have the doctors' clinical experiences with them. Unfortunately, the American Medical Association (AMA), FDA, and associated organizations don't recognize clinical outcomes (or patient experiences) as valid indicators of a treatment's effectiveness. Double-blind, placebo-controlled studies are valued over the actual results that doctors get with their patients. Whenever front-line, practical studies have been conducted in doctors' offices to evaluate alternative treatments, their results have often been disregarded and trivialized by the medical establishment.

In writing this book, I didn't intend to address cancer politics, but I quickly learned that it's impossible to talk about cancer without mentioning the politics behind it, because politics have limited people's access to beneficial treatments and brainwashed much of society into thinking that full-dose chemotherapy, radiation, and surgery are the only effective treatments for cancer, when in reality, there are safer, better alternatives for many people. People often don't know about these alternatives unless they research them, because they aren't actively promoted by the FDA, AMA, insurance and pharmaceutical companies, or the media, which is heavily subsidized by the pharmaceutical industry. However, the doctors in this book, as well as their patients, will attest to the fact that these treatments have been used by thousands of people, and that they work. Patient success stories can be found on the doctors' websites, and elsewhere. The purpose of this book is to help people with cancer access important information that would otherwise be difficult to find.

Politics aside, those who read this book will find a wealth of information on cancer treatments that have either successfully put many people's cancers, even terminal cancers, into remission, or have allowed patients to live functional lives for many years, even though tumors may still be present in their bodies. Advances in medicine have transformed many kinds of cancer from a terminal disease into a malady that can either be cured or managed successfully for years, like other non-fatal chronic illnesses.

It may seem improbable that a person could live for years or decades with a tumor present in the body and yet not have symptoms. Nevertheless, some doctors, such as those found in this book, are accomplishing that with their patients. Of course, these doctors are also putting many cancers into remission. In both cases, their outcomes are far more positive than what is typically seen in conventional medicine.

A plethora of treatments are described in this book, from Insulin Potentiation Therapy (IPT) to gene-targeted therapies, pancreatic enzymes, mistletoe, dendritic cell vaccines, nutrients, botanicals, and other proven therapies. No one doctor's protocol is exactly like another's, and by studying the similarities and differences among them, readers may find it easier to discern the treatments that may or may not work for them.

A multitude of alternative cancer treatments are promoted on the Internet, in support groups, books, and elsewhere, and it can be challenging for the average person to know which treatments to pursue. My goal in writing this book has been to diffuse some of the confusion by presenting options that have worked for many people, based on the authoritative clinical experience of licensed doctors, rather than anonymous Internet websites. You may feel over-whelmed by the tremendous amount of information contained herein, so I suggest that you highlight those sections that seem most beneficial or relevant to you, and take note of the treatments that are mentioned multiple times throughout the book. Chances are, if several doctors are using the treatment, it's because it has worked for many people. The opportunity to make comparisons between alternative treatments based on different doctors' percep-tions is one of the benefits of this book.

As a survivor of chronic Lyme disease who was severely disabled by symptoms for more than seven years, I have learned that similari-ties exist between Lyme disease and cancer. People with these diseases must do more than just take a drug or receive six rounds of an intravenous treatment to get well. The desire to get well power-fully influences healing, as do people's beliefs and emotional support systems, attitudes, diets, daily habits, and nutritional protocols, in addition to other factors. While this book describes medical treatments for cancer, it also discusses other factors that influence healing. This is to provide a comprehensive perspective on attaining and maintaining health, so that the factors which caused people to be sick in the first place are minimized or eradi-cated from their lives. The importance of a holistic approach to healing, which takes into consideration all aspects of a person's life and biochemistry, shouldn't be underestimated.

I am not the author of the information in this book. The authors are the fifteen doctors who agreed to devote their time and energy to interview with me and then revise their interviews several times after I transcribed and re-wrote them. I have provided medical definitions and clarified the doctors' perspectives throughout the book, but only in a grammatical sense, so that the information would read like a book, rather than a conversation, and readers would fully understand the doctors' information and the medical concepts contained herein. I have done my best to act as a conduit of information between the doctors and my readers. This book, if I have done my job, should get readers as close as possible to a face-to-face conversation with these doctors.

Yet, because the information has been taken from my conversations with the doctors, it won't read exactly like a textbook or any other type of medical book. In fact, readers may notice that my writing style differs somewhat from chapter to chapter, according to the doctors' manner of expression and how they shared information with me. Maintaining these stylistic differences was necessary and desirable in order to preserve their information.

Also, the information is intended to provide an overview of each doctor's treatment approach, rather than an in-depth dissertation on every aspect of their protocols. A highly detailed explanation of each doctor's protocol would have required that a separate book be written for each doctor. Having suffered from a chronic disease myself, I understand the value of obtaining a bird's-eye view of a complex topic, and this book was written partly for that reason. Those who want to learn more about a specific type of treatment can do further research on their own. I believe that readers will find that the book offers an informative and comprehensive overview of the best cancer treatments available in integrative medicine. These provide a solid foundation upon which to conduct more detailed research.

Finally, while each doctor who participated in this work provided a unique viewpoint, I noticed two common themes in all of the chapters. First, there is no such thing as a "one-size-fits-all" treatment for cancer in integrative medicine. "Cookie cutter" protocols don't work for most patients. Every patient is unique and requires an individualized, customized treatment approach. Second, healing from cancer isn't just about eradicating tumors and cancer cells. It's about addressing the multiple systemic dysfunctions and factors which caused the cancer to establish a foothold in the body in the first place. It's about healing the immune system, removing toxicity from the body, establishing healthier habits, balancing hormones, replenishing nutrients, healing past trauma (emotional and physical), and dealing with various other problems, biochemical and otherwise.

May this book provide you, the person with cancer, hope, healing, and the prospect of better days ahead, and may it provide you, the cancer doctor, with new and innovative ways of treating your patients. And to everyone else who picks up this book, may it enable you to better understand the disease that we call cancer, so that you may know how to prevent it in your own life, and better support others in their quest for healing.

A Note from the Publisher

This book contains a tremendous amount of information, and readers may become overwhelmed if they are not prepared to assimilate it.

While reading the book, you are encouraged to employ an "information organization strategy," so that you can keep track of the information that is most relevant and important to you. It is recommended that you have at your side a highlighter marker and a notepad. You can use the highlighter to mark information that you feel is important, and that you wish to return to in the future. You can use the notepad to write down the names of treatments, tests, or procedures that you want to integrate into your treatment plan or discuss with your doctor.

• CHAPTER 1 •

Stanislaw R. Burzynski, MD, PhD
HOUSTON, TX

Biography

Stanislaw R. Burzynski, MD, PhD, is an internationally-recognized physician and biochemist-researcher who has pioneered the development and use of biologically active peptides for diagnosing, preventing, and treating cancer since 1967.

In 1967, at the young age of 24, he graduated with distinction from the Medical Academy in Lublin, Poland with an MD degree, finishing first in his class of 250. During the same year, he identified naturally-occurring peptides in the human body which he concluded controlled cancer growth. He found that there is a marked deficiency of these peptides in cancer patients.

The following year, in 1968, he earned his PhD in Biochemistry and became one of the youngest candidates in Poland to ever hold both an MD and PhD degree.

From 1970 to 1977, while a researcher and Assistant Professor at Baylor College of Medicine in Houston, his research was sponsored and partially funded by the National Cancer Institute. At Baylor, he authored and co-authored sixteen publications. Five concerned his research on peptides and their effect on human cancer, and four others were co-authored by other doctors associated with MD Anderson Hospital and Tumor Institute and Baylor College of Medicine. It was at Baylor that he named these peptides "antineoplastons" due to their activity in correcting and normalizing neoplastic or cancerous cells.

In May 1977, Dr. Burzynski received a Certificate of Appreciation from Baylor College of Medicine, commending him for five years of dedicated service to the college and acknowledging him for the contributions that he made to the "advancement of medical education, research, and health care."

That same month, Dr. Burzynski founded his clinic in Houston, where he has since treated over 15,000 patients. He is also President of the Burzynski Research Institute, where he continues to pursue scientific research on antineoplastons.

Dr. Burzynski is a member in good standing of many renowned medical associations, including the American and World Medical Associations, American Association for Cancer Research, Society for Neuroscience, Texas Medical Association, Royal Medical Association (U.K.), and the Society for Neuro-Oncology.

Dr. Burzynski is the author and co-author of over 300 scientific publications and presentations. Throughout his career, he has received numerous prestigious awards from various medical, educational, and governmental institutions. As of January 2007, he holds 242 patents related to proprietary scientific inventions.

Other groups of scientists have expanded Dr. Burzynski's work, including researchers at the University of Kurume Medical School in Japan. Several hundred publications on antineoplastons and their active ingredients have been written by scientists who work independently of the Burzynski Research Institute.

What Cancer Is, What Causes It, and How to Treat It

Cancer can be defined as the uncontrolled growth of abnormal cells, which is caused by cancer genomes (a *genome* is all the genetic material contained in an organism, including its DNA, or deoxyribonucleic acid). The cancer genome is a special combination of genes which conspires to produce cells that successfully compete for survival with normal cells of the body, and which are able to survive better than these normal cells. Scientists have now identified genomes for about 100 different types of cancer, so they can tell how many genes are abnormal in various types of cancers and what those specific genes are. Modern scientists are finally accepting that it's the abnormal, malignant genomes which cause cancer and that these genomes are more complex than normal genomes. Cancer genomes are very complicated and there is much we have yet to understand about them. There are multiple factors which cause abnormal genomes to develop, but it's a very difficult task to try to identify what all of these are.

Regardless of the factors that trigger the development of cancer, in order to effectively treat it, doctors must identify and then control the abnormal genes that are causing it. This is a very difficult task, since the average cancer has about 80 abnormal genes but can have over 500 abnormal genes. The average number of abnormal genes involved in most people's cancers ranges from 40 to 200. These abnormal genes hijack and suffocate a much larger number of normal genes—approximately 600-1,000.

In addition to normal genes, the body also has silent genes; that is, genes that have been switched off (by environmental and other factors), and which no longer help the body to protect itself against cancer. Turning these silent tumor-suppressor genes back on again is very important for defeating cancer.

So, controlling gene expression is a complex task, made even more difficult by the fact that the 80 or so abnormal genes that cause cancer can end up creating a deregulated network of over 3,000 genes in the body—all of which cause and spread malignant disease.

The Role of Antineoplastons in Controlling Cancer Cells

Two things must be done in order to control abnormal genes. First, the genes which cause cancer cells to grow in the body, called oncogenes, must be turned off. Second, the genes which fight cancer, called tumor-suppressor genes, must be turned on. In order to accomplish these goals, molecular switches must be used. As an analogy, consider a switchboard that has different switches for turning on and off a piece of machinery. You can turn off certain switches to make the machinery stop, and turn on other switches to turn it back on.

The human body has similar molecular switches, some of which turn off oncogenes, and others which turn on tumor-suppressor genes. These switches are called antineoplastons, which are naturally occurring peptides and amino acid derivatives in the blood and urine that the human body naturally uses to control cancer growth. They comprise a biochemical defense system that controls cancer without destroying normal cells. The name "antineoplastons" comes from their function in controlling neoplastic or cancerous cells: i.e., anti-neoplastic cell agents.

Hence, treating cancer involves using biochemically synthesized antineoplastons that will both turn off the activity of the genes which cause cancer and turn on the activity of genes which suppress cancer.

Since the function of antineoplastons is to bring gene activity to a normal level, they affect only abnormal genes in the body. They turn off the genes which are hyperactive and turn on the genes which are inactive. They do nothing in normal cells, because the activity of a normal cell doesn't need to be affected. As an analogy, suppose that you need to adjust the temperature in various rooms of your house. You turn up the thermostat in the rooms that are too cold, and you turn it down in the rooms that are too warm. The too-hot and too-cold rooms represent the body's abnormal cells, and the thermostat represents the antineoplastons, which either turn up the temperature or turn it down (or turn off hyperactive genes and turn on silent genes). The room where the temperature is normal represents the normal cell that isn't affected by antineoplastons.

How I Discovered Antineoplastons

I discovered antineoplastons a long time ago, in 1967, when I was a medical student. In addition to being a medical doctor, I am also a chemist. Through my research as a chemist, I discovered that cancer patients had a deficiency of certain peptides in their blood; peptides which we all have and which protect our bodies against cancer. I isolated these peptides and tested them together with scientists at the MD Anderson Cancer Center and learned that many of them would kill malignant cancer cells, but not harm normal cells. After isolating the peptides, I characterized their chemical structure and reproduced them synthetically (in the typical manner that all pharmaceutical agents are developed for use on cancer patients). Thus began my work with antineoplastons.

Using Antineoplastons and Gene-Targeted Therapy to Treat Cancer

At my clinic, my fellow doctors and I have been given permission by the FDA to use antineoplastons, mostly in clinical trials. The anti-neoplastons we use in these trials affect approximately 100 different genes which have been instrumental in the formation of our patients' cancers. I have discovered that if I can turn off around 100 genes which are causing a cancer to grow, then I can stop the growth of that cancer, or even eliminate it. To achieve this in our patients, we must determine the proper combination of genes for each one.

The entire world is moving in the direction of gene-targeted thera-py for cancer treatment by creating its own gene-targeted therapies. However, the current gene targeted therapies on the market are quite primitive: most, like Avastin, only work by affecting a single gene. So while these therapies can work for awhile, they are insufficient for treating cancer because cancer has a gene-signaling network of thousands of genes (on average 2,400) and will eventually overcome the effects of any therapy that is targeted to affect only one of its genes. At our clinic, we are really a decade or two ahead of others who use gene-targeted therapy because our medications (antineoplastons) work on close to 100 different genes and are comprised of naturally-occurring chemicals that don't harm the patient's body, unlike other gene-targeted therapies which often have adverse effects upon normal cells.

If doctors use a therapy that works on just one gene (the targeted gene is typically called the "driver" oncogene), then it's possible for their patients' tumors to shrink. Unfortunately, those tumors will eventually find a way to subvert that gene. Also, there are about twelve main gene signaling pathways in cancer (gene signaling is part of a complex system of communication that governs cellular activity and which coordinates cell action), which means that, in order for gene therapy to work, doctors must influence not only single genes, but their entire pathways, which are also comprised of numerous genes. And that's still not the end of the story! In addition to this challenge, they must get rid of their patients' malignant stem cells, which multiply and produce new cancer cells. Further complicating matters is the fact that these malignant stem cells are practically immortal. So treatment requires finding special combinations of antineoplastons that will also influence the gene signaling pathways and kill malignant stem cells without harming normal stem cells. Once doctors are able to do this, then their patients can be cured.

At our clinic, we have antineoplastic medications that address all of these areas. Nevertheless, every one of our patients is different, and because cancer can alter its DNA, we are always working with a moving target. Currently, scientists have discovered that there can be up to 3,152 different abnormal genes in cancer, and that count will increase over the next year or two as they continue to discover new genes. My average patient has approximately 80 of these, so there are a tremendous number of abnormal gene combinations which can result in a patient. Since every patient has a unique genomic signature, we can't use the same treatment for everybody.

It's important to emphasize that although patients may be diagnosed with the same type of cancer, the abnormal genes which cause their cancers will be different. We have to identify the particular genetic signature of each one of our patients and then put together the best combination of medications that will neutralize their cancer-causing genes.

Treatment Process

Before new patients come to our clinic, we review their medical records to make sure that we can treat them. Many people come here from other states and countries and we don't want them to travel long distances if we are unable to help them. That's the first step in our assessment process. Then we do an initial consultation, and after that, we're usually able to start them on a treatment regimen. We also collaborate with their local doctors, since they will ultimately do most of our treatments at home. After they have been on a regimen for two or three months, we may then ask them to come back to the clinic for a day so we can make any necessary adjustments to their treatment plans. We try to get their oncologists to cooperate with us, so they can also work together with them on this.

Our initial consultation involves testing the cancer cells in the blood, the results of which enable us to determine the activity of our patients' most important oncogenes. We are usually able to get the information we need from these tests in just two days, and can begin treatments soon thereafter. In some cases, though, we need to revise patients' treatments after further testing of their specimens.

Doing a tumor biopsy is a good way to get a sample of a patient's cancer cells, but it takes a few weeks to get biopsy results back. I would prefer to do biopsies over blood tests, but they aren't practical because most of our patients need treatment right away. In any case, blood tests can sometimes be more useful than biopsies, because in metastatic cancer, every tumor in the body has a different genome. Taking a sample from one tumor won't necessarily tell us what's going on in the rest of the body and how to treat the other tumors.

Eventually though, we try to take a biopsy of the entire cancerous genome in all of our patients and we conduct tests of the proteins that are produced by the most important oncogenes found in their blood. Both the patient and the patient's cancer must be properly profiled at the molecular level in order to specifically identify the genes and characteristics that are causing the cancer to grow.

The most sophisticated methods of gene testing involve isolating actual cancer cells from the blood instead of just studying the products of the oncogenes within the patient's blood sample. We aren't using this technology yet, but are likely to adopt it in the near future because it would allow us to test not only mature cancer cells, but also malignant stem cells, which have a different genome than the mature cells. So for the time being, we take a regular blood sample, test cancerous tissue (do a biopsy), and then test for genetic compatibility between the patient's oncogenes and our antineoplastic medications. Then we prescribe medications that we know will kill the malignant cells which carry these oncogenes.

The accurate selection of gene-targeted medications depends upon all of the following: knowledge of which medications were proven in clinical trials to work on specific cancers, results of the patient's cancer genome analysis from tissue and blood tests, knowledge of what the patient's chief cancerous genes are, access to up-to-date clinical trial algorithms for comparison and disease matching, and properly evaluating the patient in order to determine the correct disease-stage diagnosis. Our clinic is currently working on a computer program which will automatically perform these required tasks. We anticipate that this new software will be ready in March 2011. Our database is updated daily and information from our database will be utilized by the new program.

As previously mentioned, we use a combination of medications that will target approximately 100-200 of the patient's genes: medications that will turn off the abnormal genes that promote cancer, while also turning on the normal genes that protect against cancer. These medications are usually sufficient to get rid of the tumors in about 80 percent of our patients. These are people who were told by conventional oncologists that nothing else could be done for them. For the remaining 20 percent of our patients, the treatment doesn't work and we have to do a genetic analysis again to try to come up with a different combination of medications for them. Sometimes, our treatments don't work because cancers continuously mutate and two months down the road, a cancer genome may look completely different than when the patient was first tested.

Determining patients' genetic signatures and designing an appropriate treatment regimen for them takes a lot of experience and practice. We must find medications which work well together and do not counteract one another. If doctors who perform gene targeted therapy take the wrong approach, they can cause their patients' cancers to spread faster. Therefore, it's important they understand cancer genetics. This skill can be learned. We have found that if we treat our patients properly, then they don't suffer adverse reactions, their tumors disappear, and their cancers don't come back. If done correctly, cancer treatment should be effective, without producing adverse reactions in the body.

Types of Antineoplastic and Gene-Targeted Medications

Currently, we use three different preparations of antineoplastons at our clinic, one of which has been approved by the FDA, and two of which are in the process of being approved. Two antineoplastons are administered intravenously (IV), and one is taken orally. The oral antineoplaston is called phenylbutyrate and the two IV antineoplastons are called Antineoplaston A10 and AS2-1.

While the oral antineoplaston is FDA-approved for use in general practice, intravenously administered antineoplastons are approved only for use in clinical trials, so we tend to use the oral drugs more often, since we have more flexibility with them.

In addition to antineoplastons, we also give our patients other gene-targeted medications that have been approved by the FDA. These are different from antineoplastons because they work on different and smaller groups of genes than antineoplastons (generally only one to fourteen genes, compared to antineoplastons, which may work on as many as one hundred genes).

When prescribing a regimen for the majority of our patients, we combine phenylbutyrate with other gene-targeted medications, which we select based on the results of our patients' genomic analyses. Our approach is to treat the combination of genes that are causing cancer. When prescribing medications, we also consider the type of cancer that patients have, but this is secondary to the gene analysis.

In practice, phenylbutyrate, when dosed orally, affects a smaller number of genes than IV antineoplastons because the dosing of oral medications is markedly lower than what patients would receive via intravenous administration. We need to affect 50-200 of our patients' genes, so we give them multiple medications to accomplish this. A woman with breast cancer, for example, requires treatment for at least 60 of her genes. Oral phenylbutyrate would affect only 43 of these, so we would add other gene-targeted medications to her regimen, such as lapatinib (which works on two genes), trastuzumab (which works on only one gene) and sorafenib (which works on fourteen genes).

Of these medications, only lapatinib and trastuzumab have been approved by the FDA for the treatment of breast cancer. Sorafenib is currently approved for kidney, pancreatic, and liver cancers (but sometime during the next two years, it will probably also be approved for breast cancer). Still, we may choose to use phenylbutyrate and sorafenib "off label" to treat breast cancer, because the patient's genomic analyses might reveal them to be the most effective medications for this type of cancer. The majority of gene-targeted medications only work on a single or small number of genes.

In the end, our patients might take anywhere from three to five different medications, but the combination that we prescribe is different for everyone because the genetic signature of each person's cancer is different.

For the rest of our patients, the minority, we use the intravenous antineoplastons, which affect 94 genes and have only been approved for use in clinical trials. While use of these agents is more tightly regulated, we are able to give them to patients who have consented to participate in these trials. Typically, we administer both of our IV antineoplastons (Antineoplaston A10 and AS2-1) to patients concurrently, without adding any additional oral anti-cancer medications to their regimens, because the FDA doesn't permit us to use them in conjunction with IV therapies. This is unfortunate because clinical trials on patients undergoing antineoplaston therapy in Japan have demonstrated that a combination of intravenous and oral antineoplastons is the most effective treatment strategy.

In an ideal world, we would use intravenous antineoplastons on all of our patients, in addition to oral gene-targeted medications, because combining two intravenous antineoplastons with additional gene-targeted agents would affect approximately 200 genes. However, we aren't allowed to do this due to FDA regulations, so we work within our operating limitations and make the best of our resources.

We evaluate our patients throughout the course of their treatment by monitoring their physical condition, measuring the size of their tumors, and checking their different tumor markers, which indicate tumor activity. If we have chosen the right medications, we usually see a substantial decrease in the size of their tumors within two months, so we would then continue with those medications until their tumors are gone. Most people's tumors are completely gone within four to six months. (Although our patients only stay at our clinic for two weeks, they continue to take the medications at home while following up with their oncologists). After four to six months, we usually find no trace of cancer in their lungs, liver, or anywhere. We have even seen some tumors disappear within three to four weeks if we find the right molecular switches. When the tumor disappears and we can't find cancer anywhere in the body, we assume that the patient has had a complete response to our treatments. We then switch them to a maintenance regimen for an additional eight to twelve months to prevent their cancers from coming back, and that's the end of the story. We have patients who have been cancer free for over twenty years.

In the majority of our patients we see very good results using this approach. Oncologists can also administer this type of therapy, because there are now close to 40 different gene-targeted medications available in pharmacies which work on cancer genes. Over the next three years, it's estimated that there will be at least one hundred different medications available. If oncologists learn the proper use of such medications, they could save the lives of many more of their patients.

The Use of Antineoplastons for Other Diseases

The antineoplaston medications that we use in our clinic can also resolve numerous other problems in the body, which means that they can heal other diseases, such as Multiple Sclerosis and Lupus. We have conducted brief clinical trials on the use of antineoplastons for different autoimmune diseases and have had some interesting results. But right now, our focus remains upon using them for cancer treatment. At some point, we may expand our work into other areas of medicine.

Dietary and Supplement Recommendations

Many of our patients have been "wasted" by their cancers and previous treatments, so we have two expert nutritionists at our clinic who provide dietary and supplement recommendations to help them build up their bodies. We design intravenous nutritional protocols for some people, which they follow at the beginning of their treatments. We also design individual diets for each of our patients, because what's good for one patient isn't necessarily good for another. The specific medications they take, for example, are an important consideration when determining their dietary regimens, because medications and supplements may interact with one another.

We have also developed a line of nutritional supplements that support our antineoplaston treatments, called Aminocare (www.aminocare.com), which can reduce the side effects of medications and improve normal body functioning. These products support the immune system, increase the body's energy, protect it against toxic insults, and aid in the regulation of normal cell division.

Preventing Cancer with Supplements

Regardless of its initial causes, cancer ultimately results from a change in the genes. Treatments that target the genes eliminate cancer, as opposed to treatments that destroy the cancer and also the body. Fortunately, some nutritional supplements can also regulate gene expression and people who are vulnerable to cancer may be able to regulate the expression of their genes by using these alone and thus may not even require medication. In the future, I believe that there will be easy methods for determining whether patients have abnormalities in their genes that could lead to cancer. Then doctors will be able to make specific dietary and supplement recommendations which will restore their patients' genes to normalcy and prevent them from getting cancer.

Some of the supplements that we recommend for cancer prevention include AminoCare A10 and AminoCare Brain Longevity, which are amino acid derivatives (small molecular peptide) gel capsules that are designed to reduce the deterioration of brain function that results from the aging process. We recommend that everyone who has reached a certain age take both of these as a preventative measure against cancer. We prescribe an easy regimen that consists of taking only a few capsules per day. We also have an after-sun lotion and cosmetic cream which protect against skin damage. The company Healthy Directions distributes all of these supplements.

Detoxification

Doing detoxification therapies along with antineoplaston treatments isn't necessary, because antineoplastons stimulate the elimination of cancer waste products through the kidneys (most cancer toxins are ultimately processed through the kidneys) so they are rapidly removed from the body. Hence, patients don't suffer from toxin-induced die-off reactions.

Treatment Outcomes

Many of our patients with most types of cancer have experienced positive results whenever we give them the right combination of gene-targeted medications. We keep a long list of the various cancers our patients have had and the response rate that we have achieved with each of them. Overall, we have an up to 60 percent response rate for many types of advanced cancers, meaning, patients' tumors have disappeared or substantially decreased. This response rate applies to all common types of cancer: breast, prostate, liver, colon, lung, and others. Some cancers have a higher response rate than others, but overall, our success rate is anywhere from 40-60 percent. These statistics represent, in their majority, people who were initially given a terminal diagnosis and who came to us after conventional treatments failed them. For certain types of brain tumors, we have an over 60 percent partial or complete response rate. For malignant melanoma, we have an objective response rate of around 40 percent. In breast cancer, approximately 60 percent of our patients have an objective response rate. ("Objective" here means that patients' response to the treatment was complete, partial, mixed, or improved.) These terms are defined in greater detail on the "Comparison of Responses in (the) Most Common Cancers" chart at the end of this chapter. Perhaps one-third of our patients who have other types of cancer have a complete remission of their tumors.

In general, we have many long-term survivors because we have been using antineoplastons for a long time and have been able to track our patients over the years. Again, these are all people who once had incurable cancers and the worst types of malignancies, which historically, nobody has been able to cure. But we have been able to cure many of them, and what I mean by cure is that they have been tumor-free, for five, ten, even twenty years. They lead normal lives and nobody can tell that they ever had a cancer that was supposed to kill them within a few months.

My work represents the first time in medical history that a treatment has been able to consistently cure untreatable, inoperable tumors. Take for instance, inoperative, malignant gliomas, which are located in the brainstem. Normally, patients with this cancer are given three months to live, but we have one patient who had this malignancy and who is still alive, twenty-three years later, and who remains in perfect health. Such people took antineoplastons for a normal period of time; say, a year, or a year and a half, before they got healed and forgot about their cancers. They are now graduating from college, having families, working, and leading happy, normal lives.

I have been practicing medicine for 44 years, and I have been doing antineoplaston treatment for 34 years. We have patients who have followed up with us 27 years after having received treatment from us, and who are still doing well today. To have this kind of thing happen isn't unusual for us.

Training Other Doctors to Use Antineoplastons

I employ 130 people at my clinic, two of whom are among the country's top oncologists and previous faculty members of leading medical schools in the United States, so I don't perform this type of work by myself. The main building of our clinic is 100,000 square feet and an additional 50,000 square foot building includes large research and pharmaceutical facilities which are inspected by the FDA. It's not a small doctor's office, but more like 21 medical offices in one. I have personally trained every doctor who works here with me.

To learn how to do this kind of targeted gene therapy requires a lot of training, but any doctor who wants to learn it can join us and work at our clinic. We guide doctors in their training and they then take that newfound knowledge back home with them to their clinics.

The idea of antineoplastons is catching on, but so far, only oncologists who are the most up-to-date on cancer treatments know about them. Bernadine Healy, MD, in her article, "Breaking Cancer's Gene Code" (US News and World Report, Oct. 23, 2008), estimates that it will take about 30 years to convince the majority of them about the benefits of using combinations of gene-targeted medications. This is unfortunate, but there are a number of prominent oncologists who are starting to embrace the idea and who are interested in our work because they see the good results that we get at our clinic. We have to convert them one by one.

We have trained many doctors from other countries, as well. For instance, doctors from Japan travel here, learn how to do the treatments, and then go back home. Sometimes we send our doctors to other countries to train people. One clinic in Japan that treats patients based on our methods has done clinical trials on its patients and found that their over five-year survival rate for advanced colon cancer with liver metastasis has increased to 62 percent using antineoplaston therapy, compared to a 34 percent survival rate using traditional chemotherapy. Antineoplaston therapy is expanding into many countries as I continue to invite doctors from all over the world to come to our clinic, so that we can teach them how to do what we do, and they can learn from us.

Improving Cancer Care

I really hope that antineoplaston treatment will become popular because it can save the lives of many, and also save a lot of money for the entire United States. Current conventional treatments are expensive and patients are all given the same, standard regimens for their cancers, but these regimens only work for a small number of people. Before prescribing treatments for advanced cancers, doctors should do tests to determine whether a particular treatment would be appropriate for their patients. Patients might spend less than a thousand dollars to do some testing (ie: to determine whether a specific chemotherapeutic drug would affect their cancer), but then they (patients, insurance companies, etc.) would save thousands of dollars per month in treatments because chemotherapy medications are very expensive.

Doctors must take the time to figure out what treatments will work for their patients, because otherwise, we as a community will continue to spend trillions of dollars for nothing and patients will continue to suffer the effects of ill-prescribed medications. Doctors must direct their resources through the proper channels and identify the patients that would truly benefit from different medications. If they could do this, then more people would have access to medical care, and the overall price tag of treatment would be much lower. In the future, I believe that all doctors will be tailoring their treatments to the individual patient, instead of taking a one-size-fits-all approach to medicine. Also, I think treatments will be designed through the computer, and that technology will be able to identify the medications that turn off bad genes, as well as those that will turn on good ones.

The Problem with Conventional Oncology

Most oncologists work like robots. They give all of their patients the same treatment, but this isn't beneficial, because every patient is unique and has different needs. Early stage cancer patients may be able to avoid chemotherapy if genetic testing supports that they not do it. But it's difficult to make blanket statements about the effectiveness of different approaches to cancer because what works for one patient may not work for another.

Oncologists have been trained to believe that radiation, chemotherapy, and surgery are the only ways to treat cancer. If they realized there is another universe out there consisting of treatments that work on the genes, they might want to do them, but most of them don't even think much about these alternative treatments. They use the same, standard treatments for everyone and see their patients respond to those treatments for short periods of time before they pass away. It's a very depressing practice. Most of them don't have the slightest idea of what I do. If they do, and they try this different approach, they are sometimes portrayed as quacks or charlatans. Once they learn the truth, however, then progress can begin to happen. I believe that we just need to bring the right knowledge to them, but we must often convert them one by one.

When to Use Conventional Medicine to Treat Cancer

Chemotherapy, radiation and surgery may have a place in cancer treatment. If, for instance, a patient has a tumor that's pressing up against the vertebrae and there is an immediate risk of fracturing the vertebrae, then radiation may be appropriate. Small doses of chemotherapy may work quite well in combination with gene targeted therapy, but as a single modality for advanced cancer, chemotherapy's effects are only temporary. If we are talking about patients with metastatic disease, its effects are short-lived and it leaves people with a lot of toxicity.

Most of our patients have already done chemotherapy and other conventional treatments and failed them all, so they don't usually do such treatments during gene-targeted therapy. If they haven't yet tried it, and would like to have chemotherapy in addition to gene-targeted therapy, anyway, then we can incorporate that into their treatment plans. We would prescribe lower doses of antineoplastons, because they work synergistically with chemotherapy. In most cases, though, our patients' options are limited and their decision is simple because by the time they get to us, they have usually already had radiation and chemotherapy and failed both kinds of treatment.

Side Effects of Gene-Targeted Therapies

Some gene-targeted therapies have side effects which are associated with a rapid response to the treatment. If people respond to their medications rapidly, for instance, they may get a skin rash. It's not an allergic reaction, but simply a rash that's associated with a fast response to the treatment. Fortunately, we have invented a special cream which can decrease such reactions, so that patients are able to continue their treatments without interruption. Other patients might experience an increase in blood pressure, which we also associate as being a rapid response to the treatment, so we may put them on a diet and medications to decrease their blood pressure. Such a diet might be low in sodium, with lots of fish oil and sardines, for example. We do this so that all of our patients can continue their therapies without interruption. Most patients don't experience any side effects from what we do, though. Any medication can cause adverse reactions, but these can be avoided by starting patients on a low dose of the medication and/or by giving them a different medication if they have a poor tolerance to the first one.

Factors That Affect Healing

Stress has a lot to do with the body's ability to heal. It's very important for patients to have strong supportive care from their families, but unfortunately, this doesn't always happen. For example, we have situations where family members subtly give off the impression that they are waiting for the person with cancer to pass away. Whenever this atmosphere is present, it's difficult for that person to get good results from his or her treatment. I might see, for example, a wealthy, 75 year-old gentleman, with a young, beautiful 27 year-old wife who is obviously waiting for him to die so that she can take his money. Of course, we don't see this scenario often, but it happens, especially in families where prominent people with a lot of money marry younger women. Initially, the wives give off the impression that they want to save their husbands, but after a few weeks, we realize that they really just want to let them go. In most cases, though, our patients receive great support from their friends and family members.

How Family and Friends Can Support Their Loved Ones with Cancer

The best way for family and friends to support their loved ones is to provide them with the same amount of care that they normally would during any other life situation. For example, they might help them to fight depression, or stay with them in Houston when they come here for two or three weeks to do treatment. Such support helps people with cancer to attain the best possible results from their treatments.

Roadblocks to Healing

One of the biggest roadblocks to healing is being able to effectively educate patients about their treatments. If we can't do that, then they won't get great treatment results. For example, people with advanced cancers need to understand that we can't usually get rid of their cancers with just a single anti-cancer medication. We need to use a combination of medications and we may need to adjust and perhaps even change those medications after a couple of months. If patients try to save money because they think, "Why should I take four meds when I can take one?" and they then decide to take only one medication, their cancers may respond for awhile to that medication, but eventually, it will be insufficient and their cancers will progress.

We have patients that visit us from all over the world. Sometimes their oncologists are supportive of the treatments that they do with us, and at other times, they aren't. If the oncologists aren't supportive, they may do things like tell their patients to take only one of the medications which we have prescribed them, instead of all four. If patients do this, then they won't get a good response to the treatment; even if they were initially responding to our protocol, they will stop progressing. This kind of thing tends to happen in Canada, where patients don't have as much medical freedom as in other countries and doctors tend to discourage them from taking all of the medications we have prescribed. This can be an obstacle to our patients' healing, which is why it's very important for us to educate them. We have three seminars every week to educate both patients and doctors about our treatments so that they know why we must use different combinations of medications. If we can educate them, and they follow through with their treatment plans, then we get very good results.

Insurance Coverage for Treatments

Many insurance companies cover our treatments, but it depends upon the patient's insurance plan. We have patients who spend zero dollars out of pocket for our treatments, while others spend a lot of their own money. We have a very good medical insurance department which evaluates these issues.

The Politics of Cancer Treatment in the United States and My Battle with the FDA

I present my successful case stories all over the world and the FDA has reviewed all of them, so my work is being carefully controlled and monitored. We have many successful cases which the FDA has documented, but it should take only one successful case to create a revolution in medicine—and at one time, it did.

Approximately 140 years ago, in France, Louis Pasteur was able to cure a boy who had a horrible brain disease called rabies. He developed a vaccine for the rabies and the boy was cured, and his vaccine changed medical history. We have many cases of so-called incurable brain disease which we have cured at our clinic, but instead of supporting us, the government has fought us from the beginning. Everyone is still trying to get rid of us, instead of giving us all the support that they can, so that we can save thousands of children from incurable brain tumors.

Can you imagine? Medicine in the United States has become totalitarian. It's controlled by bureaucrats. Doctors have no say in their patients' treatments. The human being is put last, and as a result, there has been no evolution in cancer treatment. The work environment for medical doctors is so suffocating and restrictive in this country that it's impossible for them to practice medicine in a manner which takes into account the best interests of the patient. This is unfortunate, but that's the country in which we live now.

In other countries, the situation is somewhat different. People say that in Japan everything is controlled, but when it comes to medicine, their doctors have more freedom than doctors in the United States. If a doctor in Japan thinks that there is a medicine somewhere in the world that can help his patients, the government of Japan will do everything possible to help that doctor get this medicine. In the United States, though, forget it! They make you try radiation and chemotherapy first, which only produce a lot of side effects.

A documentary entitled: "Burzynski, The Movie," details my experience with the FDA and is being shown at major movie theatres all around the country. (Author's note: the logline of the documentary on Facebook reads: "the documentary *Burzynski* reveals how a pioneering doctor and PhD biochemist discovered the genetic mechanism to cure most human cancers—and exposes our corrupt medical industry's failed attempts to imprison him while trying to steal his life-saving discovery"). This production has already received some awards at documentary film festivals. It reveals all of the persecution that I went through by the FDA when they discovered that I had developed a cancer treatment that works. Nobody in medical history has ever gone through as much persecution as we (in my clinic) did, because the government realized that we had something which could completely change the course of cancer treatment forever. They knew I was providing effective cancer treatment because they were supervising the clinical trials and they saw that it worked. But instead of approving my treatments, they (the people in the FDA) conspired with the pharmaceutical companies to put me in prison for life so that they could steal the patent that I had on antineoplastons. My battle with the federal government lasted fourteen years, but in the end, I won the war.

Now, we have managed to establish a working relationship with the FDA, and fortunately, those who tried to persecute me in the FDA are no longer part of the administration. They found some "wee" (insignificant) positions in pharmaceutical companies (so nothing bad happened to them), but we still face harassment at the state and local levels. This is because other oncologists don't understand what we do. They see us as competitors and so would like to get rid of us, because we are getting results that they can only dream about. Again, I believe that we will win in the end, because medicine is changing in the entire world, and more doctors are learning how to do this kind of therapy. In a few more years people will say that what I am doing is obviously effective and antineoplaston treatment will no longer be "alternative" medicine. The persecution I suffered for so many years from the FDA is unfortunate, but I have always believed I was right, so I never gave up. I thought, why should I cave in to people who only want to steal from me and make a lot of money? Ultimately, I believed that the right idea—mine— was going to win. I have always believed that. Now, the question is how to convey my message to the American people. It's difficult, because in general, people are tired and have a lot of problems, so getting them to think about new ideas isn't easy. But once we are able to explain the idea of antineoplastons to a majority, I think it will just be a matter of time before we win.

Unfortunately, at the present moment, not just anyone can come to see us. Federal regulations require that early stage cancer patients comply with the conventional "standard of care." This is partly why we don't see many early stage cancer patients; we don't have much flexibility with their treatment options. Doctors can be easily sued for malpractice if they don't recommend the standard of care to their patients (basically, chemotherapy and radiation), so this creates a difficult situation for us. They don't have much freedom with what they can do, treatment-wise. The medical bureaucrats say, "This is the type of cancer, this is how you are to treat it, and if you treat it any other way, you will be punished."

At my clinic, we are only allowed to use antineoplaston treatments on patients that can't be cured by standard, conventional approaches. These people have already been told that nothing else can be done for them. But if an early stage cancer patient doesn't want to do chemotherapy and instead prefers to receive treatment from us, it can be a difficult situation for us. In some cases, we have to get legal advice to determine whether or not we can treat them. There are ways to scientifically identify whether or not they should have chemotherapy. If they can do this and prove that chemotherapy wouldn't benefit them, we might be able to treat them. For example, at our clinic, we can test the oncogenes of women who have early stage breast cancer and determine through their oncogenes whether or not chemotherapy would benefit them.

Thus, if you are a patient in this country with an early stage of cancer, I would have to advise you to see your local oncologist first. If your cancer is metastatic (which most cancers are) then that's a different story, because metastatic cancers typically can't be cured by conventional medicine.

The Future of Cancer Treatment

These days, everything is changing rapidly in medicine. If you look into the business reports for the pharmaceutical industry, within five years, it's estimated that seventy-six percent of cancer care will be occupied by medicine which works on the genes, and only one-fourth of the market will be occupied by radiation and chemotherapy. Chemotherapy and radiation are gradually going away, and being replaced by more effective treatments, regardless of doctors' wishes. Of course, oncologists would like to be able to use the therapies and medicine that they have learned, but the economy may dictate that they use other types of medicine. Right now, it seems to be clear that over the next few years, chemotherapy and radiation will recede in use, and will eventually occupy only approximately 25 percent of the cancer treatment market. This is what economists have predicted, so it's most likely going to happen. In any case, radiation and chemotherapy should only be used for easy, treatable cancers for which these therapies are likely to result in cures. But every year, about two million people worldwide are dying from just three types of cancer: colon, lung, and liver cancer. How many of these two million people can be saved with chemotherapy and radiation? Maybe just one hundred! If patients have one of these advanced cancers, conventional treatments won't be very helpful for them, anyway. But the future is changing in front of our eyes and that's what's important.

Last Words

People should know that many advanced cases of cancer can be cured now. It's very important for patients to be educated about their diseases. It's also important that they have doctors who are up-to-date on the latest developments in cancer research. For people who currently have incurable cancers, it's possible that in the near future there will be cures available for them. In the meantime, if they are able to at least stabilize their cancers, they may survive until a new cure becomes available.

Useful Websites

Dr. Burzynski's cancer clinic: www.cancermed.com
Burzynski Research Institute: www.burzynski.com
Documentary film: www.burzynskimovie.com

Contact Information
Stanislaw Burzynski, MD, PhD

Burzynski Clinic
9432 Katy Freeway
Houston, Texas 77055
Phone: 713.335.5697
Toll-Free: 800.714.7181
Fax: 713.935.0649

Scheduling & Information (USA): info@burzynskiclinic.com
International Patients (outside USA):
patients.int@burzynskiclinic.com
Marketing and Public Relations: marketing@burzynskiclinic.com
Cancer Information Specialist: 800.714.7181
International Callers: +1.713.335.5697

Comparison of Responses in the Most Common Cancers

Personalized Treatment at Burzynski Clinic
(as of January 3, 2011)
[by highest rate of Objective Responses (OR)]

Diagnosis	No. of patients	OR (%)	SD (%)	PD (%)
Non-Hodgkin's lymphoma	100	64	27	9
Breast cancer	287	60	25	15
Ovarian cancer	59	59	22	19
Carcinoma (unknown primary origin)	38	58	34	8
Colon cancer	164	52	29	19
Prostate cancer	280	51	40	9
Pancreatic cancer	35	51	37	12
Skin cancer	8	50	38	12
Small intestine cancer	6	50	33	17
Leukemia	11	46	54	0
Multiple myeloma	11	46	27	27
Urinary bladder and urothelial cancer	27	45	33	22
Head and neck cancer	63	44	35	21
Uterine, cervix, vulvar, endometrium cancer	28	44	23	33
Kidney cancer	30	43	37	20
Esophageal and stomach cancer	41	42	29	29
Malignant melanoma	49	41	22	37
Lung cancer and mesothelioma	141	39	40	21
Hodgkin's disease	11	36	46	18
Neuroendocrine tumor	9	34	33	33
Biliary tract	15	33	47	20
Liver cancer	15	33	20	47
Brain tumor	114	27	46	27

Data as of January 3, 2011 based on medical records of the first 1652 evaluable patients. The table shows response rates for 23 selected, common cancer types treated at the Burzynski Clinic (by highest rate of OR - Objective Responses).

Definitions:

OR: **Objective Response.** This includes CR, PR, MR, & IM.

CR: **Complete Response.** Complete disappearance of all signs of cancer in response to 4 or more weeks of treatment.

PR: **Partial Response.** More than a 50% decrease in the size of the tumors (the sum of the cross-sectional area of the tumors), in response to 4 or more weeks of treatment.

MR: **Mixed Response.** A significant decrease (more than 25%) in the size of the tumors with a simultaneous increase in the size of some of the other tumors.

IM: **Improvement.** A decrease in the size of the tumors, but which hasn't been confirmed yet by the second follow-up radiological measurement.

SD: **Stable Disease.** No decrease or increase in the size of the tumors, but no progression, in response to 12 or more weeks of treatment.

PD: **Progressive Disease.** More than a 50% increase in the size of the tumors (the sum of the cross-sectional area of the tumors), in response to 4 or more weeks of treatment.

EP: **Evaluable Patients.** Patients who remained on treatment long enough to enable an objective evaluation of their response.

• CHAPTER 2 •

Nicholas J. Gonzalez, MD
NEW YORK, NY

Biography

Nicholas J. Gonzalez, MD, graduated from Brown University, Phi Beta Kappa, magna cum laude, with a degree in English Literature. He subsequently worked as a journalist, first at Time Inc., before pursuing premedical studies at Columbia. He then received his medical degree from Cornell University Medical College in 1983. During a postgraduate immunology fellowship under Dr. Robert A. Good, considered the father of modern immunology, he completed an intensive research study in which he evaluated an aggressive nutritional therapy involving high doses of pancreatic enzymes for the treatment of advanced cancer. Originally discovered in the early 1900s by the English scientist Dr. Beard, a dentist named Dr. William Donald Kelley further developed it in the 1960s and 1970s and had been using it on his patients with great success. Years of studying Dr. Kelley's methods and the extraordinary outcomes that he had with thousands of patients convinced Dr. Gonzalez to pursue further research on the therapy, which, over the years, received substantial financial support from Procter & Gamble, Nestle, and the National Cancer Institute. Results from a pilot study he completed on this therapy, published in 1999, yielded the most positive outcomes for the treatment of pancreatic cancer than any data described in the medical literature. [1]

Dr. Gonzalez's research and experiences also led him to write a book based on the therapy, entitled *One Man Alone: An Investigation of Nutrition, Cancer, and William Donald Kelley*. This monograph, completed in 1986 and published in 2010 by New Spring Press, describes his investigation of Dr. William Donald Kelley's work and has been generating interest in the alternative and conventional medical world for over two decades. He also wrote a book entitled *The Trophoblast and the Origins of Cancer*, a work which he co-authored with his colleague, Linda Isaacs, MD, which discusses, from the perspective of contemporary molecular biology, the pioneering research of Dr. John Beard. It provides a scientific rationale for the anti-cancer effects of pancreatic enzymes and their efficacy in the treatment of cancer, and includes case reports from Dr. Gonzalez and Dr. Isaacs' practice. Since 2000, Dr. Gonzalez has also been writing a series of books detailing the history, theory, practice, and success of the therapy in his own practice.

Over the years, Dr. Gonzalez has regularly contributed as a guest on health-related talk radio programs such as Robert Scott Bell, LIME radio, Deborah Ray, Ron Hoffman, and Robert Atkins. His work has been positively featured in many consumer oriented venues, including *Prevention, Total Health, Alternative Medicine, Life Extension, Longevity,* and *New Yorker,* among others.

He has received many awards, including the following:

- Teagle Scholar award from Cornell University Medical School (1982).

---

[1] Gonzalez NJ, Isaacs LL. Evaluation of pancreatic proteolytic enzyme treatment of adenocarcinoma of the pancreas, with nutrition and detoxification support. Nutr Cancer, 33 (2):117-124.

- Ernst L. Wynder Award from The Center for Mind-Body Medicine in Washington, D.C. (2000). (Dr. Wynder was the first scientist to confirm the link between cigarette smoking and cancer).

- Distinguished Pioneer in Alternative Medicine Award from the Foundation for the Advancement of Innovative Medicine (2000).

- Integrity in Science Award from the Weston A. Price Foundation (2010).

Dr. Gonzalez has been in private practice in New York City since 1987, treating patients diagnosed with cancer and other serious degenerative illnesses.

What Cancer Is and What Causes It

My approach to cancer; what it is, what causes it, and how to treat it is similar to that of the early 1900s English scientist John Beard, DSc, who developed a ground-breaking theory on cancer over 100 years ago. Conventional medicine believes that cancer develops from mature, healthy cells that go "berserk," mutate, and turn cancerous. Dr. Beard believed that cancer didn't come from mature cells, but from residual trophoblast cells that remain in all of us and which are scattered throughout our tissues and organs. Embryonic trophoblast cells are the earliest precursors to the placenta; the scattered trophoblast cells in the mature organism serve as stem cells, regenerating new tissues as replacements are needed. They sit quietly most of the time, but can, at some point, start growing just like the placenta, as the result of a stimulus, such as an infection or inflammation, but unlike the placenta, they grow in the wrong place and at the wrong time. And just as the placenta grows and invades into the uterus, cancer cells grow fast and invade local tissues and organs.

When Dr. Beard's view that cancer was caused by misplaced tro-phoblasts (which are the type of cells produced by the placenta) growing in the wrong place at the wrong time was published in a book nearly 100 years ago, in 1911, people thought that he was crazy, even though he was an eminent university professor who was nominated for a Nobel Prize in 1906 for his work in embryology. Indeed, he was a prominent embryologist, but people thought he had gone off the deep end when it came to cancer.

His theory, however, is similar to what molecular biologists are saying today; that cancer cells resemble misplaced trophoblasts (or placental cells) in many ways. They grow fast like placental cells, produce their blood supply in the same manner as placental cells, and are invasive like placental cells. Much of their molecular biology is identical to placental cells, and they use exactly the same invasive techniques in the body that placental cells use when they invade the uterus. Additionally, their transcription and other factors are similar so biologists are now beginning to study Beard's early tumor model. (Transcription factors are molecules that are involved in controlling gene expression). So Beard may not have been that far off in his thinking, but it's sad that 100 years of research have been lost in the meantime. If researchers had listened to Beard back in 1911, knowledge of cancer biology today would be more extensive. At my office, we look at cancer as Beard did.

The second component of Beard's hypothesis was that while the placenta initially grows, develops, proliferates rapidly, invades tissue, and develops a blood supply like a cancer, at some point, it changes completely and stops doing all of these things. The mature placenta is a very benign tissue, and is a necessary link between the embryo and the mother's blood supply in mammals. Cancer is different from placental cells in that it never stops growing and invading—and ultimately kills us, whereas placental cells, at a predetermined point, suddenly change completely and stop behaving like a cancer. Beard spent years trying to figure out what the signal was that caused the placental cells to stop acting like invasive cancer cell tissue, and one day realized that that it was when the embryonic pancreas became active. This led him to formulate his thesis that pancreatic enzymes control trophoblastic destiny, and since trophoblasts are like cancer cells, and enzymes control trophoblast activity, pancreatic enzymes are useful for controlling cancer and can therefore be used in cancer therapy. So these enzymes became the essence of his therapy.

Interestingly, a lot of molecular biologists, such as Max S. Wicha, MD, at the University of Michigan, also now believe that cancer doesn't develop from mature cells gone "berserk" but from stem cells. Stem cells are used to replace cells that are lost through normal turnover, aging, disease and injury, and their role in cancer development is a hot topic in modern research. We think that these cells are what Beard really identified, because he described the misplaced trophoblasts that he found as being microscopic, primitive, undifferentiated cells that are scattered throughout our tissues, which basically also describes stem cells. So we believe that stem cells were discovered by Dr. Beard in 1902, even though they weren't officially recognized as such until 1960. In summary, Dr. Beard's misplaced trophoblasts are what we today call stem cells, and these are the source of cancer.

The incidence of cancer has increased dramatically in recent years. I have been in practice for twenty-three years and I have seen things change a lot. When I was in medical school in the early 1980s, I was taught that cancer was an old person's disease. When I started out in practice, I didn't see twenty year-olds with cancer; now I see them almost routinely. Back then, if I saw young adults with cancer, it was usually because they had twenty years of smoking under their belts. But today, I see young adults with breast, metastatic lung, and other types of cancer and these cancers are far more aggressive than they were ten, twenty, or thirty years ago, and I think the reasons are environmental. Just recently, I consulted on a twenty-four year-old patient with metastatic breast cancer, and a twelve year-old with pancreatic cancer. This is happening because the world is more polluted than it used to be, and each year, it gets worse.

Assuming that Dr. Beard's theory about cancer is correct, why would these toxins affect the development of cancer in a person? He wrote in his book 100 years ago that any type of inflammation, irritation or toxic exposure could cause these immature trophoblast cells to start dividing. So, whether you believe that cancer is caused by mutations of mature cells or by trophoblasts, there is no question that environmental toxins stimulate cancer growth. And it's for this reason that younger people are now getting cancer.

There are all kinds of toxins in the environment, both appreciated and unappreciated. Recently, I read that over 75,000 chemicals have been approved for industrial use in the United States. One of my European doctor friends told me that artillery shells are now coated in inactivated uranium. Uranium is among the heaviest of metals and can penetrate walls, tanks, and artillery. It's also 98% radioactive, so no matter what anyone's politics are, every time the military utilizes one of these artillery shells, in Iraq or Afghanistan or wherever the place may be, they are increasing environmental radiation. Over the past ten years, tens of thousands of artillery shells have been discharged in war, which has added a significant load of unappreciated radiation toxicity into our environment.

So there are a lot of toxins in the environment that weren't even there ten years ago. Many of these toxins are mutagenic and carcinogenic, so whether people believe in Beard's theory or in a more traditional origin of cancer, there's no question that chemical toxins in the environment are stimulating cancer development in humans.

Treatment Protocol

Although my treatment protocol is complex, it can basically be simplified into three components: diet, nutrient supplementation (including pancreatic enzymes), and detoxification.

Diet

The first component of my protocol involves putting patients on a specific diet, which in our practice, we individualize. We (my colleague Linda Isaacs, MD and I) differ from a lot of other alternative health care practitioners in that we don't just have one cancer diet for everyone. We have ten basic diets that range from pure, raw vegetarian nut and seed diets, to red meat Atkins' diets in which people eat fatty red meat a couple of times per day. We then have ninety different variations on each of the ten basic diets. So we have balanced diets that involve a combination of plant and animal foods, as well as more extreme vegetarian and carnivorous diets, with lots of variations in-between.

Food is fuel for the body, and because our bodies are the most sophisticated engines on earth, they require the most sophisticated types of fuel. Humans aren't like white rats, that all look the same and have the same nutritional requirements. Our requirements differ, depending upon many factors, including our ancestry. For instance, the Masai in Africa traditionally subsisted on raw milk and blood. The Eskimos lived on red meat while the Polynesians consumed fruits and fish. The Pygmies in the Congo ate plants, and the Indians in the Eastern United States consumed over 1,000 edible plants in the woods where they lived. All of these different groups thrived on different diets which satisfied their nutritional needs. If you give the wrong diet to the wrong person, it's like putting water into your car's engine. The proper fuel must be put into the right engine. And humans have variable needs, because their ancestors adapted to a lot of different ecological niches with different available food supplies. The Masai, Eskimos, and other groups were very healthy when they stuck to their traditional diets.

So I must first determine for my patients what diet they need to be on, because food is fuel for the body, and every molecule that comprises us, everything that we are, comes from our food. It doesn't come from anywhere else. If I put a vegetarian on a meat diet, "all hell is going to break loose" in that person's body. If I put a meat eater on a vegetarian diet, that person will get sicker. It's important to give the body the right fuel. It works better when we do. The same is true of nutritional supplements. My patients' diet protocols are formulated based on their biochemistry.

Biochemistry also determines the type of cancer people will get. Those who, genetically, should be vegetarians and on a plant-based diet, tend to get solid tumors of the breast, colon, pancreas, lungs, liver, intestine, stomach, uterus, ovaries, and so on. People who, genetically, should be meat eaters tend to get immune cancers: leukemias, myelomas, and lymphomas, as well as connective tissue cancers like sarcomas. Omnivores, or balanced people, fall somewhere in-between, but in general, they don't tend to get cancer as often as the other two groups. Most cancer develops in those who genetically should be extreme meat eaters or extreme vegetarians. Their biochemistry determines what kind of diet they need to be on, as well as what kind of cancer they are susceptible to.

Nutrient Supplementation

Along with a specific diet plan, I recommend individualized nutritional supplement plans to my patients. Some require a wide variety of high-dose supplements, but not all, since each patient's protocol is individualized. I find, for instance, that vegetarians need different supplements than meat eaters. Vegetarians tend to do well with potassium, magnesium, a lot of the B-vitamins, and Vitamin C. They don't do well with Vitamin E. Meat eaters have great results with calcium, zinc, selenium, and Vitamin E, but don't do well when they take magnesium and potassium. They also don't do well with most B-vitamins (except for B-12 and a few others), large doses of Vitamin C and D, manganese and chromium, whereas vegetarians tend to do well with the latter minerals. Balanced people are somewhere in-between and do well with all kinds of vitamins, minerals and trace elements.

The approach that conventional medicine takes to researching nutrients and their effects upon people is nonsensical. The conventional approach yields results that are "all over the map." For instance, when testing the effects of selenium upon the body, researchers will give the same dose of the same type of selenium to everyone, but a vegetarian needs a different dose of selenium than a meat eater, so the results will be skewed because of this factor. Also, doing tests this way doesn't take into account a person's entire system. In my practice, we prescribe different forms of calcium, depending upon the patient's metabolism. Nutrients facilitate every reaction in the body, and they are extremely powerful, for good and for bad. The wrong dose of the wrong nutrient to the wrong person will cause chaos in the body, which is also why the "one-size-fits all" studies are crazy. They also don't make sense because their results are assessed independently of the impact that the particular tested nutrient has upon other nutrients in the body. Thus, the overall effect of a given nutrient upon the body cannot be accurately determined in isolation. Nutrients work together with other nutrients; for example, Vitamin E protects selenium and selenium protects Vitamin E; Vitamin C protects both Vitamin E and selenium, so if I give a patient Vitamin C with selenium and vitamin E, I don't need to give high doses of any of these nutrients, because they are preserving the effects of each other. There are very complex interactions between all of the nutrients, and vegetarians need different supplements in different doses than meat eaters do, so it's important to give the right supplements to the right people. When this principle is respected, and patients are prescribed a proper diet, every system in the body works better, from the neurological system, to the endocrine system, to all the others.

It's important to support the entire body and all of its systems, so that it can better fight cancer, and we do this in our practice. Conventional oncologists don't do this though. They don't care if their patients eat ice cream, but we do. We worry about everything, because we want every system in our patients' bodies working well and functioning as close as possible to 100 percent capacity. Only then can they effectively fight cancer.

The supplements that I prescribe to my patients include a variety of vitamins, herbs, anti-oxidants, trace minerals and glandular formulas. We are big on glandulars, which are comprised of concentrated animal glands and organs that contain minute amounts of hormones and other beneficial factors to heal and balance the body. All of our glandular formulas and other animal products come from New Zealand, a country that has never had mad cow disease and which remains the cleanest, most unpolluted place on earth. New Zealand has the strictest cattle-raising laws in the world, so they have been able to avoid mad cow and other diseases. Some of the glandular formulas that we use include freeze-dried heart, adrenal glands, dried ovaries, and lungs, which are effective for supporting the body in a variety of ways. For instance, if patients have weak lungs, I might give them a lung glandular formula. Some of my colleagues laugh at me for doing this kind of therapy, but I tell them that it really works, because, for instance, there are growth factors in the freeze-dried lung of an animal that heal human lung tissue. In the 1940s, doctors used to treat heart failure with beef heart, and it worked. Then, after World War II, pharmaceutical companies began to really push drugs and everyone forgot about these old folk remedies, but they really work! So we use a lot of glandular products in my practice, along with vitamins, minerals, and trace elements.

In summary, we try to get every system in the body to work right, by giving our patients the right diet and supplements, and by making sure that they aren't taking the wrong ones. It's just as important to get the wrong supplements and foods out of the diet as it is to bring in the right ones.

Pancreatic Enzymes

While we use dietary, vitamin, mineral, and other supplements to help our patients function at top physiological efficiency, we use pancreatic enzymes to directly attack their cancers. My average patient takes anywhere from 90-110 enzyme capsules per day, which are spread throughout the day. We really load them up on enzymes, but this is necessary in order for them to overcome cancer. Overall, my average cancer patient takes over 175 pills a day, most of those being enzymes.

In orthodox medicine, pancreatic enzymes are thought to have just one function: to help digest food. They are excreted by the pancreas into the intestinal tract, where they break down carbohydrates, fats and proteins arriving from the stomach. Orthodox medicine doesn't recognize Dr. Beard's theory that pancreatic enzymes represent the body's main defense against cancer, which is how we use them at our office. Again, pancreatic enzymes control placental growth, and since cancer cells result from misplaced placental cells, pancreatic enzymes also control cancer cell growth. We treat cancer according to Dr. Beard's theory, which was developed over 100 years ago, published in the mainstream scientific literature, and then totally ignored.

Detoxification

The third component of our treatment plan, and also the most controversial, is detoxification. When cancer cells die, a lot of toxins get released in the body, so it's important for people with cancer to detoxify themselves. Detoxification is also important during cancer treatment because the body is repairing itself, and a lot of toxins get released during that process.

We are all exposed to thousands of chemicals every day: heavy metals, pesticides, and so on. There are thousands of chemicals in our water, air, and food, and many of those toxins are stored in our cells, where they remain like a ticking time bomb. In addition, cancer cells produce all kinds of foreign molecules, such as abnormal enzymes and proteins, which are toxic to the cells. Now, when the body repairs itself and tumor tissue is broken down, all kinds of toxic wastes get released into the bloodstream. The liver and kidneys filter out these toxins, but these organs get overloaded, so we have a series of procedures at our office which we recommend that our patients use to mobilize, neutralize, and excrete all of this toxic stuff out of their bodies.

One of these is the infamous coffee enema, which, paradoxically and ironically, and despite all of the criticism against it, came from conventional medicine. Up until the 1960s, most nursing textbooks recommended them for patients. The Merck Manual, which is a compendium of orthodox treatments, listed coffee enemas as a treatment up until the 1970s. My eccentric and brilliant mentor, Dr. Kelley, who was a dentist and the first person to revive Dr. Beard's work, incorporated coffee enemas into his patients' protocols because they came out of the Merck manual and they help the liver to function better, which is also why we incorporate them into our protocols.

In addition, we recommend intestinal cleanses, juicing, skin brushing (which is an old technique used to stimulate lymphatic drainage), as well as other things to assist the detoxification organs with the process of toxin removal. All of these strategies can be done at home, including our five-day liver and intestinal cleanses, and juice fasts. We have patients who come to us from all over the world, and we teach them how to do everything here so that they can do our protocols at home.

Considerations in Treatment

Before we take on new patients, we determine whether or not we will be able to help them. If they contact us from Memorial Sloan-Kettering, half-conscious and with a breathing tube, we know that they aren't going to be able to do our program, because they have to be able to swallow the pills that we give them. Patients also have to have the motivation to want to do it. Just because their cousin or grandmother wants them to do it, isn't good enough. They have to be interested in it. So we select patients who can physically do the program and who want to do it. I also do the program myself for general prevention against cancer. I have taken a lot of pills for 29 years, but it's no big deal to me. It's a question of mindset. If people think that taking pills and drinking carrot juice is going to be a nightmare, then it will be. Most of my patients are enthusiastic, appreciate the program, and want to be here, so they just dive in and do it. Usually compliance to the regimen and ability to do it are a non-issue.

Many of my patients had health problems before getting cancer, including typical epidemic degenerative diseases like heart disease, diabetes, allergies and high cholesterol; basically, all kinds of problems. So when they come to my office for treatment, we give them the full package. We treat all of their problems, not just their cancers. Often, when we give them the nutrients that they need, their other health problems resolve. And people do come to us for treatment for other diseases besides cancer or along with cancer. We just accept it and do what we have to do. People are afflicted with a lot of health problems. That's just the reality of life today.

Treatment Outcomes

If you look at my website, you will see that, overall, most of our patients do well. However, this includes only those who comply fully with the program. The success rate for pancreatic cancer is lower because it's a very aggressive disease, but many do well over the long term, as evidenced by the case reports on my website. Usually those that don't do well have a really advanced stage of cancer.

So what do I mean when I say that my patients "do well?" The current drug that is used to treat pancreatic cancer, and which was given FDA approval, extends the patient's life by a month, on average, and this is definitely not what I mean by "doing well!" If I only extended my patients' lives by one month; if that was the best that I could do for them, I would quit my job. I would go sell shoes, literally! What I mean by "doing well" can be defined by the testimonials that are on my website. For example, I had a patient who was diagnosed in September 1991 with metastatic pancreatic cancer that had spread to his adrenals, lungs, and bones. He also had four tumors in his liver, and he was seventy years old at the time. The man lasted until he was seriously injured in an automobile accident and died in a rehab center. He didn't die of cancer. All of his tumors disappeared and he lived for fifteen years beyond his diagnosis. His case is how I define "doing well," and represents the average improvement and survival rate that we see and expect at our office.

I receive oncology journals here at my office. Recently, I read about a supposedly miraculous new immune therapy for melanoma. The results of its use show that, on average, it extends the patient's life by one or two months, which increases the two-year survival rate statistics for metastatic melanoma from 10-12 to 20 percent. It's an improvement, but it's not the same as having most of your patients still alive after a minimum of five years—which are the typical results that we get at my office. But the medical community gets hysterically excited over new drugs that provide small, incremental increases in average survival rates. To me, this is sad, not a great victory.

I started practicing medicine in 1987, and at that time, I had a patient who had an aggressive, metastatic, stage four breast cancer. She came to see me after having done chemotherapy, and is still alive and well today, with no evidence of cancer in her body. She has so far lived for 23 years past her original diagnosis. There are many people like her who have come to see me, and who are now living normal, healthy lives, after having had terrible, terminal cancers.

Other Doctors Who Do Pancreatic Enzyme Therapy

There are other doctors who claim to treat cancer with pancreatic enzymes, but I don't know them or what the quality of their work is. They, and others, know about Dr. Beard's work, and there are other scientists who have rediscovered his work, but I'm not sure what similar therapies are out there, or how good they are. I'm not saying I'm a genius. Dr. Beard was the genius. I was just smart enough to realize that he was right.

The Role of Stress, the Mind and Spirituality in Healing

I first met Dr. Kelley (the dentist who first introduced me to Dr. Beard's work) when I was a medical student, hoping to spend the rest of my life at the prestigious Memorial Sloan Kettering Cancer Center in New York. I watched Dr. Kelley perform miracles with his patients, and I asked him how much healing depends upon nutritional factors, and how much of it depends upon biochemical, psychological, and spiritual factors. Being the bright young medical student that I was, I expected him to say that it's all nutritional, but instead, he said, "Healing is 100 percent biochemical." He waited five seconds and then said, "It's also 100 percent nutritional." After another five seconds, he said, "And it's 100 percent psychological and spiritual." He added, "Someday, you are going to appreciate that." Well, it took me awhile to appreciate his perspective, because I was very biochemically-oriented at the time, and thought that healing meant giving patients a pill. I now know that it's not that simple, and that psychological and spiritual aspects play an important role in healing, too, because we aren't just white rats running around in a cave; we are far more sophisticated than that. Our minds influence our biochemistry, and our biochemistry influences our minds.

Stress is a great enemy to our health, and if people have constant marital stress, for example, that stress can undermine the physiological repair of their cells. Hans Selye, MD, a Canadian endocrinologist, dedicated 50 years in Montreal to studying the physiological effects of stress upon humans, and came to the irrefutable conclusion that psychological stress has enormous effects upon the body. Doctors who don't address the issue of stress are going to miss opportunities to help their patients, but it can sometimes be a tricky matter. If a patient with breast cancer is married to an abusive alcoholic, for instance, it will be tough for her to find peace and healing at home. As her doctor, I would want to guide and help her through that situation, because this kind of constant psychological stress could be really physiologically debilitating and impact her healing.

Healing isn't just about taking some enzymes; patients have to adjust their lives as necessary, and do what they can to get them in order. Some patients might need just a bit of counseling, while others require serious marital counseling. Emotional detoxification, along with the right nutritional protocol, is important.

When it comes to making spiritual recommendations for people's healing, everyone has different needs. I have Muslim patients from the Middle East, as well as evangelical Christians, so any recommendations that I make for their spiritual health must correlate with what's suitable for their particular mindset. I have to tailor it to their background and needs, and just as one diet doesn't work for everybody, so one type of spiritual practice doesn't work for everyone, either. That said, many people who come to my office have already addressed the spiritual side of healing, because they tend to be holistically oriented anyway, and understand the role that spirituality plays in health.

Belief patterns also play an important role in healing. The man that I mentioned earlier, who in 1991 had stage four pancreatic cancer, was quite intelligent; he had a master's degree in archeology, and was an expert in 19th century French art. He knew that he had stage four pancreatic cancer, in his liver, lung, bones, and adrenals, but he believed that chemotherapy wasn't going to work for him and that it would be a waste of time. He was given eight weeks to live. This was in 1991, when I had only been in practice for four years and wasn't yet famous. This man had read about me in some alternative medicine journal, and when he walked into my office, there was something about me that just "clicked" for him, and he said to me, "I know this (my condition) is serious. I'm going to do the best I can, and having met you, I know that you are going to do the best that you can (for me). I believe I'm going to get well, and if I don't, I'm still going to do the best I can." He wasn't afraid or in a state of panic. I don't know that I could have been so calm had I been in his shoes. But he got well. It was amazing. He didn't care that his doctor had said, "You are wasting your money on quackery and you're going to die!" ...along with all the usual stuff that conventional doctors say.

I have other patients who will contact my office and say, "My doctor says that this is quackery, so why should I do this?" When this happens, I know that we are in trouble. Such patients aren't operating out of faith, and that is a problem. The man with stage four pancreatic cancer had faith, but it wasn't an irrational faith. He chose to see me, based upon what he had read about me and his initial interactions with the staff at my office. He wasn't into magical thinking; he was far too smart for that. He just had faith that he was going to get well, and this belief helped him to get well. He read about what I did, decided that my treatments were his best option and had no fear or anxiety about his decision to come see me.

Anxiety kills. Stress turns on the sympathetic nervous system, and when this system turns on, the body breaks down. When this physiological-stress nervous system (sympathetic nervous system) turns on, it breaks down tissue that's needed for energy at the time of stress. Stress is antithetical to healing. The man with pancreatic cancer was told that he was going to die, but he chose to handle the situation without fear. He wasn't naïve, but he wasn't afraid. He dealt with it. If people with cancer can't get over their fears, that's going to affect their healing. At our practice, we think fear and anxiety are our greatest enemies. Patients that don't have faith in what we do can't get well. Their brains are more powerful than our therapies, and if they are being treated by a doctor that they don't have faith in, that's scary for them. If I was being treated by a doctor that I had no faith in, I would be out the door of his office so fast—no, I would be crawling out of his window! Even if patients do my treatments, if they don't believe in them, their brains will override anything that I can do biochemically for them. The brain is powerful. In order to heal, people need to have faith in the type of treatment that they are doing.

That's why we are selective about the patients we treat. It's not for our benefit, but for theirs. There's no point in taking in a patient who would rather be at Sloan-Kettering Clinic, doing conventional treatments. I have patients who somehow got talked into coming to my office, but they would really rather not be here. So we try to "feel them out" beforehand. I can tell if they would rather be in the conventional medical world, and if so, I must tell them, "You really shouldn't be here." Whenever I do that, they almost look relieved. But I have to tell them this, even though I know that conventional medicine isn't going to work for them, because receiving conventional care is what they need in order to feel okay emotionally. American conventional medicine may not be the best for treating cancer, but it's still the authority, and some people need that, along with the fancy facilities and expertise that conventional medicine provides. We are on the fringe of medicine, and that makes some people nervous.

It may not always be the patient who's nervous, either, but the patient's cousin who's a nurse and who thinks we are crazy. There are usually plenty of relatives who think that their loved ones with cancer should be going to the Mayo clinic, instead of to the "crazy doctor in New York who does enemas." People with cancer have to have faith if they are going to go the alternative route with their treatments, because they aren't going to get support for this kind of medicine from their local doctors and families. In fact, they usually get the opposite and they have to be strong enough to stand up to that.

Patients who have a lot of fear and anxiety are always tough to heal. Everyone who comes in for cancer treatment is scared, yes, but they have to have faith to get over that, and believe that they are going to get well, even though their local doctors may have told them that they are going to die. The people who believe that they are going to get well, no matter what, are those who have the best outcomes.

I believe that attitude is the single most important determinant of success for any type of treatment, although if patients don't believe in the therapy that they are doing, they won't ultimately comply with it, anyway. Even if they do, their brains will sabotage it, because they don't believe in it, and their brains can shut it off, but if they are able to reverse their thinking, their physiology completely changes for the better.

Some people are so driven by fear that they can read the case reports on our website and still ask questions like, "How come there isn't someone like me on there?" No single person is exactly like another, yet a person operating out of fear and anxiety will find a way to minimize or undermine the power of those successful cases. They will say things like, "Well, (that person who got healed) is a man rather than a woman." Or, "I'm from Toledo, but this other person who got well is from Cincinnati, so how can I relate to that?"

People shouldn't underestimate the power of fear and anxiety, because it can undermine most anything.

In any case, people with that level of fear about my treatments don't belong in my office, because the experience would be difficult for them. I would prefer that they go to Sloan-Kettering, if they are more comfortable there. Most of the patients that we accept would rather die than go to a major cancer tertiary treatment center, though. They don't care what the doctors think. Those that have "Sloan-Kettering syndrome" (and I say that with respect because I was going to spend my life there) are patients who need the authority and support of the medical community behind them, so places like Sloan-Kettering are where they belong. I don't do what the doctors there do, but they are still smart people.

You know, nobody trusts what politicians say anymore. People are even skeptical about religious authorities. But the one great authority that they still respect is doctors and conventional medicine. I have seen journalists who don't believe what any politician or religious authority tells them go to Sloan-Kettering or the NIH (National Institutes of Health) and take what they are fed there as if it were the Word of God. They don't question it nor understand it, but perhaps due to the influence of pharmaceutical companies, or ego, they tend to believe that medicine is comprised of wonderful, dedicated scientists searching objectively for the truth, not people with prejudices and egos like everyone else! So medicine remains, in our culture, one of the last great bastions of authoritarian control that people bow down to and don't question too much.

The Problem with Conventional Cancer Care

Statistically, the success rate of conventional treatment for most cancers hasn't changed much over the last 50 years. Most patients who have been cured had cancers that were localized at the time of their diagnosis and which were cured by surgery. Chemotherapy and radiation can do nothing for most solid tumors of the lung, breast, pancreas, ovaries, liver, colon, and uterus, especially when they are metastatic. Like Suzanne Somers said in her book, *Knock-*

out, few cancers today respond to chemotherapy. Those that do are the same ones that responded to chemotherapy nearly 30 years ago; the childhood leukemias, testicular cancers, choriocarcinomas, Hodgkin's disease, and certain lymphomas. So for the great majority of cancers, chemotherapy and radiation still do nothing, just as they did nothing 50 years ago! The only way that conventional medicine can cure these cancers is if they are caught early and can be surgically removed, but most of the time, they aren't caught early. So for the great majority of cancers, the standard approach, including immunotherapy, doesn't do much at all. There has been very little progress despite all of the claims.

Why Oncologists Use Conventional Medicine, Even When It Doesn't Work

I've often asked myself this question. Some oncologists may do conventional treatments for the money, but I think most are well-intentioned. However, if they are experts in pancreatic cancer, for instance, then they know that their patients just don't get well. What kind of expertise is that? If I was an oncologist who was an expert in pancreatic cancer, I would get so discouraged. I mean, I'm supposed to be an expert and I can't get anyone well? And year after year, these "experts" are treating patients who are dying. I guess they hope that there will be some effective new treatment on the horizon. That's the cheerleading approach to medicine—that there will always be some new remedy down the road that works, but in conventional cancer care, there haven't been that many new remedies and those that have been invented aren't that great. Take the new drug, Avastin, for example. I read in the Wall St. Journal that it has earned five to six billion dollars in revenue. It's supposed to stop cancer angiogenesis (new blood vessel growth), and has been heralded as a miracle drug. All cancers were supposed to respond to it, but not only does it not do anything for breast cancer, for which it was highly promoted, it also has serious side effects and the FDA is thinking of yanking it for breast cancer, after millions of dollars have already been spent on its development. It made the front page of the New York Times, but it just doesn't work well for breast cancer.

Managing hundreds of very sick patients is a lot of work for a physician, and my wife will tell you that I work seven days a week. I also have to keep up with all the new research, but I don't regret my decision to become a doctor. It's a choice I made, and it's a lot of fun because I see most of my patients get well. If I was an oncologist and most of my patients didn't get well, it would be a depressing job for me. Then again, most oncologists don't interact much with their patients. They work with nurses, who administer the chemotherapy to their patients. Here at my office, I work one-on-one with my patients. I have also seen a lot of oncologists detach from their patients when they don't do well. As their patients get worse, the oncologists come to see them in their hospital rooms less and less, and most of their care ends up being through orders which they give to their nurses. I think that emotionally detaching from their patients helps them to do their job.

The Politics of Cancer and How It Affects Treatment Options

One of the problems with getting our treatment approach into mainstream medicine is that enzymes and nutritional supplements can't be patented, and therefore, aren't studied and promoted because drug companies don't want to fund anything that can't be patented. I understand the position that the drug companies are in, but there needs to be a change in our governmental policies, too, and the government is in collusion with the drug companies. There are a thousand full-time drug company lobbyists in Washington. That's two for every congressman and senator! They are all working full-time, making six figure incomes and trying to influence medical legislation. Right now, drug companies are happy about the new health care legislation under President Obama, because their drugs will all be covered by the new health care laws. This is because their lobbyists have cut special deals with congressmen in the back rooms in Washington. The drug companies will make billions of dollars under these new laws. There is nothing in medical legislation that favors alternative medicine. That's why drug companies aren't fighting Obama's health care plan. Their drugs are going to be paid for now, by taxpayers—to the tune of billions of dollars in profits per year. There is so much collusion between government research institutions like the NCI (National Cancer Institute) and the drug companies. I know because I worked with the NCI for ten years and it's like the Harvard business school for the drug industry! You go to work for the NCI, FDA, NIH (National Institutes of Health), and after five or ten years, you can go to work as an executive for a drug company and earn 1.5 million dollars per year. These government institutions are training ground for drug company executives. And for them, scientific truth is secondary to profit.

One of the nice things about living in a relatively free country is that people can still raise their voices and protest such injustices, but the fact that no drug company opposes the Obama Care health plan is detrimental to the work of people like me, because we receive no support, no insurance coverage, and no research funding for our treatments. It all goes to the drug companies.

Sadly, politicians don't understand medicine, and if the information that they receive about it doesn't come from a drug company lobbyist, then they don't hear about it, don't care, and aren't interested in any other type of medicine. So the only way that people like me survive is because of word of mouth. People hear about my office and the successful results that we have here, and they come. Or they hear about it through books, like this one and Suzanne Somers'. The interest in alternative, or natural, medicine is driven strictly by the American population. It's a wonderful thing to see. This interest persists despite the enormous antagonism of the NCI, NIH, government research groups, and the drug companies that would rather get rid of supplements and doctors like me. We survive only because of public demand, because the voice of the people demands that we exist. The support for what we do isn't going to come from the government or the drug companies—that I promise you. They couldn't care less about successful cancer treatments in alternative medicine. They actually think the world would be better off without supplements and "alternative" medicine.

My Greatest Challenge as a Practitioner

My greatest challenge as a practitioner is helping my patients to get over their fears. They are facing death, so of course they are afraid, but they have to get over it. In terms of changing the world, I don't think globally, but instead work on a one-on-one, personal level with people. This is a patient by patient battle, and each battle must be fought differently and I must think fast in order to determine how to best fight each one. So my greatest challenge is the next patient who will walk into my office on Monday morning and how I will work with them to get them better. Every patient who comes to see me is an adventure. Every battle has to be fought in a slightly different way. So as for changing the world, for me, it's one patient at a time.

How Friends and Family Can Support Their Loved Ones with Cancer

Friends and family can support their loved ones by just doing that; loving and supporting them, and not being critical of their choices. Whether they choose to visit my office or Sloan-Kettering, the job of friends and family is to support the decision of the person with cancer. The last thing that people who are fighting death need, for example, is eight cousins whom they haven't seen in twenty years suddenly giving them advice about what they should do. But a strange thing happens. When people get cancer, suddenly, everyone around them becomes an expert: the mailman, the health food store owner, and the cousin from Topeka that they haven't spoken to in ten years. All of a sudden, they know what the person with cancer should do, even though they have no idea and should really keep their mouths shut. Their job, if they really want to be helpful, should be to answer any questions that the person with cancer has, but otherwise, they should keep their opinions to themselves. If they want them to go to Sloan-Kettering or another clinic, it doesn't matter. The patient is the boss of his or her treatment. Friends and family must learn to say to their loved ones, "That (treatment) wouldn't be my choice but I will love and support you, no matter what you choose to do." This is their disease and their body. The single most important piece of advice that I could give to friends and family of the sick would be, "Don't be critical. Keep your opinions to yourself, and just support the patient in his or her decision." When people are fighting cancer, the last thing that they need is to fight half a dozen family members. I have had patients who have literally had to ask their so-called friends to stop calling them because they were hostile about their choice to see me. I tell patients to cut friends and family off if they aren't going to be supportive of them. They don't need extra stress; they need love and support. So sometimes, the patients have cut them off and it is the best thing that they could have done. Discussions with family members over treatments can lead to battles and control issues in relationships, and people with cancer need to be supported.

Last Words

There are ways to treat even the worst of cancers successfully, such as through what we do here. When you, the patient, make a decision out of fear, you make the wrong decision. So first, take a deep breath and relax, and realize that you can get well. Make decisions out of relaxation and faith. Decisions that are made out of fear and anxiety are always panic-driven and are usually bad decisions. You don't need to be afraid. You can get over this. Just get rid of the background noise; leave it behind, and you can do well!

Contact Information
Nicholas Gonzalez

Nicholas J. Gonzalez, MD PC
36A East 36th Street
Suite 204
New York, N.Y. 10016
Phone: (212) 213-3337
Fax: (212) 213-3414
www.dr-gonzalez.com

• CHAPTER 3 •

Robert Zieve, MD
PRESCOTT, AZ

Biography

Robert J. Zieve, MD, is one of the most experienced and well-trained physicians in integrative medicine in the United States. He is the director of the Pine Tree Clinic for Comprehensive Medicine in Prescott, AZ (www.pinetreeclinic.com) and is supervising physician at the EuroMed Foundation integrative cancer clinic in Phoenix, AZ (www.euro-med.us).

Dr. Zieve graduated from the Ohio State University College of Medicine. He has practiced holistic and integrative medicine for over thirty-five years, and worked for over twenty years as a Board Certified specialist in emergency medicine and as the director of an emergency department at a small hospital. He has lectured to groups in both orthodox clinical and holistic medicine, both locally and nationally, for over twenty years. He has taught classes at the university level as well as at physician education forums. One of his teaching assignments was at the Southwest College of Naturopathic Medicine in Tempe, AZ. Additionally, he was President of the Arizona Homeopathic and Integrative Medical Association for two terms, from 1998 to 2000, and during 1999-2001, he was Medical Director of Paracelsus Fox Hollow Clinic, which was the United States affiliate of Paracelsus Klinik in Lustmühle, Switzerland, near Louisville, Kentucky.

Dr. Zieve is trained in many different medical disciplines, including homeopathy, nutrition, herbal, anthroposophical, and European biological medicine, as well as conventional allopathic and energy medicine. He is able to practice medicine in these diverse areas due to the extensive training he has received over the past twenty years. Examples of his extensive training include: a graduate course in homeopathy, a two-year physician course in anthroposophical medicine, training in nutritional medicine, ten years of ongoing study with Dr. Dietrich Klinghardt, MD, of the American Academy of Neural Therapy; a two-year course with The Biological Medicine Foundation that included training with Dr. Rau at Paracelsus Klinik in Switzerland; a two-year course with Lee Cowden, MD, in Bio-energetic Medicine; extensive training with Gerard Geunoit, MD, the well-known French homeopathic physician; a two-year course called Clinical Herbal Medicine Training in Cancer Therapy with Donald J. Yance, CN, MH (AHG); a one-year course in Hellinger Family Constellation Therapy with Mark Wolynn at the Hellinger Institute of PA, and a year of training in Recall Healing with Gilbert Renaud of Canada.

Dr. Zieve is the author of the 2005 book, *Healthy Medicine: A Guide to the Emergence of Sensible Comprehensive Care*, as well as the 2006 book, *Beyond the Medical Meltdown: Working Together for Sustainable Health Care* (Bell Pond Press). He has also been interviewed by the Huffington Post's health and wellness expert. That interview can be found on the Internet at the following address: www.huffingtonpost.com/nalini-chilkov/healthy-medicine-a-new-mo_b_809753.html

Dr. Zieve is the founder and director of the Center for Healthy Medicine (www.healthymedicine.org), a non-profit organization that has developed a plan for the transformation of health care in the United States, which includes strategies for developing effective and affordable care for all Americans.

Dr. Zieve is also Chief Medical Consultant to the Healthy Medicine Academy (www.healthymedicineacademy.com), and host of the weekly radio show, Healthy Medicine, which can be downloaded online from the Healthy Medicine Academy website. Many national cancer physicians have interviewed on this show, including Bernie Siegel, MD, and Donald Abrams, MD, Director of the Osher Cancer Center at the University of California, San Francisco, as well as others.

As an integrative medicine doctor who focuses on cancer, Dr. Zieve takes on different roles with his patients. Sometimes, he's their primary care physician who treats their cancers, and at other times, he's their primary care physician who works in collaboration with their oncologists. At other times, he is the consulting physician to their primary care doctors.

What Cancer Is and What Causes It

There are many different ways of looking at what cancer is. To me, cancer is the illness of our times, and has really taken off in the 20th century. Physician reports from one hundred years ago show that doctors could work their entire careers without ever seeing a cancer patient. So it's really a disease of the 20th century, even though it's occurred throughout history, and it's especially an illness of Western civilization. As other cultures have taken on various illness-generating elements of Western civilization, the incidence of cancer in these cultures has increased, too. So when I describe what cancer is, I think it's important to set the stage, not only in terms of what happens on a physical level in the body, but also what happens in our lives today. Some of the key elements which are associated with cancer and why it's an illness of our time can be compared in many ways to Western civilization itself; in fact, we are all part of a cancer-like social and economic milieu.

Cancer is uncontrolled or unlimited cell growth. The body has a natural way of killing or putting to death cells that are pre-programmed to die. This is called apoptosis. For instance, red blood cells are destined to die every 120 days. Those rhythms exist in every type of cell, organ, and tissue line in the body. When natural cell death, or apoptosis, is disrupted, there's uncontrolled growth of a particular type of cells in the body, and this is what constitutes cancer. This ideology of uncontrolled growth parallels what has happened in Western civilization over the past 50 years: our house values have grown, our bank accounts have grown, our debt has grown—everything has grown exponentially. There isn't a sustained rhythm of birth, adolescence, growth, maturation, decline, and death; the natural rhythm that has always been a part of civilization (until recently) has been disrupted. Instead, we have developed a civilization of uncontrolled growth without boundaries. Similarly, the loss of natural cell death, or apoptosis, which occurs in cancer cells, can be compared to the growing fear of death in our civilization and to a glorification of the physical world.

When there is strong, healthy cell-to-cell communication, and normal apoptosis, then people are less likely to develop cancer. The body's cells are constantly communicating with each other, on a biochemical and photonic (light) level. These communications go on instantaneously and continuously, and hundreds of thousands of them happen throughout the body, every second. The body operates on the basis of community. It doesn't operate on the basis of egotism and individualism. When it does, what results is the same thing that happens in a civilization when individual interests become more important than those of the community: there is chaos and destruction. When it occurs in the body, it is cancer.

Another element that's associated with cancer development is a loss of rhythm in a person's life and body. There's a tremendous loss of rhythm in people's lives today. We see this on a societal level, as well. This is evidenced by the conditions that many suffer from, such as insomnia, digestive difficulties, Attention Deficit Disorder (ADD), and Attention Deficit Hyperactivity Disorder (ADHD). In addition, millions of people have a deficiency of rhythm in their daily activities. That loss of rhythm contributes to and sets the stage for uncontrolled growth, a lack of communication and of any sense of community, both in their bodies and in their lives. In such an environment, the various triggers that are traditionally thought to cause cancer become activated.

So the development of cancer isn't just about environmental contaminants, but also the way that we live and think. I dialogue with my patients about this, because it's important to put cancer into the context of the greater milieu, and examine it in terms of the terrain in which we live. It's also important to examine cancer in terms of the internal terrain, or milieu, of the individual patient, as we examine the factors in his or her life which may have triggered the cancer to develop in the first place.

I will often spend fifteen to twenty minutes talking to my patients about the lifestyle aspect of disease alone. During this discussion, I may ask them, for instance, what happened in their lives in the two years leading up to their cancer diagnoses. I often find that there has been some significant life event: a loss of money in the stock market, the death of a spouse, or another traumatic event, which probably triggered the sudden growth of their cancers, which in reality, had been developing slowly in their bodies over a period of ten or more years. Other practitioners who ask their patients this question notice a correlation between their patients' life events and their development of cancer, as well. Even though it takes five to fifteen years for a microscopic cancer to develop into a detectable cancer, it has generally been observed that most people with cancer have had a significant event happen in their lives within the two years prior to their cancers becoming detectable, which accelerated the development of those cancers so that they eventually became detectable.

It's also important to understand what cancer is on a physical level. Basically, what happens, regardless of the factors that stimulate its growth, is that somewhere in the body, microscopically, there has been a loss of natural programmed cell death, so certain cells in an organ or tissue start to grow, initially without nerves or a blood supply. This is called the first stage of cancer, also referred to as cancer in-situ. At this stage, the cancer can grow from a single cell to many cells, as it obtains its food locally, at the site of its manife-station. It can remain that way for many years, and people can live with it for the rest of their lives and never have it progress beyond that stage if they have a strong immune system that effectively carries out its surveillance. This process of carcinoma development in-situ goes on in everyone's bodies all of the time. For example, many people have carcinoma in-situ in their breasts or colons, which never develop into full-blown cancers, because they have strong tumor suppressor genes. This initial stage of cancer is often not detected by any known diagnostic method, unless the patient has a Pap smear, biopsy of a polyp (an abnormal growth of tissue projecting from a mucous membrane), or a suspicious appearance on a mammogram.

Sometimes, though, cancer can change from the in-situ phase and move into what's called the locally invasive phase. In this phase, the cancer basically says to the organism (or the body), "I need more food to grow." It will then invade locally through tissues to get that food. Even then, it may not be visible on a scan or blood test. At some point, though, it will start to invasively grow, and depending on the type of cancer, it will start to be palpable and/or visible and detectable in the body. It may remain as a small, localized growth, which can be managed, or it may become metastatic.

During the third, or metastatic, phase, the cancer not only invades local tissues, but is also able to stimulate the formation of new blood vessels which help it to migrate through the body. It also starts to put out chemicals that disrupt the immune system's cancer detection radar, and simultaneously, puts out chemicals that stimu-late the growth of new blood vessels around it.

If this continues unabated, at some point, the cancer will be able to steal so much of the body's vital forces and nutrients that the person will develop cachexia, a condition whereby the body be-comes unable to utilize its nutrients from food, because many of those nutrients are instead feeding the cancer. At this stage, cancer becomes irreversible in most people, and leads to death.

It's important to note here that cancer isn't a local disease. It's always a systemic disease. Even when a local breast cancer or melanoma is discovered and diagnosed via biopsy, there are usually cancer cells from the "mother ship" circulating through the body and making new homes elsewhere. One of the big mistakes that modern medicine makes is that it doesn't recognize the fact that by the time a local cancer is discovered, there are already metastatic cells from that particular cancer floating around the body. This is true even before the cancer is officially considered to be metastatic. Studies on bone marrow biopsies in breast cancer patients have revealed that many breast cancer patients with localized cancers and whose lymph node biopsy results showed no cancer didn't just have cancer in their breasts. They also had micro-metastatic breast cancer cells in their bone marrow, even when they had normal bone and PET scans, and just a small lump in their breasts. So no cancer is local, and the problem with modern medicine is that it approaches cancer as if it was a local disease, and this is one important reason why modern oncology has a lot of failures.

People who have been diagnosed with an early stage of cancer, who get a tumor removed and go into remission (according to modern standards of diagnosis), may still have cancer cells circulating or deposited in their bodies. These can later re-establish themselves and cause active cancer again in other organs. Published studies, even out of major university centers, describe how people may have an increased risk for developing metastases after they have had a breast lump or local tumor removed, if the surgeries to remove their tumors are done at an inappropriate time.

The Role of Emotions in Cancer Development and Healing Emotional Trauma

I like to hear a patient's story. Most people with cancer initially have a lot of fear, so it's important for me to listen to their stories; to watch their gestures, mannerisms and expressions; to observe the lines on and the color of their faces, and the look in their eyes. Over the years, I have learned that the look in people's eyes can give me important clues about how well they will do with their treatments. If I see that fear, depression or anxiety are predominant in their expression, for example, then I will have to work a lot harder on treating their emotions, or hidden problems in their family dynamics or psyche that could get in the way of their treatments working.

The typical cancer personality has been described and discussed in many books. It encompasses people who are excessively caring, highly conscientious, hardworking, responsible, and who have a strong tendency towards carrying others' burdens. Such people are considered to be more prone to cancer. If I detect these characteristics in my patients, I may probe deeper into their psyches to find out more about their lives. I don't usually do this during their first several visits with me, but perhaps during the first or second month that I work with them, and only if they are open to discussing their lives with me. I will try to discover answers to certain questions, such as: How much are they worrying for others? For instance, how much is the woman with breast cancer worrying about her children and not taking care of herself? How much is the man with prostate or colon cancer feeling or worrying about a sexual secret that will be discovered, or feeling sexual shame? I ask these questions because such worries sometimes contribute to different types of cancer. Colon cancer, for instance, has also been linked to people not being able to let go of something; anal and rectal cancer have been linked to people feeling deep disgust about certain issues in their lives. So I will look for these links, or correlations, and see if patients want to resolve the underlying emotional issues which may be contributing to their cancers' development and survival. At our clinic, we have a well-trained therapist, as well as others that we can refer our patients to, and with whom I may work indirectly as part of our patients' care.

In my discussions with patients, I also observe how they respond to stress. Chronic stress raises cortisol levels, which in turn weakens the immune system. For instance, if it seems they are resentful towards their mothers, fathers, husbands, or wives, at some point, this may have been a contributing factor to their illnesses. Or if a woman loses a child, and isn't able to resolve that conflict on a psychological level, her breast may open up or widen its ducts, as if she were reaching out for her deceased son. The body's attempt to repair this widening may lead to the development of an intraductal breast cancer, which is the most common type of breast cancer in women. Of course, such processes happen on an unconscious level, so I try to help patients become aware of potential connections between emotional events and disease, so that they can let go of the traumatic conflicts that have been downloaded into their psyches, and be healed of their cancers.

I learned about these types of correlations, which are described in German New Medicine, from the international teacher Gilbert Renaud, PhD, who teaches a system called Recall Healing in Vancouver, Canada. According to his website, Recall Healing is a process that involves unlocking the secrets of illness by identifying and resolving the emotional trauma that causes disease. More information can be found at: www.recallhealing.ca. Doctors can take courses on Recall Healing and learn to identify such correlations in their patients.

Healing emotional trauma is an individual, personal process. Sometimes people aren't ready to address their issues. I am careful not to impose my agenda on my patients. Sometimes they are so full of fear that at first, I must work with them exclusively on a biochemical and physiological level and do things like build up their energy, run tests, start IVs, do low-dose chemotherapy and other treatments; in short, put together the best biological program for them that will increase their strength and improve their sleep and overall functioning. As they start to feel better, they begin to gain confidence in our treatments, and at that point they might be ready to look at the psychological factors which contributed to their diseases in the first place. Other people are ready to do such conflict work from the "get-go." In any case, whenever patients are ready, I will schedule a session with them to focus solely on this aspect of their healing.

Not all cancer doctors are trained in these approaches, so I would advise the patients of such doctors to see a Hellinger practitioner or a therapist trained in Recall Healing, who understands cancer personality issues and can focus on the emotional aspects of healing with them.

Treatment Approach

In my experience, successful cancer treatment involves addressing five main areas, which are summarized in the diagram below:

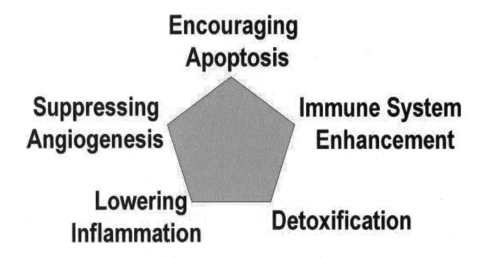

1. Immune system enhancement

2. Detoxification

3. Lowering inflammation

4. Suppressing angiogenesis, or the capacity of cancer cells to make new blood vessels so that they can spread

5. Encouraging apoptosis, or the natural death of cancer cells

CHAPTER 3: Robert Zieve, MD

My treatment approach has evolved organically through many years of being blessed to study with other experts in the field, both nationally and internationally, as well as from my experience of treating patients. I have evolved in being able to work with patients in a way that is intelligent, and which is backed by good science and common sense. I go beyond just treating people; I encourage them to actively participate in healing their cancers and their lives.

My treatments include botanicals, homeopathy, IV solutions, and nutrient and detoxification therapies to address all of the above components of healing. (Note: while "botanicals" refers to herbs, it also includes plant parts that aren't strictly herbs, such as bark, seeds, roots, and stems.) Because cancer is a systemic disease, and we see many patients with stage three or four cancers, chemotherapy plays an important role in helping them to heal or have a longer and better quality of life. For such situations, I prefer to use low-dose, high-frequency chemotherapy in an Insulin Potentiation Therapy (IPT) format. This is frequently effective even for metastatic cancers, though it isn't recognized as a valid treatment in modern oncology. Sometimes, patients choose not to do IPT. Whenever that's the case, I will work with them and their oncologists to help design an alternate program that will produce a promising outcome. These treatments and specific examples of how I use them are described in greater detail in the following sections.

Where I start people in their treatments depends upon the phase of disease that they are in. For instance, I won't have lengthy initial conversations with patients who are really sick and come into the EuroMed Foundation clinic in a wheelchair. We will instead start them on a nutritional IV right away, to build up their strength, as we initiate low-dose chemotherapy and a program of oral botanical remedies and nutrients. The IVs that we give may consist of Vitamin C (which has been well-researched in the medical literature for its usefulness in cancer care) along with minerals and other vitamins.

Sometimes, people who have come into our clinic in wheelchairs have been able to walk within days after having received a nutritional IV and low-dose chemotherapy treatment, and this gives them hope. They are also usually feeling better, and the color has come back into their faces.

For a woman with an early stage of breast cancer, my treatment approach would be different. We would sit down and dialogue and my goal would be to present her with different treatment options. I would explain to her what cancer is and let her know that we obtain the best results by individualizing our patients' care. This is very important, whether we have patients who aren't in pain and have good vitality, or who come into our clinic in wheelchairs. The key thing people must understand is that one size treatments don't fit all.

Individualizing my patients' care involves focusing on three main areas. First, I determine how I can best strengthen their core energy and vitality. This includes developing a well-thought-out nutritional and botanical protocol for them. Second, I identify the weaknesses in their bodies' terrain, which can be discerned through blood tests. The body's terrain essentially refers to its biochemistry and physiology. I determine factors such as patients' levels of acidity, their inflammation and mineral deficiencies, as well as whether they have heavy metal toxicity, lymphatic blockage, or blood that clots too easily. The objective is to get their bodies and internal terrain to self-regulate better. The third area involves looking at the specifics of their cancers and finding out where they are vulnerable. It may include doing chemo sensitivity testing on biopsy slides at nationally recognized labs. No matter how ill our patients are, we want to identify early on where their cancers are weak and then attack them from that angle, in ways that don't weaken the body.

The more that doctors build their patients up with good botanical, nutrient, and homeopathic programs for a month (if time permits) before those patients start chemotherapy, or while they are doing chemotherapy, the better their outcomes will be. The core of a good treatment program involves looking at patients' biochemistry, and asking questions like, "Are they diabetic? Do they have high blood pressure? Do they have inflammation? How well do they detoxify? How strong are their immune systems?"

The treatment approach that I just described is called the Eclectic Tri-Phasic Medical System (ETMS), which is taught by Donald Yance, Jr. CN, MH, RH (AHG). He teaches and collaborates with oncologists, integrative medical doctors, naturopaths, acupuncturists, nutritionists, and other health care professionals on how to restore a balanced biochemistry and physiology to the body, how to build up the immune and endocrine systems, and how to do detective work to find out where people's cancers are weak, and where they are strong. Again, the more we individualize our patients' therapy, the better are their outcomes.

It's important to recognize that not all cancers, even those of the same type, are the same. For example, the past few patients that I have worked with who had pancreatic cancer required different treatments, because their cancers evolved in different ways. Gemcitabine is the number one chemotherapeutic agent used for pancreatic cancer in conventional oncology, and it's very toxic. By doing chemo sensitivity testing, and using low dose chemotherapy in an IPT format (IPT will be explained in the following section and elsewhere throughout the book), we can give several agents to our patients which are better suited to their particular cancers.

Some patients benefit greatly when we do chemo sensitivity testing using either their tumor pathology slides (which we take from their biopsy procedures), or live tumor tissue which we send by overnight mail to nationally reputable labs. These tests can show us where their cancers are weak, and what treatment agents and regimens would be most effective for them. Patients with stage three and four cancers greatly benefit when low-dose chemotherapy agents (used in an IPT format) are combined with a nutritional protocol to build them up. Even those with early stages of cancer are likely to have metastatic cells, and may also benefit from such a protocol.

Sometimes, we add other types of pharmaceutical drugs, such as Herceptin, to our patients' protocols if their test results suggest that they will have improved outcomes with these. Other prescription drugs, which we administer in low doses, such as the diabetic medicine Metformin, or aromatase-inhibitor drugs like Aromasan (which we use in estrogen-positive cancers), as well as low dose naltrexone, can also add to our patients' success.

When we have success in treating people's cancers, it's amazing how their other conditions, such as diabetes and hypertension, improve. This is because the factors which contributed to these conditions in the first place: inflammation, chronic infections, poor detoxification, and/or a weakened immune system, have been addressed. Unfortunately, we have a specialty-based medical system where every specialist is off in their own little corner, learning primarily about only one area of the body, and too often, they get "stuck out on a branch." But it's not the branches that matter—it's the trunk of the tree, and the roots.

IPT—Insulin Potentiation Therapy and Metronomic Chemotherapy

Note: IPT is explained in Chapter Five and other chapters throughout this book, so the specifics about how it works won't be discussed here. Please refer to the IPT section in Chapter Five for more information.

We do IPT, Insulin Potentiation Therapy, at our clinic in Phoenix (but not at our clinic in Prescott). At our clinic in Phoenix, we see patients from all over the country. In fact, 80 percent of them are from different parts of the country.

It takes well-trained people to properly administer IPT. We have a very able and caring nurse (who was originally a thoracic surgeon from Poland) who does our treatments, as well as a highly skilled physician's assistant. We hold weekly group meetings at a big round table with our physicians, nurse, physician's assistant, patients, and their families, to discuss our patients' progress and answer any questions they might have. There are many issues involved in doing IPT, such as the timing of its administration, the type of agents being administered, the role of insulin in the treatments, and a thorough knowledge of chemotherapeutic drugs. Those who do IPT need to be good at it. We have a lot of confidence in the nurse and physician's assistant who work at our clinic.

I recommend IPT as part of most patients' protocols, because it makes good sense. It's less toxic than traditional chemotherapy, and often works well, even though the drug dose is only one-tenth of that which is normally used in chemotherapy. That said, even low-dose chemotherapy can affect the bone marrow, and consequently, the body's white and red blood cell counts. This means that patients might become slightly anemic during their treatments. We recommend bone marrow soup and botanicals (herbs) to support their bone marrow and white blood cell production. Most people tolerate the low-dose chemotherapy well, though. Another great thing about low-dose chemotherapy is that we can combine several chemotherapy agents together at once without overdosing patients, making it more likely that at least one or two agents will work well on their cancers, especially when we have chemo sensitivity lab test results to help guide us in our decisions.

A new approach to chemotherapy, called metronomic chemotherapy, has been growing in popularity in conventional oncology. This involves giving patients one-third of the dose of some of the drugs that they would be given in a normal chemotherapy regimen, and on a weekly basis instead of once every three weeks. Like IPT, I believe its success is enhanced by doing chemotherapy sensitivity testing to identify the one or two chemotherapy agents that the cancer will be most sensitive to. Unlike IPT, however, both metronomic and full dose chemotherapy require that doctors give their patients just one agent at a time.

Regardless of the chemotherapy method that's used, the most important thing when making treatment decisions is to apply good science and not make decisions out of fear. It's important for patients and their doctors to take the time to develop a good treatment plan together. And of course, it's important for doctors to help their patients maintain a positive mental attitude. Bernie Siegel, MD, has an intriguing approach to this. He teaches art and does group therapy sessions for people with cancer, which are very effective for helping them to stay positive.

One of the challenges facing patients who choose to use IPT is finding oncologists who will support them in it. Patients who come from out of state may have problems getting approval for it from their oncologists, because most oncologists think it's unproven.

While it's true that million dollar research studies haven't been completed on IPT (for a lot of reasons that I won't go into here) there is good outcomes-based evidence on it from our clinic and other participating clinics. Still, many people who are in the early stages of cancer get a lot of pressure from their oncologists to do certain treatments. Many of my patients have told me that they are scared to death of going against their physicians, so doing a therapy that is outside of the box takes courage.

Finally, if patients with early stage cancers don't want to do chemotherapy, we can put together a treatment protocol for them based on dietary recommendations, botanicals (herbs), lifestyle changes, Vitamin C and magnesium IVs, and mistletoe therapy. They can sometimes get good results from doing just these treatments alone. Recently, I had a female patient whose tumor mass shrunk 40 percent after six weeks, with just the use of natural medicine. It is, however, difficult to predict whether natural therapies alone will be sufficient for patients.

Chemotherapy Sensitivity and Other Types of Testing

If patients have already had biopsies done by the time they come to our clinic, then we will send their pathology slides to a lab here in the United States to determine which chemotherapy agents their cancer cells will best respond to, based on the results of their biopsies. Ideally, tests should be done using tumor tissue, so biopsies are very helpful. This is my perspective, although I know that some physicians have a different opinion. If patients want to do live tissue testing (which is done when the tumor sample is freshly removed from the body) we help them by working with their surgeons to get their live tissue sent overnight to one of two labs in Southern California. However, this type of testing isn't practical for many people because of the location of their cancers. So the second best option, which works well for the majority of our patients, is to do chemo sensitivity testing using pathology slides from their biopsies.

In addition to chemotherapy sensitivity testing, we do many other types of tests to help determine what our patients need. Everyone needs to have intermittent but extensive blood tests for levels of C-reactive protein (C-reactive protein is an inflammatory marker), fibrinogen and D-dimer (proteins which play a role in blood clotting), along with other factors. For example, knowing the amount of fibrinogen in the blood is important because doctors can be treating their patients successfully for cancer, but if they have high levels of fibrinogen, they can suddenly develop a blood clot or embolism and become worse. Cancer, in general, predisposes people to blood clots, and some chemotherapy agents can contribute further to this tendency. Blood clotting factors such as fibrinogen are high in people with non-small cell lung and pancreatic cancers. Systemic enzyme products such as Lumbrokinase, and sometimes Heparin injections, can remedy this problem.

Testing hormone levels is also important. We check our patients' thyroid function, because low thyroid function is associated with breast cancer. We also check estrone sulfate, which is a storage form of estrogen, in patients whose cancers are particularly affected by hormones. If their estradiol levels are high, we may recommend the herb chrysin, which is a natural aromatase inhibitor that blocks the effects of estrogen upon cancer, or add a pharmaceutical aromatase inhibitor to their regimens. We always test estrogen and dihydrotestosterone levels in our prostate cancer patients, since high estrogen promotes prostate cancer growth. Then we use the appropriate botanicals and pharmaceuticals to treat those hormones.

We test our patients' hemoglobin, A1c (A1c measures the body's average blood glucose over a period of time) and fasting insulin levels. High insulin and A1c levels impair healing from cancer, and also lead to many other chronic illnesses. We help normalize our patients' blood sugar with minerals, including chromium, zinc, and magnesium. We also use good botanical (herbal) tincture combinations that include Gymnema sylvestre and celery root. Other herbs help to normalize blood sugar function, as well. Usually, patients' blood sugar problems correct over time when we use a well-thought-out combination of botanicals, nutrients and minerals. Of course, making significant dietary changes is also crucial for helping the body to better regulate its blood sugar.

Additionally, we always look at blood tumor markers. When initially elevated, these tumor markers are important for determining our patients' progress on a particular treatment regimen. We also look at their ferritin levels (ferritin is the body's storage form of iron), because high levels of iron feed cancer. We have to work intelligently to get the body's chemistry to normalize. In a subsequent section, I mention the importance of testing Vitamin D levels.

Finally, we test copper levels and levels of the copper-carrying protein ceruloplasmin, because copper is a cancer stimulant, and is involved in tumor blood vessel formation. We can give our patients all of the immune support in the world, but if they have high copper levels, new blood vessels will get created and their cancers will spread. A drug called TM (Tetrathiomolybdate) reduces copper levels and thereby shuts off the cancer's ability to spread. Zinc supplementation is also very helpful for reducing copper levels.

Addressing Growth Factors in Cancer

Growth factors are substances made by the body which govern cellular behavior. It's important to address these in some types of cancer. For example, if a woman has a HER-2 positive breast cancer, we (as well as oncologists) may use other type of drugs such as Herceptin to suppress the growth factors on the receptor sites that are on the surface of the cancer cells. We may give these drugs in addition to chemotherapy. By testing our patients' cancers, we can discover whether there are markers on the surface of their cells which would respond to these types of medications. In addition, we look at their pathology test results to determine whether there are factors in their cancers that could prevent the Herceptin or other medications from working as well. If so, we give them botanicals and sometimes drugs to help counter those factors.

Note: HER-2 positive breast cancers test positive for a protein called human epidermal growth factor receptor 2 (HER-2), which promotes cancer cell growth. Herceptin is a biological pharmaceutical drug (not a chemotherapy agent) which stifles the growth of this particular HER-2 protein, and which has fewer side effects than some of the other drugs of its type. Other drugs target growth factors in other types of cancer in a similar manner.

Building Up the Body with Botanicals, Vitamins and Other Nutrients

At our clinics, we have many different approaches to nutritional supplementation. We formulate our protocols according to good research, clinical experience, and common sense. We start our patients off with nutrients and adaptogenic or normalizing herbs, to support the body's foundations. If you have a building that's falling apart, you have to gird its foundations, so we use herbs for this purpose. The most common adaptogenic herb that we use is eleutherococcus, or Siberian Ginseng. Thousands of published studies demonstrate the benefits of eleutherococcus for people with cancer, even those who are currently doing chemotherapy. Rhodiola, astragalus, knotweed, schizandra, and ashwaghanda, as well as many medicinal mushrooms and other primary and secondary adaptogenic herbs, are likewise useful.

Herbs are amazing plants that, when used properly, have multiple ways of correcting the same problems that led to the body's development of cancer in the first place. They modulate hormones and immune function; improve cell-to-cell communication, reduce inflammation, down-regulate cancer pathways, and so on. In addition, the body needs anabolic agents to build up its tissues, and help counter its tendency to tear them down, so we make sure that we provide our patients with this foundational support early on in their treatment programs.

Improving Cellular Energy and Immune Function

As part of a good foundational support program, botanicals are also important for improving the body's cellular energy, as are certain kinds of whey protein, amino acids, and an abundance of minerals. Almost everyone in this country, whether or not they have cancer, has depleted levels of magnesium, chromium, zinc, iodine, and Vitamin D. Many physicians now routinely measure their patients' Vitamin D levels. Rarely do I see anyone with a 25 (OH) Vitamin D level that's higher than 50 ng/ml, even in people who are taking Vitamin D supplements. Yet people with serious illnesses need to have a Vitamin D level that's between 80-100 ng/ml. We just saw a colon cancer patient whose Vitamin D level came back at 4 ng/ml. Unfortunately, when I prescribed him a high dose of Vitamin D for a month, his regular doctor thought he was going to poison himself with Vitamin D. It's important for practitioners to be aware of the risks of low levels of Vitamin D, because one in two, or perhaps one in three people, are getting cancer today, and increasing Vitamin D levels can dramatically lower the risk of developing many types of cancer. Michael Hollick MD, at Boston University, and Soram Khalsa, MD, at UCLA, among others, have published research about the effects of Vitamin D upon cancer and its role in preventing cancer.

rent herbs and nutrients in our practice to in-
and improve immune function. Thousands of
nonstrate the beneficial effects of herbs and
...er. Unfortunately, most oncologists are telling
patients not to take them while doing conventional treatments, because they believe that they can interfere with their
treatments. However, one oncologist did a study that was published
in 2007, proving this to be a myth, and that not only do herbs and
nutrients not interfere with conventional treatments, but they
actually enhance their effectiveness. I am hoping that more doctors
will recognize their benefits, but until they do, one of the main
messages that I impart to my patients is that they should interview
their physicians. A one-size-fits-all approach to medicine doesn't
work, and it's important for patients to put together their own team
of competent practitioners who can help them to get better.

Building a Treatment Protocol in Layers

We usually build our patients' treatment plans in layers; meaning,
we start them off with a few treatments and then build upon those.
For most, we first prescribe a medicinal smoothie, which they drink
once or twice a day. This consists of a high quality whey protein
powder, combined with magnesium and creatine to support muscle
mass, colostrum for immune function, and high doses of astragalus,
eleutherococcus, and organic blueberries to build cellular energy.
They can choose to flavor the smoothie by adding unsweetened
almond milk or fresh flax seed powder to it. I wish we could come
up with another name for it, though, because "smoothie" in most
people's psyche means a very sweet tasting restaurant drink that's
full of sugar. It's possible to prepare these medicinal smoothies so
that they taste good, though. Our smoothies are a good way to get
nutrients into the body.

Following the smoothie, we add additional layers to the regimen;
anything from liver-protective herbs like broccoli and cabbage
sprouts to liquid iodine (if people are deficient in iodine), to minerals and high doses of Vitamin D. After checking patients' blood
levels of Vitamin D, we will prescribe a minimum of 10,000 IUs of

Vitamin D daily, regardless of the stage of cancer that they are in (unless they were taking Vitamin D before they came to see us, in which case we may adjust the dosage). We also start them on herbs that modulate the immune system, and will frequently add other nutrients and herbs, according to their needs. For example, we may give gotu kola for glioblastomas, licorice root for people on dexamethasone, urtica seeds for kidney support, and milk thistle during chemotherapy to support the liver detoxification pathways. If men have prostate cancer, we may add herbs like saw palmetto and pumpkin seed oil to their regimens. If they aren't sleeping and their muscle mass is low, then we may give them certain amino acids, such as melatonin, L-arginine, and L-lysine. My goal is to build a program that addresses the whole body, the particular cancer that my patients are dealing with, and their biochemical abnormalities.

Our patients all have different needs. One may have nausea. Another may have low energy, and yet another may not be sleeping. We need to highly individualize their treatments, as whenever we don't, we end up alienating them and not having satisfying outcomes.

The Multi-Faceted Benefits of Herbal Remedies for Treating Cancer

Herbs have multi-faceted beneficial effects upon cancer and the body. For example, people with cancer often have significant inflammation, as a result of chemotherapy agents, radiation, and the cancer itself. High doses of herbs such as curcumin and boswellia, as well as good quality fish oils with adequate amounts of EPA, can reduce that inflammation. But they, as well as many other herbs and natural agents, don't just lower inflammation. They also potentiate chemotherapy, increase glutathione levels (which is important for detoxification), improve immune function, repair damaged cells, get liver detoxification pathways working better, downregulate many cancer pathways, modulate hormones, and protect the bone marrow, among other things. It's just beautiful, and the science behind them is incredible. I have learned so much about them from wonderful teachers like Donald Yance of the Mederi Foundation and his associates at the Centre for Natural Healing in

Ashland, Oregon, and have d.
racle.

To cite some other examples (
toe increases tumor necrosis
chemical produced by white l
but which also acts in a variety or otiici ...
death; the vinca alkaloids of the Madagascar periwinkie
not only to disrupt cancer cell microtubules, but also to directly kill
cancer cells, and Camptotheca inhibits a certain enzyme within the
cancer cell which enables it to replicate itself. Some of these herbs
form the basis of commonly used chemotherapy agents today, so,
for example, if doctors give the herb Camptotheca in conjunction
with the chemotherapy agent Irenotecan, it can act synergistically
with that agent to lower the capacity of the cancer cell to multiply
by inhibiting its DNA replication. The Pacific Yew, from which the
taxanes are developed (taxanes are chemotherapy medications used
to treat breast cancer), disrupts tubulin in cancer cells so that they
die (tubulin is a constituent protein of the microtubules of cells,
which provide a skeleton for maintaining cell shape and are thought
to be involved in cell motility). In addition, pawpaw increases
apoptosis, as do fish oils, which is one reason why it's good for
people with cancer to take significant amounts of a quality fish oil
product containing at least 1500 mg of eicosapentaenoic acid
(EPA). Most of the brands out on the market aren't good, because
they are often are contaminated with mercury or not well-prepared,
so it's important to do research in order to find the best one.

When selecting supplements, patients should remember three
things. First, more isn't necessarily better. Secondly, great variations in quality exist among the herbs and nutrients that are out on
the market. Third, taking natural agents that are designed to be
synergistic with other therapies often yields better treatment
outcomes.

Many of the above-mentioned herbs are cytotoxic, and practitioners
have discovered that if they add low doses of cytotoxic herbs, like

the Madagascar periwinkle, to their patients' herbal protocols while they are doing chemotherapy, then their chemotherapy becomes more effective.

Also, most of the time, when a cancer grows, it invades the body's connective tissue. So it's important for doctors who use cytotoxic botanical remedies to simultaneously build their patients' connective tissue with other herbs like Gotu Kola, which support and repair it.

Finally, many tumors, not just breast cancer, have estrogen receptors on them. If we do chemo sensitivity testing, we can discover whether a patient's cancer has a lot of estrogen receptors on the surface of its cells. If it does, herbs such as chrysin and drugs such as Aromasin or Arimidex are excellent estrogen blockers. If we don't address this aspect of treatment, the patient's cancer cells will continue to grow, no matter what treatments we are doing.

In summary, herbs can act directly upon cancer in a myriad of ways: some increase tumor necrosis factor; others affect DNA replication, increase apoptosis, disrupt biochemical pathways in the cell, or prevent cancer cells from forming tubulin. Most disable cancer in a variety of ways and therefore are of great value when treating it.

A growing number of our patients arrive at our clinic with large bags of supplements that they are already taking and which they have acquired as a result of their cancer research. Many take fish oils and curcumin. Some take immune-supportive herbs and mushrooms. We are very happy to see this, because we believe that cancer care will evolve and produce good outcomes as a result of patients being proactive about research and doing treatments on their own. It isn't the integrative oncologists who are going to evolve cancer care; the demand will come from the public understanding the importance of a low toxicity lifestyle and individualized care.

Detoxification

When cancer cells are killed, their toxic material has to be transported through the lymph, out of the body. Botanicals, minerals, and homeopathic remedies help to keep the liver, lymph, kidney, and other detoxification pathways open so that toxins can better exit the body. We recommend a wide variety of other treatments for detoxification, including castor oil packs, coffee enemas, infrared saunas, and homeopathic, botanical and Traditional Chinese Medicine (TCM) remedies. We use a myriad of substances to support the body's major detoxification pathways, including the lymphatic system and biliary pathways. We want the skin to become a third kidney, because, like the kidneys, the skin is important for helping the body to rid itself of toxins.

Dietary Recommendations

Author Michael Pollan has three axioms regarding diet. He says, "Eat food, less of it, and more vegetables." These three quick phrases comprise the prescription that I give my patients.

We put all of our patients on some version of the Mediterranean diet, which is comprised of small amounts of animal protein, such as wild fish and free range fowl, or goat's cheese, along with lots of vegetables and small amounts of grains and fruit. This is our foundational diet. We then further individualize the diet according to our patients' needs.

I base some of my dietary recommendations upon the principles of Traditional Chinese Medicine. In TCM, the body is organized according to organ systems, and foods are thought to affect those systems in different ways. There are, for example, certain foods, such as eggs, walnuts and some fruits, which build kidney energy and in turn affect the health of the entire endocrine system. In TCM, the spleen network builds the immune system and helps the body to extract its nourishment from food. Wild salmon, halibut, yams, cooked cabbage, peas, and certain grains such as pearled barley, are examples of foods that support the spleen network and build immune energy. Foods such as watercress, endive, some bitter herbs, and cilantro support the liver's detoxification energy pathways. If patients are low on energy, this is often due to a deficiency in their kidneys' energy network. Horseradish, mustard, nettles, dandelion greens, and artichoke can help build the body's overall energy system.

I'm not big into a diet of exclusively raw foods. Certain people, for example, those who are thin and who would be considered as "yin" types in Chinese medicine, need to eat more cooked—and especially steamed—food. Other people, who have bone marrow problems as a result of chemotherapy, need to ingest bone marrow broth and add some astragalus to it. This can be prepared in a Crock-pot or other slow cooker using big cow bones and lots of vegetables.

I may recommend specific foods based on the type of cancer that my patients have, but in general, the above are my recommendations. We live in a society that is anxious about food, and this isn't helpful, either. When patients follow our guidelines, and are able to stay on the medicinal smoothies, herbs, and other treatments that we recommend, and can tolerate these along with their low dose chemotherapy regimens, they generally have good outcomes. Fortunately, most patients tolerate both quite well.

There are four levels of food: the unhealthy, healthy, high quality, and super medicinal (like the smoothies). People with cancer should aim to get as many of the high quality and super medicinal foods as they can into their diets.

Treatment Outcomes

Our treatment outcomes don't just depend upon the stage of cancer that patients have, but also the type of cancer, their mental and emotional state, and a variety of other factors.

Our goal with all of our patients is full remission, so that there is no longer any evidence of cancer in their bodies, and that they would remain this way for years, and enjoy a good quality of life. Of course, some people with stage three or four cancers aren't able to attain remission, but with our approach, they are able to live high-quality lives, even though they still have cancer. To illustrate, one of our colleagues has a patient who has lived with a stage four lung cancer for over ten years past her original diagnosis. Her doctors had told her that she was going to die within months, but she has been alive for a long time now and you can't tell by looking at her that she has cancer. Only by looking at a chest x-ray or blood tests would you know. Of course, she takes a lot of botanical and nutrient capsules and tablets every day, but she doesn't do chemotherapy anymore. I have a patient with multiple myeloma, who has so far survived and thrived for eight years beyond her initial diagnosis. She's on an extensive, targeted, natural medicine program, and must take many pills and liquids daily. She also takes a drug called Thalidomide. When taken in low doses, this drug can be effective for some people with specific types of cancer. It's important for her to take her medication because her myeloma was so advanced when she first came to see us that we couldn't put it into remission. So while Thalidomide keeps her cancer in check and allows her to live a normal life, it also prevents her from going into remission. But again, she looks and feels good. She still has high immunoglobulin levels and abnormal cells in her blood that are characteristic of her cancer, but she is a healthy, strong, functioning, multiple myeloma patient who has been living for years, with no kidney damage, and who could continue to live for decades with her cancer.

Yet another patient of ours with stage four ovarian cancer, who had lots of fatigue and routinely had to have fluid drained from her abdomen, went into full remission after doing high frequency, low-dose IPT. After six months of treatment, she is now cancer-free. That means her scans and lab tests are normal. Why did she go into remission when another stage four patient didn't? Many reasons exist, and it depends somewhat upon the type of cancer that patients have, the particular characteristics of that cancer, as well as their biochemistry and physiology. Ovarian cancer is susceptible to the right chemotherapy agents, but we find that if patients aren't also put on a good natural treatment regimen, and if they don't continue with regular but infrequent IPT chemotherapy sessions, then this type of cancer will often come roaring back.

We never tell our stage four patients that they will go into remission. It would be great if that happened, but most often, it doesn't. Fortunately, we can help them to manage their cancers like a chronic illness so that they can have longer, better lives, even if their cancers are still present to a degree. I don't use the word remission with my patients anyway, because it's too much of a buzz word today. Remission means different things to different people. The reason I don't use it is because helping people to live long, quality lives is what matters, whether or not their cancers are present on a scan.

With my treatment approach, many of my cancer patients' other conditions also often improve, so that they no longer require pharmaceutical drugs. The practical treatment outcome can be the same for the person who still has cancer as for the one who is in remission, in that both can live long, high quality lives.

Some of our patients have no detectable cancer cells left after they finish their treatments here, but there is no wishful thinking, either. If they had a stage three or four cancer, they can't just take a few curcumin tablets and maintain a good diet and think that will be sufficient. They have to really stay on top of it for years, and address it from multiple angles, so that the cancer doesn't manifest again.

Recently, I saw a woman who had some discomfort on the right side of her chest. We thought she might have shingles. Thirteen years ago, she had a lumpectomy for breast cancer. We ran some tests on her, and discovered that three of her breast cancer markers were once again elevated. Her scans now show that she has metastases to her lungs as a result of her initial cancer. This was proven through a biopsy. This scenario isn't common but it can happen.

It's important for patients to be diligent about their treatments. If you have a condition like herpes, you take 1500 mg of lysine daily for the rest of your life, because you know that the infection can come out at any time. If you have chronic rheumatoid arthritis or multiple sclerosis, both of which can be due to Lyme disease, you have to take care of yourself, because you will have Lyme organisms in your body for the rest of your life, and by taking care of yourself, you will keep them from causing you symptoms. It's the same thing with cancer; you have to be diligent and monitor it, as you maintain a good, healthy diet and nutritional protocol. Often, we suggest that our patients who have been successfully treated with IPT, and whose cancers are no longer detectable on a scan or via other lab indicators, return twice a year for the same low-dose therapy, for at least a few years, and stay on a rigorous oral natural medicine program in the meantime.

The extent of our maintenance program is different for everyone, depending upon the level of cancer that's still present and detectable in the body. The woman whose ovarian cancer is in remission, for instance, probably takes half the amount of nutrients on a daily basis than the one who still has a detectable stage four lung cancer. Ovarian cancer is sensitive to various herbs, like knotweed, or devils' claw, so I may, in addition to a core or baseline nutrient protocol, recommend these herbs as part of a maintenance program for patients with this type of cancer. Herbs, as well as immune strengthening supplements, enable the body's surveillance system to maintain control of the cancer, as do healthy lifestyle practices, such as getting good sleep, eating healthy food, exercising regularly, and keeping the mind clear of persistent emotional conflicts.

Once they have finished an initial treatment regimen at our clinic, our patients may come back twice a year to get two IPT treatments for a period of time. We have a number of patients who have been able to manage their late stage cancers for a long time, like any chronic illness. By normalizing their biochemistry, getting them to take supplements that disrupt cancer cell pathways, and working with their diet and emotional conflicts, we end up with patients who have good treatment outcomes that last. Regardless of whether they are in remission with a cancer that can't be detected on tests, or still have cancer, yet are doing quite well on a maintenance regimen, they still require support and good follow-up.

Patient/Practitioner Challenges to Healing

Tailoring my patients' treatment regimens to their biological characteristics and internal terrain is a challenge. But it's probably not my greatest challenge. I feel pretty comfortable with my knowledge and expertise, and also with the team of people that I work with. So I think that my greatest challenge as a practitioner is dealing with my patients' fears and the pressures that they face from other doctors, the media, and their families, which generally have to do with their oncologists telling them what to do. Another challenge is finding oncologists who will continue to see and evaluate our patients while they are doing our natural medicine programs and low-dose, high frequency chemotherapy. Also, some patients may require biological monoclonal antibody therapies, which involve the use of monoclonal antibodies (or mAb), that specifically bind to cancer cells and stimulate the immune system to attack those cells. These therapies can be very expensive, so getting oncologists to prescribe them can be a challenge.

Getting patients to stay the course with their treatments, and to understand the importance of actively participating in their recovery process is also a challenge, for both me and them. We live in a society that encourages passivity. If people are faced with an illness that could take their life, they have to become proactive in multiple ways so that, by the time they come out of it, and their cancers are either not detectable anymore or much improved, they are different people. They have to work on multiple levels to heal, so that they can become more aware and confident in life. They must have a good reason to live, understand the role of food in health, and strive to maintain a healthy diet. Those that do well in their recovery are transformed people by the end of their treatment course, because they have realized that they needed to change some fundamental things in their lives in order to get better, and not just in their physical bodies, but also in their souls. Their personalities, spiritual life, relationships, lifestyle, and food habits all end up changing.

Another challenge for my patients and me is what is called "the curse of the diagnosis." I have had patients who were making good progress with their healing, but who were thrown off track by the bad advice of others. For example, one of our patients with pancreatic cancer had received two weeks of IPT and nutritional IVs, including Vitamin C and magnesium, and as a result, his tumor markers fell by 75 percent. We also gave him mistletoe and detoxification therapy. But he got somewhat anemic from the IPT treatments, which is not an uncommon side effect. So we sent him to the hospital to get a blood transfusion and he came out a totally different person. His confidence was gone and he was complaining, even though he was better. In the hospital, they had asked him a bunch of questions, like, "Why are you seeing these other doctors? You're going to die if you continue to do that IPT therapy." In the end, he didn't do well with his treatments. It broke my heart. I clearly saw why this happened: his will had been weakened, and his faith in what had been for him an effective therapy, had dissipated. It's important for people with cancer to trust their instincts, stay the course, follow their intuition, and build a good advisory team, which may include an oncologist and practitioners of natural medicine. On the other hand, it doesn't help patients to be angry at the medical profession; in fact, staying away from negative talk is important for healing.

That's why we're here to advise our patients. We tell them, "This is what we offer. We feel that our treatments provide better results than the one-size-fits-all approach of conventional oncology. But do your research and put together a plan. Don't be in a hurry to get started on a treatment unless it's urgent." Even saying this, though, some people aren't going to get it, although a lot of them do. Increasingly, more people are acquiring the common-sense understanding that the one-size-fits-all approaches to healing don't work, and that cancer treatment approaches that aren't tailored to their specific needs may not be the best. Those are the people that we often work with. They take charge of their health, and are determined to do whatever it takes to get better. It's a real joy to work with them.

Risky Cancer Treatments and What Constitutes Good Science

Increasingly, more people are concluding that much of regular oncology is ineffective and responsible for causing more harm than good.

I don't define "good outcomes" as simply the elimination of a primary cancer, which can happen with conventional chemotherapy. It also means longer survival, a higher quality of life, and fewer incidences of metastases for the patient. From this perspective, modern oncology is, in many ways, a failure. Indeed, many chemotherapeutic agents are approved when studies show that they only prolong life by four months or so. Our goal is to prolong our patients' lives for years to decades, and for their quality of life to be good. For the most part, modern oncologists know how to diagnose cancer and they understand chemotherapeutic agents. But conventional treatments are largely ineffective for significantly prolonging the patient's life, except for in a small handful of cancers, such as Hodgkin's lymphoma and testicular cancer. They are effective for reducing tumor load, but not for helping people to survive with a good quality of life for many years without metastases and/or recurrences.

Our focus is on true science. I want to see outcomes-based studies, or evidence-based studies, and not just the double-blind studies that are held up as the "gold standard." Even mainstream medical publications are now acknowledging that the measurements that we have used and which are considered to be the "gold standard" for determining a treatment's success are flawed. I recommend the book *Wrong: Why Experts Keep Failing Us and How to Know When Not to Trust Them*, by David H. Freedman, to those who want to understand this concept more. People are attracted to treatment approaches in integrative oncology because they build up the body rather than weaken it, are safe, often more effective, and people incur less pain and suffering with them.

Not all non-allopathic (alternative and complementary) approaches to cancer treatment have good evidence for their effectiveness, but many do, so we try to find and use those in our practice. Good, outcomes-based research studies have been done which demonstrate the effectiveness of botanicals, homeopathy, and different nutritional supplements for the treatment of cancer. Such research studies and evidence also exists for Recall Healing. There is ample evidence which demonstrates that resolving psychological conflicts reduces tumors and/or improves the effectiveness of current allopathic or integrative treatment programs. And again, the reason we call this type of medicine "integrative" is because at times, chemotherapy can be beneficial, especially when given by low dose, high frequency methods such as IPT. Other modern oncology approaches, such as monoclonal antibody administration, can also be helpful. We rarely recommend surgery unless: there is a risk of obstruction, a tumor needs to be de-bulked or made smaller because of the pressure that it's exerting on adjacent body structures, or it would be beneficial to obtain a larger tumor specimen (which is required for doing live tissue testing).

The effectiveness of coffee enemas and castor oil packs hasn't been established by double-blind, placebo-controlled studies. But I recommend them to my patients because there is good outcomes-based evidence proving their success. Similarly, hyperthermia and infrared saunas have been shown to be very effective supportive therapies for cancer, as has injectable mistletoe therapy and intravenous Vitamin C.

There are other natural therapies that I can't speak about from experience, and I don't know if they are as effective as people claim. My concern is that if a treatment becomes a belief system, and a patient or doctor develops a blind spot because of that belief system, it can lead to worse outcomes. Belief systems can be dangerous if there is no good evidence to support them. For the most part, allopathic oncology is based on a one-size-fits-all approach, which often isn't backed by good science. Good science doesn't mean proving something in a lab. It means looking at treatment outcomes, seeing a patient's C-reactive protein levels, tumor markers or PET scans improve, identifying the factors that caused those things to happen, asking questions with an open, inquisitive mind, and applying those conclusions to each patient. Good science means individualizing a patient's program as much as possible. I'm aware that many oncologists are overwhelmed, and that the time required of them to do this for their patients is more than they have, but I'm also aware that there's a mindset in oncology, a way of thinking, that blocks many oncologists from taking a more integrative approach to treatment, and that's unfortunate.

In the future, there will be energy medicine approaches to treating cancer which go beyond infrared saunas. They will involve working with things like color, sound, and lasers. Currently, some practitioners are getting good empirical results by using energy medicine modalities, but I don't know enough about them to comment on their effectiveness. A lot of good work is being done with photodynamic therapy and hyperthermia in other parts of the world. However, even though these are effective treatments, I have seen practitioners using them to the exclusion of other therapies, which can be a problem.

An excellent guide for laypeople with cancer is a book called *You Did What?* by Hollie and Patrick Quinn. Hollie developed breast cancer at age 22, while she was eight months pregnant. Premenopausal breast cancer is much more dangerous than a postmenopausal breast cancer. Yet Hollie decided not to do conventional therapy, and instead chose a different path in order to get well. It has now been eight years since her diagnosis and she has had no recurrence of her primary cancer. She hasn't done any chemotherapy or other drugs. This is a coaching-type book that will empower people to say, "Yes, I need to put together a healing team and think my options through." A physician who's very knowledgeable and experienced in oncology ought to be part of this team. I try to help my patients move out of the fear state that they may be in, and get on the right program, which always involves natural medicine, and sometimes, chemotherapy and surgery, and rarely, radiation therapy.

Similarly, it's important for practitioners to be in a supportive environment where they can work in a collaborative spirit with colleagues. This isn't easy to achieve in today's world, but we have managed to do this at the EuroMed Foundation in Phoenix. We regularly discuss our patients and stimulate one another to develop treatment plans that will produce the best outcomes for them.

Why Oncologists Aren't Open to "Alternative" Cancer Treatments

My experience is that most oncologists are good people who care for their patients. Yet they aren't open to alternative treatments because of the "group think" factor which dictates that things must be done a certain way. This has blinded most from thinking outside of the box and asking inquisitive and open-minded questions, and has prevented them from being true scientists. This "group think" mentality is backed by a lot of money that goes into research and therapies. Good science doesn't mean double-blind studies. If a treatment keeps a patient alive for four months, is that good science? At our clinic, we aim to keep our patients alive for twenty years.

Besides the lack of scientific curiosity and thinking, some oncologists fear losing their professional status, and social and economic pressures cause them to pause before going beyond a certain boundary in their practice of medicine. We have had many patients who were supposed to die but who instead returned to their oncologists alive and thriving. When this happens, most oncologists don't ask their patients what they did in order to get well, and they don't explore their situations more. An attitude of inquiry should be present in a scientific mind, but in general, it's very lacking in modern oncology and modern medicine.

How Friends and Family Can Support Their Loved Ones with Cancer

If I had cancer, I would want people around me who were compassionate towards my experience and who would be willing to help me work through my fears. I would want to be surrounded by people who would encourage me to look at all of my treatment options, but who wouldn't pressure me to go in any particular direction, and who would instead encourage me to do my research and think things through. I would like to be around others who would encourage me to laugh, and who would ask me questions about my life such as: Who am I? Who am I intimate with? How do I feel about this cancer?

When people with cancer have others around them who can encourage them to look at their fears and express what they are going through, and support them in making wise treatment decisions, this takes them out of a state of sympathetic dominance, or a fear-based "fight or flight" response. Thinking from the heart is important. When we think mostly out of our heads, which we all do, our thoughts are almost always fear-based. When people with cancer have family members who pressure them and say things like, "You must go here, and do this or that therapy," it makes them anxious. Helping them to rest and laugh, or doing things like preparing meals for them and taking them to their therapies, is a better way to support them.

Who Heals From Cancer?

People who become proactive about their health have a much better chance at healing from cancer. Part of the answer to the question of who heals also involves looking at the "cancer personality." People with a "cancer personality" are often described as having a history of a lack of closeness with one or both parents, which results later in life in a lack of closeness with other people. That in itself provides a big clue about who might have an easier time healing. Some people have noticed that better outcomes happen when practitioners can help their patients resolve the conflicts that they carry about their mothers and fathers.

I can sometimes see in people's eyes, very early on during their visits with me, whether they are depressed. If so, I may try to help them build a support system, prescribe St. John's Wort, (which is an herb that aids in healing depression), or use combinations of amino acids to heal the brain. I may also suggest that they work with a practitioner who is trained in conflict resolution, or color therapy. People that I know who have healed their cancers or who have done well over the long term, are those who have taken charge of their emotional healing and moved beyond a fear state. They have resolved their anger and grief, so that even if they were in great pain initially, they learned to work with that pain and are now doing well.

There's a certain inner quality about people who heal. Almost all of them have some kind of support system. They really work on resolving their conflicts, or they let us work with them to help them do this. They realize that they must make significant and transformative changes to their lives and lifestyles. They know that in order to heal, they must take a break from their "normal" lives. They are the kind of people who can say, "I accept that I have this cancer, and I'm going to work with it, because I know that I can get well again and move on with my life in a better way." They need to have a good reason to live.

When people can do all of these things, their confidence builds. They want to live, not just survive, and are willing to do whatever it takes in order to accomplish that. They stay focused and don't give in to their fears. They know that their job is to stick with the program, find people they trust to spend time with, and do whatever it takes to get better. Healing happens when they find other people who can support them in getting better, and when they find the will within themselves to heal. It takes courage to do this.

Emotions and attitude are more important factors in healing than finances. Many people don't have a lot of money for treatments. That's the reality today. But I've seen people attract funds when they really want to get well. Part of this involves them focusing more on the present, directing their resources towards therapies that will help them get better, and trusting that the future will take care of itself. I have discovered that, as a society, when we can change and shift internally, even in the face of adversity, we attract people and resources that we would not have otherwise attracted had we stayed stuck in fear.

Last Words

The financial cost for treating advanced cancer is estimated to be close to $500,000 per patient. Many of these costs are hidden from patients because third parties, either government or private (such as insurance companies) pay for them, although increasingly, more people with cancer are incurring these costs and are declaring bankruptcy for medical reasons. As a society, I think we can do better with cancer treatment, and achieve not only better outcomes but also significantly lowered costs, if we adopt the approaches outlined in this chapter. That means incorporating the principles and practices of integrative cancer care into mainstream medicine, and by encouraging people with cancer to be proactive and responsible for their own lives.

If you have cancer, and can find the right treatment path to take, there is great reason to believe that you will have a good outcome. This either means seeing your cancer disappear, or living well with your cancer for many years. Find the practitioners who are right for you and form a team that will help you to get better. If you don't have cancer, take positive preventative steps by working with an integrative or holistic practitioner.

Treatments within integrative oncology have much to offer. It's my hope that these successful, intelligent, scientific, and common sense approaches will gain wider acceptance within conventional oncology, as well as within the worlds of business and government, in the same way that they are gaining acceptance within the public mind.

Be involved and proactive in your life, decide that you are going to improve and heal, and be willing to do the work required to attain these goals. Keep your heart open and your mind receptive. Discover a fuller life.

Contact Information
Robert Zieve, MD

EuroMed Foundation
34975 N. North Valley Parkway, Bldg. 6, Suite 138
Phoenix, Arizona 85086
Phone: (602) 404-0400
Fax: (602) 404-0403
www.euro-med.us

Pine Tree Clinic for
Comprehensive Medicine
843 Miller Valley Road, Ste. 204
Prescott, Arizona 85301
(928) 778-3500
(928) 717-0712 fax
www.pinetreeclinic.com

•CHAPTER 4•

Colleen Huber, NMD
TEMPE, AZ

Biography

Colleen Huber, NMD, is a naturopathic medical doctor and primary care physician who currently practices in Tempe, Arizona. Dr. Huber focuses on herbal and environmental medicine, nutrition, and intravenous therapies. She received her naturopathic medical degree from Southwest College of Naturopathic Medicine. Dr. Huber has published numerous articles in Dr. Joseph Mercola's bi-weekly natural health newsletter, *eHealthy News You Can Use,* as well as in other publications, including *The Lancet.*

Dr. Huber's clinic has worked extensively with over 120 cancer patients. She and her staff have spent countless hours with every single patient. Dr. Huber is a founding member and Secretary of the Naturopathic Oncology Research Institute.

What Cancer Is and What Causes It

Cancer is a growth in the body that's outside of the body's control and which operates on its own agenda. It's unique among other tissues in that it doesn't recognize itself as part of the body. Every normal tissue acts cooperatively with the rest of the body, but not cancer. It will grow, invade and metastasize, as it takes everything that it needs from the body to do that. And all at the body's expense.

A number of things contribute to the development of cancer. The most well-identified causes of cancer, in the scientific literature, are genetic instability and DNA damage. The cause of DNA damage has been traced most reliably to environmental toxins and radiation, but a diet void of nutrients and high in refined carbohydrates and poor quality fats, such as hydrogenated fats, also damages DNA. Trans-fatty acids, for example, have been known to alter DNA. So it's not necessarily just about industrial toxins, but also denatured food. There's a lot more cancer today than there was 50 years ago, as the quality of food deteriorates.

Treatment Approach

The treatments that I do at my clinic are multi-faceted. There's a popular delusion among oncologists and practitioners of natural medicine that cancer can be fought with one well-chosen substance. Nothing could be further from the truth. Many agents are needed to fight cancer, primarily because it arises after several normal mechanisms in the body have broken down. Cancer preys on the body in numerous ways simultaneously, and no single agent, whether chemotherapeutic or natural, has yet been found to have enough anti-neoplastic (cancer-killing) effects to reverse all of those abnormalities in all patients and be "the cure" for cancer.

At least seven events must happen in the body before cancer can occur, so when formulating a treatment protocol for my patients, I take into account and address all of the ways in which cancer has attacked their bodies in order to reverse those events and thereby, their diseases.

Following are the seven events which lead to cancer and some of the solutions that I use in my practice to address them. These seven events were first identified by cancer writer John Boik, who has a PhD in Biomedical Sciences and a Master's degree in Oriental Medicine, among other credentials.

1) **Genetic instability and DNA damage** are some of the first problems that allow cancer to develop in the body. Medical research has shown Essiac tea to be beneficial for correcting and reversing this damage. It's one of the oldest natural treatments for cancer and has helped many hundreds of people. It was developed by a Canadian nurse, René Caisse, together with the Ojibwe people of Canada. It's a combination of four herbs: burdock root (Arctium lappa), Turkish rhubarb (Rheum palmatum), sheep sorrel (Rumex acetosella), and slippery elm inner bark (Ulmus fulva). Later versions of Essiac use additional herbs that have pro-estrogenic effects which have been linked to breast tissue proliferation, so I don't recommend those altered formulas. Essiac has been found to have cytotoxic effects specifically against neoplastic cells (cancerous cells), which means it doesn't damage normal cells. It protects against DNA damage and seems to keep cancer from proliferating, so I include it my protocols. It's time-consuming to make, but it can also be purchased in various prepared forms from the health food store.

2) **Altered genetic expression** produces proteins that either facilitate or don't prevent cancer, and which result from DNA damage. Substances that are known to reverse gene expression include: dimethyl sulfoxide (DMSO) (which can be administered intravenously), turmeric, and astragalus.

3) **Abnormal cell signal transduction** starts with a signal to a receptor, and ends with a change in cell function which allows cancer cells to grow through self-stimulation, rather than depending on growth factors from other cells. (Author's note: Cell signal transduction refers to the relaying of molecular or physical signals from a cell's exterior to its intracellular response mechanisms).   Research suggests that abnormal cell signal

transduction can be corrected with alkalinizing agents, such as sodium bicarbonate, the benefits of which have been described by Tullio Simoncini, MD, an oncologist from Rome. Sodium bicarbonate isn't well-appreciated in the medical community, but it's very effective. I also use other alkalinizing agents in my practice.

4) **Abnormal cell to cell communication** sets a tumor apart from its neighboring cells by allowing cancerous cells to act in the best interests of the tumor rather than the body, and ignore the body's needs. Medical literature shows that Vitamin D improves cell to cell communication.

5) **Angiogenesis** is the creation of new blood vessels from pre-existing vessels. These blood vessels feed the tumor and allow it to hoard disproportionately large amounts of nutrients. Vitamin D is helpful for preventing this, as is avoiding copper intake. Copper can be a problem for patients with cancer, and is a mineral that I don't use because it's implicated in angiogenesis. I allow slight copper deficiencies to develop in my patients, but not to dangerously low levels.

6) **Invasion and metastasis of the cancer** results not only from the aggressive nature of the tumor, but also the low integrity and too friable (crumbly) nature of the surrounding normal tissue and basement membranes. (Basement membrane refers to a thin sheet of fibers that lines the cavities and surfaces of the organs, including the skin). Vitamin C controls the metastasis and invasion of cancer into different parts of the body in a variety of ways. It's cytotoxic; that is, it kills cancer cells (how it does this is described later in the chapter), and also strengthens and rebuilds the body's collagen. The latter is necessary for maintaining tissue integrity so that the cancer can't push through the tissue, reach down, dig in, and establish itself in new places in the body as it grabs onto new blood vessels. Turmeric is also good at preventing cancer invasion and metastasis.

7) **Immune system evasion** occurs when cancer camouflages itself and hides from the immune system, while disabling some of its functions. Vitamin A can help to restore immune recognition, as can Vitamin D, although the role of Vitamin A in immune recognition remains under-appreciated among cancer practitioners.

Once established in the body, cancer seems to thrive and reproduce despite the heroic efforts employed against it by oncologists, and without necessarily requiring that all seven of the above pro-cancer events remain in place. Therefore, without knowledge of the precise mechanisms governing any one patient's cancer, any therapy that targets fewer than all seven disturbances will leave cancer patients potentially vulnerable to the continued growth of existing tumors. Shortchanging patients of a diverse range of available, effective, well-tolerated, well-targeted, compatible, complementary, and feasible treatment options will also allow too many of the conditions that gave rise to their tumors in the first place to persist. For this reason, successful cancer therapy requires that practitioners use multiple and multi-purpose agents on their patients, many more than what most oncologists use.

In our practice, we use exclusively natural therapies for cancer treatment. Because of my naturopathic medical training and extensive training in the use of natural agents, I am skilled at choosing appropriate combinations of natural therapies for my cancer patients which address all of the conditions that gave rise to their cancers. I can also take advantage of the fact that there is greater compatibility, and fewer interactions, among natural substances than among numerous pharmaceutical drugs.

I can't emphasize enough that treatment selection needs to be made on a case-by-case basis. Two people who have the same cancer on paper may vary widely in the treatments that they need, and we are in a race against time to figure out what those are.

IV Treatments

I administer a lot of natural substances intravenously, and for practical purposes, I put as many agents as I can into my patients' IVs, so that they don't have to swallow a lot of pills. Also, it's important to attack cancer aggressively, and higher doses of anti-cancer substances can be given in an IV. Often, practitioners of natural medicine who treat cancer and don't use IVs, end up having to give their patients dozens of pills to swallow, and this can become intolerable for some patients. Not only that, but IV treatments are necessary if doctors want to get high amounts of certain substances, such as Vitamin C, into their patients. Even ten percent of a normal IV dose of Vitamin C taken orally gives some people diarrhea, but if doctors put that dose into an IV, it's well tolerated and doesn't cause diarrhea or damage to normal tissue. Of course, for logistical reasons, some substances have to be taken orally. For example, mixing oil-soluble or fat-soluble substances into a water-soluble IV that goes directly into the bloodstream doesn't work well.

Vitamin C

Intravenous doses of ascorbic acid (Vitamin C) have been found to produce from 25 to 70 times as much plasma (blood) concentration of the substance than what can be attained by oral dosing. Research has confirmed that Vitamin C in such high concentrations kills cancer cells while leaving normal tissue unharmed. The cancer patients whom I treat rarely experience side effects from these treatments, with few exceptions.

Vitamin C kills cancer cells because one of the byproducts of Vitamin C, when it's broken down, is hydrogen peroxide, and tumors don't tolerate hydrogen peroxide well. It can be tricky to have hydrogen peroxide in the veins, because it can cause phlebitis (or swelling of the veins), but Vitamin C doesn't convert into hydrogen peroxide until it goes from the bloodstream into the fluid that surrounds cancer cells. There, it harms the cancer cells without harming the body.

This is the principal beneficial action of Vitamin C against cancer, as established by a landmark study by the National Institutes of Health. So Vitamin C's ~~~~~ cytotoxic (or cancer-killing) effects have to do wit~ ~~~~ ~ave hydrogen peroxide within the vicinity of ~~~~ one mechanism that we know for cert~~ ~~~~ iously mentioned, Vitamin C helps ~e with greater tensile strength, so ~oothold. This is one of its second-

~ding Sodium Bicarbonate

~ low pH (acidic) environment, ~~portant. I use alkalinizing agents to ~l signal transduction.

(~ ot these substances is intravenous sodium bicarbonate, in sterile liquid form. Tullio Simoncini MD, first demonstrated the beneficial effects that sodium bicarbonate has upon cancer, and I find that I get better results when I use this substance as part of my patients' therapy. Those that choose to have sodium bicarbonate in their IVs do much better than those who choose not to have it. It's beneficial for most types of cancer.

The Gerson Clinic in Mexico operates under the belief that potassium is beneficial to the body, and that sodium isn't. Basic biochemistry, however, teaches us that we have a sodium-potassium pump in our cells, and that we need both sodium and potassium in those cells at all times. Unfortunately, we've had patients who, out of deference to the Gerson Clinic's protocol, don't want to have sodium bicarbonate in their IVs. These patients don't tend to do as well as other patients.

Vitamin A

Vitamin A is a generally less appreciated but crucial part of our treatment protocol for its immune-stimulating effects and ability to help the immune system identify cancer. Another very important quality of Vitamin A, with regard to neoplastic cells, is its ability to introduce differentiation. This means that Vitamin A forces cancer cells to mature into more benign, stable types of cells. It has also been shown to induce apoptosis (programmed cell death) in cancer cells, and to inhibit their proliferation. Recent objections have been made about Vitamin A for its allegedly competitive and detrimental effects upon Vitamin D, but older research supports dosing Vitamin A and Vitamin D together as part of an effective anti-cancer regimen.

Considerations in Treatment

Naturopathic training emphasizes individualized, comprehensive treatment of the patient's symptoms. Therefore, there is no specific formula that I prescribe in cookbook fashion to all of my patients, or even to the same patient from one day to the next. Treatments vary from person to person, depending upon their symptoms, signs, and type of cancer. For example, I generally recommend a different list of herbs and supplements to my breast cancer patients than to my lung or colon cancer patients. Also, a breast cancer patient with high blood pressure would be treated differently than a breast cancer patient with normal blood pressure. My recommendations are based upon the preponderance of research about different agents and their effectiveness for treating cancer. With colon cancer, for instance, I often recommend IP-6 (Inositol hexaphosphate acid, also known as phytic acid, which is a powerful antioxidant that's naturally present in whole grains and high-fiber foods), because studies have shown that it has beneficial effects against colon cancer and especially adenocarcinoma, which is often the form that colon cancer takes. For breast cancer, I have found artemisia, Co-Q10, and astragalus to be useful. These treatments are all supported in the medical literature for these purposes.

Patients who come to my clinic generally prefer to receive only natural treatments. They usually come to me because they don't want to do chemotherapy and/or radiation. Almost all of them reject chemotherapy and most of them also reject radiation. Only half, or fewer, would do surgery, so sometimes, I am expected to do the heavy lifting of tumor removal with natural treatments alone. That's a tall order, indeed.

I fight tumors as aggressively as I can, and with every means possible, but with one abiding principle in mind: whatever I do can't weaken or sicken the patient. My treatments must make people feel as good as they did when they first came to my clinic, or better. Otherwise, we have to keep working to troubleshoot their conditions until we find the right mix of treatments for them. This requires that they schedule a consultation with me prior to each treatment to make sure we always get it right. I don't charge my patients for these office consultations, only for IV treatments. Given that they generally come in three times a week for treatments, I sometimes end up doing a lot of consultations. During the consults, I want to know how they are feeling. I ask them, for example, if they have had any reaction to their last IV. Through these conversations, I can generally figure out what we need to eliminate from their protocols and still have good success at treating their cancers.

Dietary Recommendations for Healing

I try to keep my patients' dietary regimens simple. Basically, I have only one strong request—that they avoid sugars and sweeteners. Much research has been done on the correlation between blood glucose and tumor growth. Studies have shown a strong correlation between blood sugar levels or glycemic load and cancer growth in people with pancreatic, breast, gastric, colon, ovarian, liver, and prostate cancers. Given this evidence, it would be reckless to allow cancer patients to assume that sugar intake is harmless.

I also try to get my patients to consume whole, natural foods as much as possible. Vegetables are important. Raw vegetables offer more value than cooked, but I don't require that people give up cooked vegetables. Fruits are mostly okay, too. I also tell my patients not to be afraid of animal protein. There are clinics that advocate vegetarianism, but I disagree on this dietary approach. Vegetarians and vegans get less protein than omnivores, which means that they consume more carbohydrates by default. And all carbohydrates, when metabolized, break down to at least some form of sugar.

Besides avoiding sugar and alcohol (alcohol turns to sugar in the body), I also discourage my patients from consuming soy because of its phytoestrogenic component, which has been linked in some studies to cancer development. Other than that, I tell people to go crazy and eat whatever they want, but to try to consume more natural foods than processed, and to get a wide variety of nutrients into their diets. My patients ask questions like, "Should I have green squash or yellow squash?" And I tell them that they don't need to be so particular; they can eat whatever they like, as long as they are consuming a variety of foods which offer good nutritional balance. Some people will say things like, "I'm only going to eat blueberries and salmon because I think those are the two healthiest foods," and I tell them that such extreme diets aren't necessary. A nice, varied, healthy diet is best.

Treating Hormonal Imbalances

I don't like to prescribe a lot of hormones to my cancer patients. Since I have a number of ways to fight cancer which are safe, tried and true, and known to not cause any new cancers, I prefer to stick with those and stay away from hormone replacement therapy, which is complicated.

Instead of prescribing hormones, I make sure that my patients have enough natural hormone precursors like Vitamin D and cholesterol. Also, low cholesterol levels are a risk factor for cancer, so if I see that my patients have a total cholesterol level of 120 (normal levels are closer to 200), I may recommend that they eat foods containing cholesterol, such as eggs, to increase their levels. Nowadays, it's very fashionable among doctors to prescribe statin drugs for high cholesterol, but I prefer not to do this. There are much healthier ways to bring cholesterol down to 200.

Peri-menopausal and menopausal women whose hormone levels are low can be especially tricky to treat because normal levels of testosterone and progesterone have anti-cancer effects. Overall, estrogen tends to be pro-cancerous; however, there are several types of estrogen, and not all encourage cancer growth. Estriol actually protects against cancer, but estradiol tends to increase cancer risk. Some types of estradiol fight cancer, but no compounding pharmacy makes the latter type of estradiol, at least in the area where I practice. So replacing hormones can be a bit of a mine-field—one that I prefer to stay away from.

The Pros and Cons of PET Scans

PET scans are still the most reliable, state-of-the-art way to diagnose cancer and determine its location in the body, and they are useful for detecting cancers from the neck all the way down to the thighs. No other imaging technique will do that. They don't work for the brain, so MRI's are used to diagnose tumors in the brain. During a PET scan, patients get injected with radioactive glucose, which goes straight to their cancer tumors, which light up for the camera because of the radioactivity. Benign cysts and tumors don't light up, because they don't uptake glucose, which enables the PET scan to distinguish between benign tumors such as fibroids or lipomas and malignant tumors. One major flaw of the PET scan is that it produces fuzzy images, so sometimes patients get a PET/CT combination instead. Because CT (CAT) scans are crisp and clear, they can more accurately capture the size of the tumor. So while the PET scan reveals the tumor's location, the CT scan indicates the tumor's size.

Despite their effectiveness, I don't recommend that people with cancer get PET scans frequently or at all if they don't have to, because every time they do, they get injected with the radioactive glucose, which feeds their tumors. In our practice, we use them only sparingly when we come to a "fork in the road" with our patients and need to decide whether, or how, to continue treatment.

Lifestyle Recommendations for Healing

I recommend that all of my patients get sunshine. Here in Arizona, we have more sunlight per square foot per hour than anywhere else in the world. I also recommend that they exercise, because it really helps their overall well-being and is a necessary component of good health.

Treatment Plan Duration

I keep track of my patients, past and present, whenever possible. As of my data from July 2009, the average time that my patients needed to do treatments in order to reach remission was 4.4 months. This includes patients who had lumpectomies. As far as anyone knows, there's usually no tumor remaining in the body after a lumpectomy, but chemotherapy is often recommended after this surgery to mop up any remaining cancer cells. Many people will choose to come to me after having had surgery, instead of doing chemotherapy. And except for one person, all those who received treatment at my clinic after a lumpectomy were fine after eight weeks, but those who didn't have surgery required, on average, six months of treatment. So if I combine these patients with those that previously had surgeries, the treatment time averages 4. 4 months.

While undergoing the active phase of treatment, some patients will choose to have a chest port placed in their upper chest, which is the same type of apparatus that is used for delivering IV chemotherapy treatments to the body. If they come to my clinic three times per week for several months, it becomes too repetitious to insert a needle into their arm veins, especially if they have few arm veins to work with in the first place. Also, all those needle pokes tend to tax their patience. After they finish their regular rounds of treatment, some patients choose to leave the chest port in for IV maintenance treatments, which they come back to the clinic to receive on a weekly, bi-monthly, or monthly basis, depending upon the person. If they have an aggressive cancer, such as pancreatic cancer, I may ask them to come in more frequently. Once my patients are in remission and after their tumor markers go down, I feel safest keeping them on a maintenance regimen for two or three years.

When patients finish treatments at my clinic, I prescribe them a non-IV nutritional protocol to follow at home, which includes dietary and supplement recommendations. Usually, when I talk to them months later, I find that they have continued on this protocol.

Treatment Outcomes

I track all of my patients' progress, and follow up with them by phone every July. That said, not all of my patients return my calls and I don't like to be a pest, which means I can't get data for all of them. The data that I do have, however, shows that overall, I have had an 87 percent success rate at treating cancer. I define success as either remission, evidence of reduced tumor load, tumor necrosis, tumor softening, or long-term stability, together with an absence of pain and general improvement in patients' well-being, as opposed to them dying or getting worse during treatment. The 87 percent represents those that have come to me with cancer, whom I have treated and who are still alive, stable, at a high quality of well-being according to their own estimation, and in better shape than when they first came to me. We don't turn anyone away, even if their prognoses look bleak. Some have been wheeled in on gurneys from hospice. Who am I to turn anyone away? I don't play God. I try to turn around every cancer case that I can, and save every life that I can. I've witnessed a good number of stage three and four patients go into remission and return to normal, active lives.

For example, I have one patient who survived a particularly deadly cancer, and she has never had a recurrence. It's called Lynch Syndrome, and it's a combination of a variety of primary cancers, including ovarian, uterine, and colon cancer. None of her older relatives who had it lived past the age of 50. It's a very brutal type of cancer. But this woman is still doing fine in her fifties, and I call her every July to check up on her.

I have another patient who is the only known survivor in the medical literature of a certain, rare type of cancer. Radiation and chemotherapy didn't work for her. She had surgery twice and after the second surgery, the surgeon said that he didn't want to do surgery anymore because her tumor just kept growing back. Her radiologist also refused her further treatment, because her tumor wasn't responding to radiation and he didn't want to burn her anymore. Her chemotherapy oncologist told her that chemo wasn't working, either. In desperation, she came to us, having never considered natural treatments. Her tumor was 13 cm, but we were able to shrink it. Now it's gone and she's doing well. She has a very active job and is coming in to the clinic for maintenance treatments every month. This case was so remarkable that a local Phoenix television station shot a program at our clinic with the patient and me in 2008, shortly before we received confirmation that she was cancer-free.

Patients who do solely naturopathic treatments have better results than those that do chemotherapy or radiation combined with natural treatments. Chemotherapy is hard on the body. People tend to come down with life-threatening conditions, like pneumonia, as a result of chemotherapy, or their white blood cell counts "bottom out" and their immune systems get so depleted that it becomes unsafe for them to go out in public. Sometimes, they end up taking a one-way trip to the hospital. A recent patient of mine was also doing chemotherapy and came down with pneumonia; I haven't seen him since. Chemotherapy, in general, makes tumors resistant to other therapies and makes treatment for these patients difficult. Those who have the least improvement at my clinic are people that previously underwent chemotherapy; however, we have been able to bring many of them into remission.

I can't always confirm cancer remissions, because some patients don't want to do a PET scan or biopsy to confirm that their tumors are gone. They may choose to risk not knowing whether or not their tumors are still there. Sometimes, they can't afford to continue treatments, and may get frustrated and ask questions like, "How long do I have to do these treatments?" I tell them that the only way of knowing whether or not their cancers are in remission is by doing a PET scan or biopsy. If they aren't willing, or financially able to do that, then they can't know how many more treatments they need to do. By the time people seek help from a naturopathic physician for any ailment, they have often rejected the conventional medical system for one reason or another, and this includes having developed a distrust and disdain for conventional imaging. Imaging tests such as the PET scan are a "hard sell" to such people. They will say, "You want me to have radioactive glucose after telling me not to eat sugar?" Biopsy can be an even harder sell. So, I often can't confirm my patients' remissions, but by the time they leave my clinic, either their symptoms have improved and/or their tumors have shrunken, necrosed, softened, broken up, or become inert. (Breast lumps, or cancerous lymph nodes, for instance, will often soften).

Everyone who has gone into confirmed remission here has stayed in remission, with the exception of four people. Of these, two began to eat sugar every day after finishing their treatments. Another one, for some reason, got bone metastases (but he's now back in remission) and a fourth didn't do treatment long enough. Her tumor markers and ultrasound results were good, but she had a bone metastasis which came back with a vengeance after she left us. That said, she had only done eight weeks of treatment, and although many people have done well with only eight weeks of treatment after a lumpectomy, I have since re-evaluated the matter and now recommend 12-24 weeks of treatment after lumpectomies. It's better to be safe than sorry.

I have pancreatic cancer patients in remission that once had stage four cancers. I also have former stage four breast, lung, melanoma, and colon cancer patients who are in remission. These have been the major ones. By far, the most common cancer that I see is breast cancer, because women tend to be more proactive about their health (and treatments) than men, and breast cancer is also a more common cancer. The next most common cancers I see are prostate and lung cancer. There are a wide variety of other cancers that I treat: colon, lymphoma, leukemia, etc.

I believe that my protocol is more effective than what a lot of doctors are doing because most doctors that I know try to keep it simple and choose just one treatment for their patients, so they can learn what works or doesn't work. However, no matter how good or what the treatment is, and whether it's a natural remedy, chemotherapy, or otherwise; maybe ten percent of patients will have wonderful, miraculous results from it. Those people will then promote that treatment as if it were "the best thing since sliced bread." But these people are in the minority. For the other 90 percent, precious time is lost, and the tumor keeps growing. That's why I fight cancer on multiple levels, and I think my approach is unique for that reason. Other doctors, whether oncologists or naturopaths, tend to not do that. So that's what's different about my clinic. It's also why I am having so much success with my patients. The results of a three-year follow-up study on my patients can be found on the Internet at:
www.natureworksbest.com/general/cancer-2010.pdf

People often learn about my clinic through word of mouth. They have heard that what I'm doing here has worked for others, so they trust my treatments. I also have a group of patients who are convinced that their other family members with cancer died from chemotherapy. These younger patients often say, "I will never get chemo!" I have another group of patients who say things like, "My quality of life is more important than the quantity, so I don't want to become debilitated and beaten up by chemotherapy. I would rather have a better quality of life during treatment, even if my life is shortened in the process." These people don't necessarily have faith that my treatments will prolong their lives, just that they will make them feel better. They often end up pleasantly surprised when they see themselves outliving those that they met in the chemotherapy room at the hospital.

Roadblocks to Healing

Some patients don't take their treatments seriously. For example, some repeatedly go on vacation before they are finished with their treatment regimens. Such people probably didn't have much confidence in their treatments from the beginning, and as a result, don't tend to do well. I wish they understood that they have to stick with the program until they go into remission.

I consider the treatment of diabetes and heart disease to be a walk in the park compared to cancer. Cancer must be fought thoroughly, aggressively, and continuously, especially when using natural treatments. Patients must be diligent, as this is their only hope for beating it. Some think that what I do to treat them is "unnecessary fluff," while others think, *Cancer isn't so bad. Look at all the people in the IV room! They all look fine. They even go to the gym.* The people in the waiting room are talking about going golfing, or to the farmer's market. They aren't acting sick, and they may not even feel sick. This is because, unlike conventional cancer treatments, people feel good when they do naturopathic treatments. However, some patients are lulled into a false sense of security about where they are at in their recovery and end up passing away when they aren't diligent with their treatments.

Insurance Coverage for Treatments

Unfortunately, insurance plans don't generally pay for my treatments. If people have to stop doing treatments, it's often because of financial limitations. Most people can only pay for this type of treatment for so long before they run out of money, and the recession has increased the financial hardship of some. Fortunately, some insurance companies are working towards establishing plans that pay for naturopathic treatments. In the meantime, a minority of patients are lucky enough to have good insurance plans which cover a percentage of their naturopathic care, sometimes up to 70 percent. Most patients have to pay for their treatments, though, so I advise such people to switch to an insurance plan that covers natural treatments.

Inexpensive Cancer Treatments

If patients can't afford IV treatments, it's difficult for them to heal. If they are able to visit my clinic for an occasional IV treatment, it's better than if they didn't do any treatments at all. If they can't afford IV treatments, I would advise them to consider Essiac tea, turmeric, and Vitamin D and hope for the best. And if that doesn't sound very promising, that's because it's not. These are among the most powerful oral anti-cancer remedies, but they are probably insufficient for winning the battle against cancer. For someone who doesn't have cancer but who's trying to prevent it, though, these substances are great and among the best preventative remedies available.

Ineffective/Dangerous Cancer Treatments

Overall, chemotherapy has a really low success rate. The average five-year survival rate is 2.5 percent for all cancers. Not to mention that it poisons the body and increases patients' risk of developing other cancers. It also makes their original cancers resistant to further treatment, so that when they come to me after having done chemotherapy, it's harder for me to treat them. Some naturopathic doctors will point out that chemotherapy is only strongly successful at treating certain lymphomas, leukemias, and testicular cancers, but I find that these types of cancers are also relatively easy to treat with my remedies. They just happen to be "slam dunk" cancers that are easy to treat with naturopathic medicine, compared to some of the others.

It's sad that the book *The Emperor of All Maladies: A Biography of Cancer,* by oncologist Siddhartha Mukherjee, MD, describes people with leukemia and the other cancers as hopeless cases. No, sir, they are not! They actually respond well to natural treatments. Mukherjee's book was just published in 2010, yet is already way outdated.

Sadly, some people end up doing conventional treatments only because they are pressured into them by their families. For example—and this is a heartbreaking story—a mother of six came into our clinic with non-Hodgkin's lymphoma. She didn't want to do chemotherapy and said, "I don't want to be sick. I don't want to lose my hair (she had beautiful, long hair). I have six kids to take care of. I'm too busy for this (to endure the side effects of chemotherapy)." But she couldn't afford my treatments, and needed her father to help pay for her treatments. Unfortunately, a so-called friend told her father that doing natural treatments was suicide, so her father refused to pay for her treatments and told her that he would only pay for chemotherapy. Prior to this, she had received one IV from me, and as a result of that one treatment alone, the lymph nodes that had been poking out of her neck flattened completely. Her response to our treatment was unusually fast, as it typically takes a while longer for lymphomas to respond to treatment, but her case represents how fast lymphoma can respond to natural therapy. Yet because this woman's father would only help her financially if she did chemotherapy, that's what she's now doing. For someone to be dragged through chemotherapy against his or her will is very sad. This woman definitely didn't want to do it and had no good reason to do it.

Finally, another problem with conventional medicine is that the treatments cost a fortune, up to tens of thousands of dollars per treatment. My treatments are a fraction of that. But because cancer is a political disease, and it's not profitable for drug companies to promote natural medicine, most people don't know about the wonderful benefits of this type of medicine and most insurance companies don't pay for it. The decades-long media blackout on natural medicine also maintains the status quo. Just look at who the media's biggest advertisers are —drug companies. A while back, *Newsweek* had a cover story entitled, "Crazy Talk: Oprah, Wacky Cures and You." (June 8, 2009) On the cover of the magazine was an unflattering head shot of Oprah looking away from the camera. The article disparaged the natural treatments that Oprah had mentioned on one of her shows without offering any evidence for its contentions. What I found to be screamingly egregious was the fact that seven of the first twenty pages of that issue were full-page drug ads. *Newsweek* couldn't have made their motives and their money trail any plainer.

There are also some ineffective natural treatments, such as some of the so-called "latest, greatest" findings in medicine. Chlorine dioxide, sometimes marketed as Miracle Mineral Supplement (MMS), is currently a hot treatment that's being promoted on the Internet. We have one patient who was doing well on just our treatments, who has insisted on using MMS and it has made him sicker. Another darling of the Internet last year was Protocel, and I haven't seen any good results from it, either. Those are the two ineffective natural treatments that come into my mind as being the "latest and greatest" fashion in cancer treatment, but for which there is no outcomes-based evidence for their effectiveness. Our IV room can sometimes become a spontaneous cancer support group, and some people thrive on talking about the latest thing that's out there, whether ozone or hyperthermia, etc., but not all of these treatments are good.

How Friends and Family Can Help Their Loved Ones with Cancer

I try to support my patients the best I can. During their initial consultations, I allow them time to "get off their chest" whatever it is they need to say. For instance, I can think of three breast cancer patients, who, when I asked them, "How does your husband feel about you doing these treatments?" all answered, "Well, he's angry at me for getting cancer." Can you imagine the moral and emotional immaturity of a man who acts like he's the victim and who blames his wife for getting breast cancer? So I try to be there for patients who are in such situations, to listen to them, because they need emotional support as well as medical support when their families aren't providing it.

My advice to the friends and family of those with cancer is for them to not act like victims when they aren't the ones with cancer, and to not blame their loved ones for getting sick. I also tell them to not eat desserts in front of them! If people with cancer are trying to stay away from cigarettes, I also tell friends and family members to not smoke in front of them (especially if they have lung cancer).

Final Words

To anyone who has recently been diagnosed with cancer, I would say:

1. Although you have to act soon, know that you don't have to do anything drastic this week. Take this week to examine, with a clear head, all of your available options. Decide what you want to do, and then get started.

2. Stay in charge of your own health care. Don't let anyone (neither family members nor professionals) bully you into doing anything that you don't agree with.

3. Many cancer patients have put themselves and their interests last. Now it's time to put yourself first.

Recommended Resources

One comprehensive website that I recommend to those who want to learn more about cancer treatments is: www.cancertutor.com.

Contact Information
Colleen Huber, NMD

Dr. Colleen Huber, NMD
1250 East Baseline Road
Tempe, Arizona
Phone: 480.839.2800
www.naturopathyworks.com

• CHAPTER 5 •

Juergen Winkler, MD
OCEANSIDE, CA

Biography

Juergen Winkler, MD, is Board Certified in Family Medicine. He completed his medical training at San Bernardino County Medical Center in 1991, and subsequently spent four years in the Air Force at two different bases. At KI Sawyer Air Force Base, he was Chief of the primary care clinic, where he improved patients' access to, and the delivery of, medical care within the hospital. Additionally, he managed its allergy and immunization clinic and also directed a headache clinic. After leaving the Air Force, Dr. Winkler went into private practice in Carlsbad, California for two years, after which time he began an eight-year career in homecare, where he made over 12,000 house calls to homebound geriatric patients in San Diego County. Since 2005, he has been working with Les Breitman, MD, in private practice at Genesis Health Systems: An Integrative Cancer and Medical Treatment Center (formerly called the Alternative Cancer Treatment Center of Southern California).

Dr. Winkler has maintained an interest in alternative and complementary medicine since medical school, and in 1996 he joined the

American College for the Advancement in Medicine. He is also a member of the American College of Osteopathic Pain Management & Sclerotherapy, Inc. He has special training in chelation therapy, Insulin Potentiation Therapy (IPT) for cancer treatment, and Mesotherapy for pain management. His treatment approach is based on nutrition, heavy metal detoxification, and immune system enhancement. In addition, he treats hormonal conditions associated with menopause, hypothyroidism, and andropause.

How I Became Involved in Integrative Medicine

While attending medical school at the University of Maryland at Baltimore, I became interested in alternative medicine, which was outside the paradigm of the conventional medicine that I was being taught at school. Consequently, there was little time for me to pursue this interest, but when I had time, I would study nutrition, and occasionally, listen to lectures at the local school of Oriental medicine. Once in residency, I learned ear reflexology, hypnosis, and other alternative treatment modalities. I also attended lectures on acupuncture whenever I could.

Learning about different types of medicine and other perspectives was helpful for breaking up the very left-brained, didactic, allopathic medical training that I was being taught. It also helped me to maintain a balanced understanding of disease and healing. Although I have received training in conventional medicine, which is vital in today's world, I have sought to incorporate other perspectives into my training, in order to have a more balanced medical background.

After medical school, I moved to California to complete a family practice residency at San Bernardino County Medical Center. Whenever I had time, I pursued my interest in alternative medicine, while sticking to the core of learning conventional medicine, which I also really enjoyed. My residency program was a lot of fun, and I learned everything from pediatrics and obstetrics, to surgery and internal medicine. After my residency, and as mentioned in my biography, I went into the Air Force and over the following four years, was stationed at two different bases.

During my last year in the military, doctors used to send me all of their chronically fatigued patients because they learned that I was effectively helping patients with Candida and other chronic conditions with nutritional remedies. Some of the doctors around me weren't happy, though. They thought I was practicing witchcraft. But any medical doctor who goes beyond the perspective of conventional medicine is accustomed to their work being referred to in this way. Still, my patients liked that I could heal them, even though my colleagues got frustrated because I wasn't practicing medicine "like I was supposed to." After the military, I went into private practice for a couple of years, and one of my goals during this time was to build upon my knowledge in nutrition, chelation, and all of the other alternative medical therapies that I had started studying in medical school and while in the military.

There's a strong fraternal order among doctors and it's especially strong among oncologists. Most oncologists are very "cookbook-like" in their treatment of patients. They have a regimented way of doing things, with no in-between. They have a book that they use to look up chemotherapy treatments for their patients, called the *Guide to Chemotherapeutic Regimens*. When prescribing a regimen, they just calculate their patients' weight and body surface area, and from those, determine what their treatments should be. That's how conventional medicine treats patients.

I wanted to break out of the cookbook model, so in 1995, after I had already been doing chelation and nutritional therapies, I joined the American College for the Advancement of Medicine (ACAM), an organization which focuses on integrative medicine (which involves combining alternative and conventional treatments, and tailoring those to the individual).

The doctors that I shared a practice with after the military didn't agree with my approach to medicine, so in 1997, I ended up practicing on my own, and doing homecare for eight years. I would see six to eight patients per day, so I probably made a total of about 12,000 house calls during those eight years. I also became the medical director for Call Doctor Medical Group, a mobile medical group, and got involved with helping the elderly. One of my goals with the elderly was to focus upon restoring their functionality so that they could do things like cook meals, get dressed, and bathe. The ability to function is important, not only for the elderly, but also for those with chronic diseases, especially cancer, so I carried this concept over into my treatment of the chronically ill.

My mother-in-law developed pancreatic cancer about five years ago, and her battle with disease provided me with the incentive that I finally needed to move out of homecare, and start working more with cancer patients. So in 2005, I joined another doctor in private practice, Les Breitman, MD, and we developed our own IPT model for cancer treatment, which we have used in our practice over the past five years. Our goal when we treat cancer is to keep the disease at bay and/or put patients into remission, so that the disease won't interfere with their lifestyles.

Treatment Approach

We focus upon treating patients individually, and addressing the particular characteristics of their cancers, as well as their ability to detoxify. This includes stimulating the immune system to help it recognize cancer, and reducing blood flow to tumors (inhibiting angiogenesis). These, as well as other aspects of our treatment approach, are covered more in-depth in the following sections.

IPT—Insulin Potentiation Therapy

Insulin Potentiation Therapy is a simple medical procedure that uses the hormone insulin, followed by chemotherapy and glucose, to make chemotherapy drugs more effective, in smaller doses, with few to no side effects.

There are no double-blind, placebo-controlled, university-based, FDA, or pharmaceutical company-funded studies for IPT, or many of the other treatments that we do at our clinic. IPT was basically developed as a result of several doctors who better understood cancer physiology and how the body works, and who felt they could treat cancer patients with less toxic methods than what's found in conventional medicine.

A Mexican doctor named Donato Perez Garcia, MD, was the first to notice that insulin, when combined with certain medications and nutrients, was useful for treating various health conditions. For instance, he and his son, also a doctor, found that insulin, when combined with low dosages of chemotherapy, was very effective for treating cancer patients. Their results were impressive and they presented their data to the National Health Institute (NIH) in the early 1960s. The NIH promptly shelved the information and has since made it difficult for physicians to get funding to study the effects of IPT. Since then, a growing international organization has been developed, which teaches IPT to interested physicians.

In order to understand how IPT works, it's important to first explain cancer cell physiology and compare it to that of normal cells. Cancer cells have six times as many receptors for insulin on the surface of their membranes as normal cells, and ten times as many IGF-1 factors, or Insulin Growth Factor-1 receptors. Insulin stimulates growth and the uptake of glucose into the cells for energy. It also transports amino acids and vitamins into the cell. Cancer has a high metabolism, and must feed itself. It prefers sugar and simple carbohydrates since it doesn't metabolize fats and proteins very well.

One reason we know that cancer cells have a higher than normal metabolism is because of PET scans, which reveal areas of increased metabolic activity in the body. These scans essentially involve injecting labeled sugar molecules into the body, which are then detected by scanners once they are inside the body. The sugar molecules go to areas of increased metabolic activity, which happen to be where the cancer is. To further understand how this works, consider the following example: Let's say you have a cage with a bunch of hamsters that are sleeping or crawling around, with the exception of one, which is very active, running on a wheel and burning a lot of calories. The active hamster represents a metabolically active tumor in a body of normal cells (which are the sleeping and crawling hamsters). Thus, tumor cells are more sensitive to sugar because they need more glucose for producing energy. So they pick up sugar by means of insulin, a lot faster and more aggressively than normal cells do.

When doctors drop their patients' blood sugar levels by giving them insulin, it creates a state in the body, called a therapeutic moment, in which the body elicits the release of adrenaline (epinephrine). This causes patients to feel hot, sweaty, and drowsy. When adrenaline and insulin are mixed together in a low blood sugar state, cancer cells and other inflamed cells become much more receptive to whatever substances are introduced to them through an IV, including chemotherapy. This means that doctors can give much lower doses of chemotherapy to their patients, and their effects will be greatly enhanced, or potentiated, by the insulin. Only one-tenth of the full chemotherapy dose is needed to obtain effective results, and it can be administered in a much shorter period of time than regular chemotherapy. In order for IPT to be effective, the patient's blood sugar levels must be dropped to 30-40 mg/dL (the normal range is 65-99 mg/dL). Despite this, the procedure is thoroughly safe. People do get a bit groggy, but after a while they get used to it, and after the procedure doctors can quickly restore their low blood sugar back to normal by giving them an infusion of glucose.

Chemotherapy Sensitivity Testing

Two patients with the same type of cancer can be sensitive to a whole different array of chemotherapeutic agents, so instead of grouping all of our patients together and giving them all the same agents, we do chemotherapy sensitivity tests. These determine the specific chemotherapy agents that their tumor cells may best respond to. There are two labs that we use for this purpose; one is in Greece, the other is in Germany. The lab in Greece is called Research Genetics Cancer Center (RGCC). Here, they extract circulating tumor cells from patients' blood samples, culture them out, and then expose them to different chemotherapeutic agents. Results are then calculated according to the percentage of cancer cells that are killed by the agents, which may be 50 or 80 percent of a culture—or none. Then they choose the agents that the cancer cells have the highest response rate to and recommend that these be used for treatment. The labs can also provide comprehensive information on the genetic makeup of people's cancers, which helps us determine appropriate therapies for our patients. Once we have this information, ideally, we will put together two different treatment regimens for each of them, with each regimen consisting of three different medications, which we alternate. The purpose of doing this is to reduce the cancer cells' resistance to the drugs. It takes ten days for the results of the Greek test to come back. Another advantage of this test is that only a blood sample is required to do it, rather than tissue from the tumor itself, so unlike some types of chemotherapy sensitivity testing, it's safe to use in those with metastatic disease.

Most doctors in the United States won't even look at this type of testing, though. But those that do, find it helpful, and are discovering that drugs that most doctors ordinarily wouldn't even think of using to treat certain types of cancer are effective for those cancers. For example, many conventional doctors use a drug called Gemcitabine to treat pancreatic cancer, but the RGCC test demonstrates various breast cancers to also be sensitive to this agent, and recent breast cancer studies confirm this. We use agents that aren't commonly prescribed to treat certain cancers and yet we find that they work.

So not only have we been able to figure out how to best treat our patients through chemotherapy sensitivity testing and the IPT process, but we have also figured out strategies to make treatments more tolerable for them.

157

Additionally, we use a bioresonance device called the Asyra on our patients, which detects areas of stress in the body, even before those areas of stress manifest as symptoms. We have found a strong correlation between the chemotherapy agents that patients test positive for with the Asyra, and the ones that they test positive for on the RGCC test. So the results that the Asyra provides help us to determine useful chemotherapy agent combinations for our patients. The medical community needs to learn more about devices such as the Asyra, but they thus far appear to be quite useful.

Pre-Chemotherapy Nutritional Protocol

In addition to IPT, we give our patients pre-chemotherapy nutritional IV's, comprised of nine nutritional supplements, which we administer prior to IPT. These substances make the chemotherapy more effective by keeping the drug(s) in the cells longer. They also prevent the cancer from repairing itself after it has been damaged by chemotherapy, and reduce its resistance to the chemotherapy. Also, while the pre-IPT nutritional IV is intended to have its greatest effects at the site of the cancer, it has the additional benefit of boosting the immune system at the same time.

One of the substances that we use in the pre-cancer nutritional IV is glutamine. We give patients this amino acid both orally and intravenously before they start treatments. Other substances that we include in the IV are L-arginine, L-proline, resveratrol, quercetin, niacinamide, acetyl-L-carnitine, and L-theanine. We also give a green tea extract known as EGCG. Each one of these substances has a different effect upon the cancer and patients' symptoms. For instance, acetyl-L-carnitine reduces brain fog and glutamine boosts neutrophil, macrophage and other immune cell counts and is a source of food for them. Glutamine has additional anti-cancer properties, and protects the GI tract against the side effects of chemotherapy.

A lot of oncologists struggle to overcome the MDR-1(multi-drug resistance-1) gene in cancer. This gene codes for a pump in the cancer cell called the Pgp pump, which removes chemotherapy drugs from the cell. Nutrition can inhibit that pump and thereby reduce the cancer's resistance to chemotherapy.

We used to have patients who would become resistant to their chemo drugs somewhere between their eighth and tenth treatments, and we found that if we switched their drugs from time to time and did pre-chemo nutritional IVs, we got better results. So now we rotate their drug regimens, and use three different chemotherapy drugs at a time, so that their cancers don't have a chance to develop resistance to them. Since we have employed these strategies, it now takes 16-25 treatments before patients might become resistant to their treatments. Drug resistance is something that all IPT practitioners, as well as traditional oncologists, must address.

Tailoring Treatments to the Individual Patient

Whether or not we recommend IPT depends upon the patient that we're treating and the type of cancer that they have. For instance, we may recommend that a twenty-year-old with lymphoma see a conventional oncologist, because conventional medicine tends to have good results with lymphomas, leukemia, and testicular cancers. Lymphoid tissue replicates quickly and responds well to full-dose chemotherapy, so doctors can get away with using higher dosages of medication for this type of cancer. For an 80-year-old with ovarian cancer, which isn't a very metabolically active cancer, we may recommend IPT treatments once per week, or even less frequently, since older patients aren't as metabolically active and therefore, their cancers don't replicate as quickly.

As another example, recently, we had a patient come to our clinic who had just been released from the hospital. She had lost forty pounds over the course of six weeks. We wouldn't immediately give this kind of person chemotherapy until we figured out what her nutritional status was. We know that patients who have a weakened antioxidant and nutritional status are set up for failure in their treatments. If we were to give this woman low-dose chemotherapy through IPT, she would wind up in the hospital for a blood transfusion, because she would be too weak to tolerate the chemotherapy, even at lower dosages. Considering patients' unique situations helps us to determine appropriate treatment protocols for them.

Determining whether IPT treatments are effective for our patients is also very important, so we do a PET/CT scan on them after they have done six weeks of therapy. We also measure their tumor markers on a weekly basis, and observe the trend in the markers, which helps us to discern their response to treatment.

Conventional Chemotherapy versus IPT

When patients' cancers respond well to conventional medicine, as in cases of leukemia, lymphoma, or testicular cancer, we refer them to a conventional oncologist. We will continue to see them to give them nutritional support, which helps them to get through their conventional treatments and also reduces the side effects of those treatments. We can do IPT for these cancers too, but the IPT organization of doctors as a whole supports conventional treatment for certain types of cancer. IPT does work on most types of cancer, though, so we will use it on patients with the above-mentioned cancers if they prefer to not receive conventional care.

When chemotherapy is given in smaller, gentler and more frequent doses we have observed that patients respond well with fewer side effects than if they had done full-dose chemotherapy. Some patients that have stopped conventional care due to its side effects have re-grown their hair while undergoing IPT. We, along with other IPT doctors, have also observed that patients have less deterioration in their quality of life than if they had done conventional treatments.

The kinds of people who walk through our door are generally very educated and don't want conventional care, anyway. Many others have already been through conventional care. Either the side effects of their conventional treatments were intolerable or they didn't respond to the treatments. They are the type of people who make their own decisions regarding treatment (rather than allowing someone else to dictate what they should do), so we don't usually have to discuss whether IPT or conventional medicine is best for them. We don't participate in any insurance plans, so patients don't get assigned to us for treatment. They are here because they want to be here. We are a cash-based practice and most doctors who do the type of treatment that we do are also cash-based, because IPT is generally outside of the health insurance system. People look for us; we don't look for them. They call us because they don't want conventional treatment. At times, I may suggest that they see an oncologist to see if they can offer them an effective treatment option that we might be unaware of or unable to provide, and I have no qualms about making such referrals. I have no animosity towards mainstream medicine. I just prefer to do things "outside of the box." Fortunately, I believe that IPT may become a mainstream type of treatment as more and more people become aware of its benefits.

Treating Hormone Imbalances

It's important for us to treat our patients' hormone imbalances, especially if they have hormonally-driven cancers, such as of the breast, prostate, ovaries, and uterus. To determine hormonal status, we do 24-hour urine tests, which provide us with a comprehensive breakdown of the body's hormone levels, and clues about what we need to do to treat them. If women have hormonally-driven cancers, it's important that we get their estradiol (and some of their other hormones) into a less proliferative state. Estradiol is one of three types of estrogen that the body produces which contributes to cancer growth. Estriol, or E-3, is a less proliferative hormone than estradiol, E-2. E-2 is a great hormone for females to have at age thirteen when they are becoming women, but women in their 50s and 60s need more estriol, not estradiol.

Unfortunately, we live in a society where all of the chemicals and toxins that we are exposed to, such as phthalates and Styrofoam (polystyrene), are mimicking and creating more estradiol in our bodies. As a result, men are becoming more feminine, gaining weight, developing insulin resistance, and getting bigger chests. The chemicals which are stored in their fat are estrogen-aggravating, which perpetuates the problem. Women face similar problems as a result of excess estrogen. Also, estrogens interfere with thyroid function, so the thyroid becomes more sluggish, and in turn makes the rest of the body more sluggish. Then the liver can't process all the estrogen and the result is a condition of estrogen dominance in the body, which worsens insulin resistance and creates a tendency for people to put on weight. This then creates even more problems in the body. For example, when women become overweight, their bodies produce more testosterone, which leads to polycystic ovarian and masculine-type problems, such as facial hair and acne.

Doris Rapp, MD, an environmental doctor who has written several books and who is still practicing in Arizona, said at a recent conference that there is such a pollution problem in some of the lakes in England that some of the male fish are now carrying eggs! The male fish are no longer male fish.

Excess estrogen not only has an effect upon cancer, but upon the immune and nervous systems, as well. We have a model that we use in our practice; a triangle diagram, which illustrates the integration and interrelationship between the nervous, hormonal and immune systems. The nervous system sits on the top of the triangle, the immune system sits off to the right, and the hormonal system is on the left. We address and treat imbalances in each one of these systems so that they work together better as a whole.

The body's hormonal system is based primarily on the thyroid, adrenal gland, and sex hormones. It's important to make sure that all of these hormones are functioning properly, because they affect cancer growth and patients' overall health. We have many patients who have low thyroid and adrenal function, and their sex hormones are also in disarray. So, for example, we may look at their thyroid function and treat them for hypo or hyperthyroidism based on their body's basal temperature and symptoms, not just their test results. If patients have a body temperature of 96.8, are freezing cold, and have a pulse of 50 bpm, but their thyroid tests are normal—sorry, I don't think that their thyroid function is normal! If I give them thyroid hormone and they perk up, then it means that they had a thyroid problem, regardless of what their blood tests showed. It's because blood tests can be inaccurate that we prefer to diagnose based on the body's temperature and functioning.

When we do use thyroid tests to support a clinical diagnosis, we don't just look at T4 values, but also free T3, free T4, and reverse T3. It's important to properly balance all of these levels. We don't give thyroid hormone to people who have depleted adrenal glands, though, because then their livers will metabolize cortisol that's produced by the adrenals too fast, and they will get tired. So we first support their adrenal glands with adrenal glandular extracts, homotoxicology formulas, and products such as AdreCor, by NeuroScience, which contains various vitamins, amino acids, and the adrenal-balancing herb rhodiola rosea. One liquid glandular formula that we use is called CF Support, by Xtra-Cell, which contains proteins and peptides, as well as other growth factors and signaling molecules from porcine adrenal and mesenchyme tissue (the latter is a type of loose, connective embryonic tissue). We use a lot of other agents for adrenal and thyroid support, as well.

Treating Immune System Imbalances and Infections

We don't just do tests to determine the status of our patients' cancers and hormones; we also look for any other problems that might be impacting their health. Through additional testing, we often find that we need to detoxify them and clean up their immune systems. For instance, in the early stages of treatment, we measure their inflammatory mediators, such as cytokines, to determine what's causing the inflammation in their bodies. We check the status of their immune cells, to see what, for example, the T-cells and natural killer (NK) cells are doing. We want their immune systems to be active and balanced, and will prescribe remedies to accomplish that. Many patients have chronic infections that weaken their immune systems and impair their ability to effectively fight cancer.

The immune system is comprised of cells that are divided into two types; Th-1 and Th-2, the ratios of which should be balanced in the body. Basically, the body starts off with a Th-0 cell, which eventually differentiates to become a Th-1 cell or a Th-2 cell. These further differentiate to make lymphocytes, B cells, and T cells, among others. Understanding immune cell differentiation is complicated, but basically, there should be balanced numbers of all the immune cells in the body. We can determine what might be affecting the immune system based on the body's balance of Th-1 and Th-2 cells. We then use a whole array of supplements to balance and activate the immune system, including homeopathy and homotoxicology remedies from GUNA and Heel, which are very helpful for this purpose. If necessary, we complement our cancer treatments with these agents.

Another remedy that we use a lot of is AVE (also known as Avemar), which is fermented wheat germ, to boost NK activity, because NK numbers tend to be low in people with cancer. AVE also keeps cancer from taking up sugar, and thereby prevents its growth. It has a lot of other beneficial properties, as well.

Intravenous germanium is another substance that we sometimes give our patients. This is an immune balancer that stimulates Interferon gamma (a cytokine that's critical for innate and adaptive immunity against viral and intracellular bacterial infections and for tumor control), reduces cancer pain, and stimulates oxygen delivery to tissues. We also use herbal supports, such as ginkgo biloba, green tea extract, marshmallow, and slippery elm. These herbs support the gut, and thereby, immune function.

In addition to supporting the immune system with nutrients, we also look for other chronic diseases that our patients might have in addition to cancer, because these weigh down the immune system. For instance, some people have chronic mycoplasma and get fevers every night. Others have Lyme disease and we have to treat them with antibiotics, or natural remedies that include homotoxicolgy formulas, which we can also do as part of their IPT treatments. By using IPT to treat infections, we are able to kill two birds with one stone, because IPT makes treatments for Lyme and other chronic infections more effective, too.

To determine which infections might be playing a role in our patients' diseases, we do tests that expose their cells to different fungi, bacterial or viral antigens, to see how they respond, which then gives us clues about what else might be triggering an immune system response. From the results of this testing, we may order more tests; a Lyme disease or stool test, for example, to see specifically why the immune system is reacting in an unbalanced manner. We find that many patients have Epstein-Barr, herpes and cytolomegaviruses, as well as other chronic viruses. In addition, some may have Lyme and mycoplasma infections, which are sometimes re-activated in the body by chemotherapy. If they have active viruses, then they usually also have heavy metal toxicity, which further weakens the immune system. Treatment at this point can become complicated, because if they have infections and heavy metal toxicity, then they also tend to have methylation and other detoxification problems. All of these issues must be addressed if they are to fully heal.

Balancing Brain Chemistry

The brain, like the immune system, has its own balancing mechanisms, which can be categorized as excitatory and inhibitory. The inhibitory mechanisms put the body to sleep; the excitatory mechanisms keep it awake and functioning during the day. It's not good to have too many excitatory mechanisms without enough inhibitory ones and vice versa, because otherwise, people would be manic or in a coma! Most of our patients are running—to quote a colleague, Denise Marks, MD—"an SUV life on a mini coupe gas tank!" They run on "empty," which means that they have no inhibitory-supporting neurotransmitters such as serotonin, so their mood is down, and neither do they have enough excitatory neurotransmitters, so they have no energy. From urine tests, we can obtain information on our patients' brain chemistry, and then determine which amino acids will correct their neurotransmitter deficiencies. Green tea with L-theanine, for example, keeps people calm and has anti-cancer effects. Supporting the body's serotonin levels, with a combination of mainly 5-hydroxy tryptophan, zinc, B6, and other vitamins, helps patients to maintain a positive mood and good quality of sleep. Serotonin also helps to activate the rest of the brain; it's the gateway to the entire functioning of the brain and its chemistry. Balancing the hormones also has a positive effect upon brain chemistry.

Other Tests and Treatments to Heal and Support the Body

One test panel that we do is based upon a recent lecture that I attended, entitled "Cancer Is a Chronic Disease," which was given by a nutritionist at the Institute of Functional Medicine. This nutritionist stressed the importance of checking hemoglobin A1-C levels to monitor patients' glycemic control on their diets, as well as checking fibrinogen, C-reactive protein, and free copper and zinc levels. Testing copper to zinc ratios is important, as well. Most people with cancer have an excess of copper, and not enough zinc, and excess copper stimulates tumor blood vessel growth. So we prescribe different supplements to deal with each of these imbalances: Nattokinase for elevated fibrinogen levels, for example. To reduce inflammation, we treat infections and also use a hops derivative known as Kaprex, by Metagenics.

We also do high dose Vitamin C and K-3 IVs, and detoxification therapy using phenyl-butyrate. Vitamin C appears to a cancer cell as a sugar molecule and is quickly taken up by the cancer. Once the Vitamin C connects with an iron molecule in the cell, peroxide is released, which injures the cells internally. Cancer cells have a difficult time repairing from such damage. Vitamin K-3 augments the effects of Vitamin C and helps to inhibit cancer growth.

Phenyl-butyrate is a derivative of the short-chain fatty acid butyrate, and is thought to have anti-neoplastic activity as well as the ability to assist with cancer cell destruction. It can be given intravenously as part of IPT treatments or a detoxification protocol.

Finally, many of our patients have low Vitamin D levels, so we often prescribe 10,000-15,000 units of Vitamin D per day, along with ox bile and other enzymes to help digest fat, if they have trouble digesting these fats (since Vitamin D is fat-soluble). Some patients have a poor antioxidant status, as a result of not being able to digest fats and proteins (and hence their nutrients), so we add enzymes to their regimens which aid in protein and fat digestion. We also give them antioxidant support in the form of supplements. We have to literally restore everything in their bodies while they are being treated for cancer, and this can't usually be accomplished in a short amount of time. Thus, we must prepare them for the possibility of doing treatments with us for an extended period of time, perhaps many months.

In summary, we look at different parameters in our patients, and if we can improve those, then it makes their bodies into a more hostile environment for cancer. We have a regimen of supplements that we prescribe, which depend upon their test results and symptoms.

Detoxification

We recently hired a nutritionist, who said to us, "Your cancer patients are springing up and down the hallway! They aren't acting like cancer patients. How can they feel that good?" When we get cancer patients that have already received conventional treatments, they do look sick, but within a month of coming to our clinic, they look like normal people again, because we revitalize them and spend a lot of time doing nutritional interventions to detoxify them and improve their quality of life.

We sometimes have to do detoxification treatments on our patients before we can start them on IPT, especially if they have had high dose chemotherapy and/or radiation prior to coming to our clinic. They may require several weeks of nutritional IVs before their bodies get built up enough to tolerate IPT. Conversely, some of our other patients have done Gerson-type cleansing therapies prior to coming to our clinic, which means that their lab values tend to be normal and we can get them started on IPT treatments right away.

Some of the agents which we use in our detoxification IVs include: high dose Vitamin C, glutathione, and phenyl-butyrate (as previously mentioned), all of which cleanse and restore the body. Phenyl-butyrate is particularly helpful for restoring immune function. It also reduces inflammation as it targets and boosts immune cell production. We can accomplish a lot of different things with phenyl-butyrate.

We also use homotoxicology remedies to clean out the cells and stimulate toxin drainage through the kidneys. Oral chelating and toxin-binding agents such as powdered zeolite are also important. What we use varies from person to person. People usually come in here with a laundry list of supplements already, so we also try to work with what they are already using, if it's beneficial for them.

Finally, we may recommend infrared saunas or far infrared mats for sweating out toxins. Infrared mats deliver heat that penetrates the body and induces detoxification of the impurities that have built up in the tissues over many years.

pH-Balancing Treatments

Since most cancers thrive in an acidic environment, we do cesium chloride therapy as part of our IPT treatments, to balance the body's pH levels. Cesium, being one of the most alkaline elements, has a high pH value and is also readily taken up by cancer cells, and raises their pH to a level at which they can no longer survive. We make sure, however, to monitor our patients' potassium levels while they are on cesium therapy, since it can also reduce potassium levels.

DMSO

We sometimes give our patients DMSO, a penetrating agent that augments the effects of chemotherapy by bringing it deeper into the tissues. It also has anti-inflammatory properties.

We use many other substances in our practice, but our choice of treatments depends upon our patients' lab test results and symptoms; whether, for example, they are exhausted, chemotherapy toxic, or emotionally depressed.

Magnet Therapy

Another type of treatment that we do is magnetic therapy, because it increases tissue oxygenation, improves immune function and re-polarizes the body. It's also relaxing. Ideally, I like my patients to have a magnetic bed that they can lay on at home, three times per day for fifteen minutes at a time. I use one myself, because I get muscle tension headaches and it quickly gets rid of them. Magnetic beds can also alleviate pain, increase energy, improve mood, and "re-set" the brain—among other things. A book written by a chiro-practor named Dr. Joel Carmichael, called *Magnetic Resonance Stimulation: Using the Field to Maximize Your Health (2009)* describes one type of magnetic bed, called the MRS 2000, which was developed in Germany and which we use on our patients.

Dietary Recommendations

During therapy, we put our patients on a healthy, low-glycemic diet that's high in fruits and vegetables. We don't recommend that they go on a raw vegan diet, except for short periods, because it's diffi-cult to get enough protein on a low-glycemic vegan diet. Even Dr. Gerson (who recommends a vegetarian diet) used to put his pa-tients on liver extracts so that they would get enough protein. That said, many cancer patients have a difficult time digesting proteins, so it's important for them to take digestive enzymes with their meals. It's also important that they get gluten and casein out of their diets. We allow them to have a little yogurt, or cottage cheese, (as prescribed by the Budwig diet), but drinking milk every day isn't a good idea. We encourage them to eat a lot of eggs, because eggs are rich in lecithin and protein. A whole live animal comes out of an egg, which means that there are a lot of healthy ingredients in eggs, including higher amounts of healthy fats and proteins. Fat is impor-tant for rejuvenating cell membranes. Seven percent of our eye cell membranes are new every day, which means that every two weeks we get a new eye cell membrane! Patricia Kane, PhD, mentions in *The Detoxx Book* (which she co-authored with John S. Foster, Domenick Braccia and Edward Kane) that the visual contrast function of the eye is dependent upon the amount of inflammatory processes in the body, because inflammation gets into cell membranes and impacts the ability of the eye to see contrast. Contrast can be measured by reading a card (which is found in *The Detoxx Book),* the results of which can reveal whether there's inflammation that's upsetting the cell membranes. If so, then it's important to get more proper fats into the body so that the cell membranes can repair themselves. So we try to make sure that our patients get a proper balance of Omega 3-6-9 fats, as well as other nutrients.

Treatment Duration

The duration and number of treatments that our patients need vary. We had one woman with metastatic breast cancer who needed aggressive treatment for three months. Once her PET scan was negative, and her bone and liver lesions were no longer active, we began to taper off her treatments. We didn't stop them abruptly, because cancer cells are still present in the body after PET scans are negative. Other patients, who are highly toxic and have other problems such as viral and bacterial infections may require treatments for longer periods of time. One patient has been seeing us on a weekly basis for two years. Two years ago, she was on a ventilator and doctors had told her husband to let her go. He wasn't ready to do that, and she was very weak when she got here, but now, she's doing well. Recently, I hosted a women's health lecture, and she came to the clinic to give a testimony of her remission.

Logistics of Treatment

A lot of people travel to see us. Many come from Los Angeles, since we are an hour and half away from central LA. Others drive from further away, but because they may require nutritional IVs or other therapies a couple of times per week, we help them to set up Vitamin C IVs and other therapies at clinics which are closer to where they live. They can then go to these clinics in-between treatments with us. We know doctors who are part of ACAM, who can duplicate our vitamin and nutritional IVs, and who may be closer to our patients' homes than our clinic. Therefore, we are able to help patients who live in many different places.

Treatment Outcomes

Our treatment outcomes are variable, and often depend upon the patient. If patients take ownership of their healing process and say to themselves, for example, "This (type of treatment) is what I want. I have researched the procedure and I think it's the best," then they tend to do well. If they think, "I'm going to die, no matter what I do," then they won't do well. If they want the IPT therapy to work, that in and of itself will have a huge beneficial effect upon their healing.

If they say, "I'm scared that I'm going to die anyway. What can you do for me?" I have to ask them, "Well what can you do for yourself?" I try to talk to them about their anxieties, fears, and unresolved anger, because it's important for them to work through these difficult emotions. It's helpful if they have a counselor, pastor, or minister that they can talk to. At our clinic, my colleague's wife comes in to pray and talk with our patients. We also know psychologists and counselors that we can refer them to see.

I have seen plenty of people who were initially given a death sentence who are still alive, several years after having done treatments with us. The results have been amazing. For example, I had one patient who didn't think that he would make it until Christmas, and nearly two years later, he's still on the planet. In conventional oncology, doctors will tell their patients that they are allowed six rounds of chemotherapy, and if that fails, then that's it—it's all that they have to offer them. At our clinic, we will keep doing treatments, while maintaining our patients' quality of life. Some of them get treatments before work, and then go to work for the rest of the week without any problems.

We have a lot of success stories, but some people pass away, too. A lot of family members are grateful towards us, though, even when their loved ones don't make it. They will say things like, "Thanks for treating her. We couldn't even get other doctors to see her, because she was so bad, but you did." And we typically find that during the time that they were alive, they had a better quality of life than they would have had if we had turned them away. It leaves tears in our eyes when family members are happy that we could do even this for their loved ones.

When people die, it's not always because of cancer. One of our patients was responding well to our treatments for metastatic esophageal cancer, but because he had a mitral valve in his heart that was deteriorating, he died of heart failure. Sometimes, patients get tired and weary of their treatments, although thankfully, nobody has ever died as a direct result of IPT. I don't think that conventional doctors can say that about their treatments. They give their patients high doses of chemotherapy, which ends up affecting their bone marrow. Then they wind up in the hospital, where they get a horrible septic infection and die. We've never had that happen at our clinic. We do see some bone marrow suppression, in perhaps ten percent of our patients (if that), but we do a lot of nutritional therapy so that they don't wind up having serious problems.

Roadblocks to Healing

The biggest roadblock to healing that we have come across is patients not being able to pay for their treatments, because insurance companies don't generally pay for what we do. If they do pay, they will often let the claims sit for six to nine months, before they bring them before a medical board to challenge our work by telling the board that what we are doing violates the "standard of care." They will do anything to not pay for treatments, and whenever they do pay, it often comes as the result of a lot of persuading. One patient of ours, a chiropractor, went and researched the beneficial effects of low-dose chemotherapy, and took the evidence that he found on IPT to his insurance company. As a result, they paid for 85 percent of his treatments! Another patient took his claim to the same insurance company, and the insurance company took his claim to the medical board. The board so far hasn't said anything to us, nor has the insurance company paid for his treatments.

If patients don't have money for treatment, they can go to church fundraisers or apply for assistance at the IPT for Cancer website: www.iptforcancer.com, where others have set up tax-free donations for people with cancer. These donations are given to treatment providers, who then invest the money in their patients' treatments.

People with cancer struggle, but somehow, most of the time they come up with funds for treatment. The greater challenge might be when family members offer to help pay for treatments, but want to dictate the treatments that the person with cancer does. For instance, they will often tell their loved ones that they want them to go the conventional route, or do the type of treatment that they themselves prefer. So getting financial help from family can become a double-edged sword, which brings up another roadblock to healing—family and friends telling their loved ones that they are doing the wrong treatments, which is hardly encouraging. People with cancer should be able to choose the treatments that they want to do.

Also, just as some friends and family members want their loved ones to do conventional treatments when they would rather do IPT or other treatments, sometimes, it happens the other way around. I have patients who are here because their family and friends wanted them to see us because our therapies are less toxic, but the patients may be very conventionally-minded and unsure about what we do, which isn't good, either.

The other roadblock to healing is closed-minded, uneducated doctors. Doctors must take care to not give uninformed opinions about treatments. I don't give an opinion about things that I don't know about, but some oncologists will give their patients opinions about therapies that they know absolutely nothing about—like IPT.

I want to say to them, "Why don't you ask us our opinion about IPT, since we are the ones doing it? We have been doing these treatments and we know what goes on with them." I wouldn't go to a patient and say, "What kind of results does your oncologist get using conventional therapy?" I would instead ask the oncologist about his or her therapy, or go look up that therapy on the Internet and learn about it myself. Oncologists shouldn't give opinions about treatments that they know nothing about, yet traditional oncologists and doctors are more than happy to do that.

Patient/Practitioner Challenges of Healing

The greatest challenge of healing, for both practitioners and patients, is creating an ideal environment where practitioners can educate their patients on the importance of lifestyle aspects of healing, such as diet, cooking, and exercise, and patients are able to comply with their recommendations.

Being able to create a mental environment that's stress-free and relaxing is another challenge to healing. For example, when people get a chronic disease, they find that they can't keep up with everyone else, so they automatically become reclusive. I mean, when you get the flu, you don't want to go out and have a social life, do you? You want to crawl into bed and wait until it's over. So if people are having chronic flu-like symptoms, it's too mentally exhausting for them to be social with others. I don't like to use a lot of antidepressants in my practice, but I find it important to build up my patients' brain chemistry with nutrients, which helps them to combat the depression that sometimes accompanies isolation. Also, exercising every day is important, because it releases endorphins. If it makes people feel good, they will want to keep doing it, too. There is some evidence that correlates exercise with an increased lifespan in people with cancer. So we encourage our patients to do gentle exercise for a half-hour daily. It's also important for them to do activities that they enjoy.

Ideally, we would put a clinic on an island, and take all of our patients there! Creating the perfect environment where patients can get well is the greatest challenge to healing.

Dangerous/Ineffective Treatments

A chemotherapy drug called Avastin has gotten much bad press, so I wonder about its safety. There have been concerns about people having strokes while taking it. I get concerned about the frequent usage of high dose chemotherapy and how debilitated patients get while doing it. I think it can be dangerous. When evaluating the benefits of any therapy, it's important for doctors to look at their patients' progression with that particular therapy, or statistics of people's overall survival with it. Oncology uses various techniques to monitor the effectiveness of conventional treatments, but there aren't good parameters for knowing whether patients should receive these treatments or not. If you look at people with cancer, you can tell whether they are healthy and robust, but there has to be some better objective criteria to determine whether or not we can treat them with chemotherapy, because we are giving them a poison. A wise doctor I know once said that poison given in small dosages is therapeutic, but in heavy doses, is dangerous. Doctors have to know what drug to give, how much of it, and when the patient is ready for it. Some of the new chemotherapeutic drugs that are coming out on the market are very expensive and carry a high risk of serious side effects, such as anaphylactic-type reactions. These drugs include Erbitux, Vectibix, and Herceptin, just to name a few. Monoclonal antibodies (MABs) often cause reactions in patients and are potentially dangerous.

Are there cheaper, safer ways to treat cancer? Probably, but in the meantime, the majority of cancer patients are spending a lot of money on dangerous treatments, and whether the overall survival rate has increased as a result of these treatments is questionable. For example, there is a medication for renal cell carcinoma that is currently being talked about in the medical journals, which is supposed to extend the patient's life from an average of 22 months to 24 months. Well, if it were me, I don't know how willing I would be to spend thousands of dollars to take a drug that has severe side effects, and to spend those extra two months of my life laying around on the couch staring at the ceiling, miserable because I am in so much pain. Such a treatment doesn't improve the patient's quality of life (in fact, it does the opposite) or longevity. Now, if they came up with a drug that extended the patient's life from two to five years, then that would get my attention. Too often, we want full-dose chemotherapy regimens to do something positive, but they really haven't proven to be all that effective.

I don't want to criticize doctors in conventional medicine. They have spent a lot of time getting to where they are, but I think they have been a bit blindsided by the pharmaceutical industry. Drugs are all that they are taught, but medicine needs to be about more than just writing prescriptions for drugs. I want doctors to understand what people are about, because every person is different and has unique needs. No two people on the planet are exactly alike.

Last Words

Our protocols are comprehensive and based on the individual person. We treat the whole person. Our patients are human and we treat them as such. We spend a lot of time figuring out what's going on with them and their bodies. We address everything that we can: from diet, exercise, detoxification, inflammation, and angiogenesis to the nervous, immune and hormonal systems. We also address spiritual and emotional issues; and even dental care, because there are correlations between dental root canals and problems with the rest of the body. Do we have the answer to all of these issues? No, but we try to put them together in the best way that we can.

Contact Information
Juergen Winkler, MD

Genesis Health Systems: An Integrative Cancer Treatment Center
2204 El Camino Real Suite 104, Oceanside, CA 92054
Phone: 760-439-9955   Fax: 760-439-6755
Email: info@ipthealing.com

•CHAPTER 6•

Elio Martin Rivera Celaya, MD with Steven Hines
Ciudad Acuña, Coahuila, Mexico

Biographies

Elio Martin Rivera Celaya, MD, is Chief Medical Officer of Hope Wellness Center in Ciudad Acuña, Coahuila, Mexico. He is a conventionally trained medical physician with more than twenty-five years of clinical experience. Over the past fifteen years, he has also received cross-training in nutritional medicine. He received his medical degree from the University of Monterrey, in Nuevo Leon, Mexico, and is certified in chelation, oxygen, nutritional, and magnet therapy.

Additionally, Dr. Rivera-Celaya is a pastor and founder of a non-denominational Christian fellowship church in Mexico. He has written several bilingual Christian books and is an international speaker. He has also founded several orphanages in Mexico, one of which is next door to Hope Wellness Center. His compassion for people is evident throughout his medical practice and ministry.

Steven Hines is the co-founder and head of research and development for Hope Wellness Center. He has received extensive training in naturopathy and endocrinology, and has functioned primarily as a clinical consultant for Dr. Rivera over the past fifteen years. He is also a master herbalist and has more than 12,000 hours of training in nutritional biochemistry, anatomy, and physiology. His deductive reasoning skills are invaluable to the patients at Hope Wellness Center. Currently, he's writing a book on gastrointestinal diseases and has co-authored a book entitled, *The Road to Health* which contains information on a gut-healing, anti-inflammatory, and anti-fungal diet that has profound healing benefits for those with cancer. Steve is also an accomplished musician and humanitarian.

About Hope Wellness Center

Hope Wellness Center takes a unique approach to clinical medicine. We treat our patients according to their individual needs, instead of giving them "cookie cutter" treatments for their ailments. Doctors in conventional medicine have given up on most of the patients that we see at Hope, but the word "incurable" doesn't daunt us. We aren't discouraged when some say, "No one has ever gotten well from this disease." Our patients routinely recover from life-threatening or supposedly incurable diseases.

Many people don't realize that diseases which are considered to be incurable in one country are often successfully treated in another using different treatments. For example, Chinese doctors successfully treat viral meningitis with intravenous garlic extract. German, Russian, and Cuban doctors use intravenous ozone to kill viruses of all types. In England, homeopathic medicine is used in lieu of vaccinations, and is also used to treat psychological disorders. In Asia, acupuncture is sometimes used as the sole anesthetic during surgery. Having a global medical perspective is critical for those who hope to recover from cancer and many other diseases. We adhere to that global perspective when treating our patients at Hope.

Hope has no allegiance to any drug company, machine, or latest gadget. We keep an open mind—but also maintain a scientific filter—to find the best possible treatments for our patients. We listen to them with a trained scientific ear, and in doing so, are able to discern exactly what they need. Statements like, "My headache started right after I got some dental work done," or "Ever since I started on that high blood pressure medicine, I just can't sleep," provide us with key insights that we pay attention to and use to determine the root of their problems.

Our core values at Hope Wellness Center include: listening to our patients, diligently searching for the latest research on all ailments, and earnestly seeking to find a cure for every patient.

What Causes Cancer

Cancer is caused by many things, including viruses, bacteria, fungi, mycoplasmas, heavy metals, genetically engineered foods, trans-fatty acids, estrogen-mimicking compounds, and electromagnetic fields, as well as other environmental toxins and factors. All of these cause inflammation in the body, which leads to excessive cell turnover and a lack of blood flow to cells, which then results in hypoxia and cells that are starving for oxygen (or gasping for breath!).

When cells don't receive enough oxygen, they must revert to a different type of energy production called anaerobic glycolysis. This system is very inefficient because it requires 40 times more glucose than normal aerobic metabolism. It also produces large amounts of lactic acid waste. When in a low-oxygen state, cells also produce signaling proteins called hypoxia inducing factors, which signal the brain to create more blood vessels in the area, in order to increase oxygen and meet the cells' elevated need for glucose. The creation of new blood vessels from pre-existing blood vessels is known as angiogenesis. Inflammation leads to cell hypoxia and angiogenesis, which ultimately leads to uncontrolled cell growth and cancer.

For example, 90 percent of people who develop primary liver cancer are those who also suffer, or who have previously suffered, from Hepatitis A, B, or C—diseases which cause chronic inflammation, and consequently, set the stage for liver cancer. Similarly, people who have smoked for many years develop chronic inflammation of the lungs, which leads to lung cancer. Men that have benign prostatic hypertrophy (prostate enlargement) and frequent urination (due mostly to infections and hormonal imbalances) have chronic inflammation of the prostate, which can lead to prostate cancer. Fibrocystic breast disease causes chronic inflammation of the breast tissue, and so leads to breast cancer.

There's an old saying, "Find the cause and the cure will be forthcoming." Inflammation is the cause of cancer, and is triggered by one or more of the aforementioned factors: viruses, bacteria, fungus, mycoplasma, heavy metals, genetically engineered foods, trans-fatty acids, estrogen-mimicking compounds, and electromagnetic fields.

These factors then cause alterations in the genes that are responsible for cell cycle regulation. The gene alterations are then what perpetuate cancer, rather than the initial triggering factors. Once the genes have mutated, they must be normalized if the cancer is to be stopped.

Testing and Treatment Approach

When patients come to see us, the first thing that we do is take a blood sample and send it to one of four different labs. The labs look for circulating tumor cells (CTCs) in the blood. If CTCs are found, they are then tested for genetic alterations, and exposed to various anti-cancer compounds, both conventional and natural, to determine the compounds to which they are most sensitive. We use this information to tailor our treatments to the individual patient. It's essential for us to know in advance what treatments will and won't work for our patients. If cancer cells don't succumb to a treatment agent in a test tube, it's not likely that they will succumb to that agent when it's given to the patient, either. And there's no use in beating up a patient's immune system with unnecessary medications, unless they have a reasonable chance of working. The labs test the cancer cell's reaction to many compounds, such as: Ukrain,

Iscador, Vitamin C, Vitamin D, peroxides, ozone, Selectox (which is our proprietary cytotoxic agent; a botanical extract that's selectively cytotoxic (lethal) to cancer cells); IR2 (another proprietary formula), as well as dozens of others.

After we receive information from the lab on the genetic makeup of the patient's cancer and to which compounds it will be susceptible, we prescribe the patient a regimen involving these compounds, which we may administer orally, intravenously, or in an Insulin Potentiation Therapy (IPT) format. We then add other appropriate botanicals, precious metals, trace elements, minerals, stem cells, and patient-specific vaccines to the treatment regimen, which help to repair the patient's aberrant genes and normalize his or her immune system function.

The vaccines that we administer are made from circulating tumor cells, tumor tissue, blood, urine, saliva, stem cells, cytokines (inflammatory messengers), immune-modulating botanicals such as Beta 1,3D glucans, and so forth. Extensive research has proven that botanical substances such as resveratrol, quercetin, licorice root, ashwagandha, and isoflavones can repair genetic material, so we use these, too.

Methyl donor substances such as folic acid, methylcobalamin (Vitamin B-12), S-Adenosyl-methionine (SAM-e), and Vitamin B-6 are essential endogenous molecules that the body uses to repair genetic damage, so they are also part of our regimens. (A methyl donor is a substance that can transfer a methyl group, which is a carbon atom attached to three hydrogen atoms (CH_3), to another substance). Many important biochemical processes rely on methylation, including lipid and DNA metabolism. Scientists suspect that adequate DNA methylation can prevent the expression of cancer genes. Some of the above methyl donor substances can also act as receptor agonists or antagonists (hydrogen or electron donors), which ultimately means they have an anti-oxidant effect upon the body. They can also alter DNA or RNA transcription, and thereby positively impact gene expression.

Controlling the Over-Expression of Estrogen Receptors on Cancer Cells

Most cancers, regardless of their site of origin in the body, over-express estrogen receptors. That means that either they have an excessive amount of estrogen receptors on the surface of their cell membranes, or their ratio of active to inactive receptors is too high. Whenever there are too many receptors, the end result is that the cell divides and reproduces more rapidly. Estrogen is a major growth factor which contributes to the proliferation of cancer.

Xenoestrogens (which are man-made, synthetic estrogens) mimic the activity of the body's estrogen and are found in pesticides, herbicides, and industrial solvents. Xenoestrogens drive the over-expression of what is called the "alpha" estrogen receptor on cancer cells. There is another estrogen receptor, called the "beta" receptor, but many scientists consider this receptor to have been misnamed. They believe that it should be called the "anti-estrogen receptor" because whenever it's filled by the body's natural hormone "2 Methoxyestradiol," for which it was designed, it actually antagonizes the alpha estrogen receptor and prevents it from being over-stimulated. This, in turn, prevents cancer cell division and reproduction. In Europe, doctors use this hormonal metabolite to treat patients with hormone-sensitive cancers. We do urine tests on our patients to make sure they are producing adequate 2-Methoxyestradiol, and if not, we treat them appropriately.

Other natural compounds also bind to the beta estrogen receptor on cancer cells and prevent over-stimulation of the alpha receptor. These include fermented soy beverages such as Haelan 951, which contain many isoflavones. It's important to note that soy beans alone don't have the active chemicals necessary for binding to the beta receptor; they must be fermented by specific fungi and bacteria to produce the proper byproduct.

In any case, we find it essential to give our patients beta-receptor agonists in order to counter the negative effects of xenoestrogens and other alpha receptor stimulators. The more that estrogen alpha receptors get stimulated, either by endogenous factors (the body's internal processes) or environmental xenoestrogens, the more beta receptor agonists must be made available to stop the cellular proliferation which results. This is a very important aspect of cancer treatment that's unfortunately missed by most oncologists. Also, we always add iodine supplementation and Di-indole Methane (a phytonutrient which controls estrogen levels) to our patients' diets because these cause estrogen to be metabolized into anti-cancer pathways (2 Methoxyestradiol) in the body rather than pro-cancer pathways.

Restoring Proper Cellular and Immune Function with Electrolytes and Other Nutrients

Every patient's internal terrain is uniquely altered by cancer, so we must evaluate and treat each of our patients on an individualized basis. We don't apply the same protocol to everyone, although we have found that whether our patients have cancer, cardiovascular, autoimmune, or other types of diseases, all of them are depleted in electrolytes at an intracellular level. So we give everybody treatments to replenish their intracellular electrolytes, which in turn restores proper cellular function.

As a society, we experience electrolyte depletion because we are all forced to consume foods that are devoid of potassium and magnesium, and overloaded with sodium. This eventually leads to intracellular depletion of potassium and magnesium. When in this state, the cell's voltage-gated sodium channels cease to function properly. This causes potassium to leak out of the cell and the cell to fill up with sodium and excess water, which then causes edema (or swelling), which cripples the cell and prevents it from functioning normally. The result is a low energy state in the body and the collapse of cell membrane potentials. (Cell membrane potentials are synonymous with electric charge, and refer to the difference in voltage, or electrical potential difference, between the interior and exterior of a cell). This is important because without an adequate electrical charge, the cell can't open and close to let oxygen and nutrients in, and waste or toxins out.

We have spent years at our clinic perfecting the art of repairing this common problem, and have created a system called "Hyper Cellular Respiration Therapy" to solve it. This involves using IPT to open the cell's glucose channels to allow glucose, electrolytes, vitamins, co-factors, and enzymes to enter into its intracellular compartments. We do this, along with pulsed magnetic coil therapy, which assists with restoring the cell membrane's electrical charge. We find that we are able to consistently accomplish this in our patients, with just four to six weeks of therapy.

We use just about every tool in the holistic toolbox to help our patients. While they stay at our clinic, we give them fresh green juices daily, put them on detoxification regimens, and provide them with pastoral counseling. Most patients receive three to four separate IV bags daily, which may contain anything from nutrients to botanical extracts such as Ukrain, Iscador, and Selectox, to various reactive oxygen species (chemically reactive molecules that contain oxygen and which are used to oxidize pathogens and toxins), anti-viral, and anti-fungal substances. It's important for us to treat viral, fungal, and other infections in our cancer patients because such infections can suppress the immune system and lower patients' energy levels. And patients need lots of energy to beat cancer!

We also make specific, individualized vaccines to relieve patients of their allergies, which in turn helps to restore their immune function so that they can better fight their cancers. Chronic allergies are a major cause of Th-2 dominant, or inflammatory, immune system responses. When patients are Th-2 dominant, their cytotoxic T-cells, natural killer cells, and macrophages, which are all important for fighting cancer, don't work like they should. Even normal programmed cell death (apoptosis) is suspended.

Additionally, we administer substances such as glycoproteins, to increase macrophage and T-cell activity, and enhance cellular communications. These are essential for proper communication among natural killer cells, cytotoxic T-cells, and macrophages. They are integrated into the cell membranes of immune system cells and help those cells to recognize cancer.

Fungal or yeast cell membrane extracts such as Beta 1,3D glucans, when injected or ingested, also stimulate the immune system so that it can better fight cancer.

The Relationship between Fungal Infections and Cancer

Often, fungal infections are misdiagnosed as cancer. Cancer and fungi look very much alike when growing in human tissue. A spore on a piece of wet wood in a forest becomes a mushroom overnight, with structure and mass that take up space and use glucose. If we were to grow a mushroom in the breast, figuratively speaking, it would look just like a cancer. Also, fungus and yeast grow very quickly, much like cancer cells—although their growth is even faster than cancer cells. Furthermore, the toxins that yeast and fungi produce can actually trigger the development of cancer.

We have discussed the possibility of fungal infection misdiagnosis with pathologists, and how it's possible to mistake a fungal mass for a cancer mass. A retired pathologist once told me that pathologists are aware that fungi are often present in tumors, but they have been trained to think that the fungi are present because the immune system has been suppressed by cancer, when in reality the fungal infections may be the cause of the cancer. All kinds of infections flourish in people with compromised immune systems, but pathologists tend to believe that when people have cancer, their fungal infections "are just along for the ride"—that is, if they have even considered a correlation at all! They aren't taught that fungal infections might be the cause, rather than the effect, of cancer. But the truth is, pathologists generally only find what they are looking for. For example, if they stain a tumor tissue block with Hematoxylin/Eosin (H&E), a testing stain that has a high affinity for cancer cells, they will only see cancer cells. On the other hand, if they stain it with Gomori Methenamine Silver, they will only see fungus in the sample. Hence, it's easy to miss the many fungi that could be present in a sample and see only instead the few cancer cells (comparatively speaking) that are there. Fungal infections are not always found together with cancer, but in a statistically relevant percentage of people, they are. Further complicating this issue is the fact that fungal infections create an environment in the body that's favorable to cancer development.

Often, after patients have been treated with chemotherapy and radiation, they will suffer from a recurrence of their cancers. The recurrence is usually assumed to be a reappearance of the original cancer. However, due to ongoing immune suppression as a result of chemotherapy and radiation, it's more likely that they have developed a fungal infection. Chemotherapy has a devastating effect upon the gastrointestinal tract. It destroys it and hampers its ability to stop fungal overgrowths, so fungi and yeast are able to easily grow. This destruction of the gut is often referred to as "Leaky Gut Syndrome." In this syndrome, a damaged GI tract allows fungi and yeast to leak into the bloodstream. After the fungi leak into the bloodstream, they find some warm and cozy tissue where they can "set up shop." They thrive particularly well in areas of weakened tissue, and once they begin to grow, they invade the surrounding normal cells and create inflammation, lactic acid, toxins, and hypoxia, as they alter the tissues' pH. This is the perfect environment for cancer to originate in.

Oncologists, however, assume that such fungal overgrowths are a return of the original cancer. And because they don't want to subject their patients to more needless biopsies, they don't do further tests to determine whether or not these "recurrences" are really cancer. It's not hard to see how this mistake can be made. Tragically, in some cases, the cancer may be successfully treated and yet the patient ends up passing away from an easily treatable fungal infection. Recently, I (Steve) had dinner with a pathologist to discuss the staining/testing of cancer and fungal tissue. I asked him what percentage of tumors he stains to determine whether fungi are also present. He said that in over thirty years of working as a pathologist, he has never tested a suspected cancerous mass for the presence of fungi. That's very telling.

It is important to note that cancer and fungi thrive on the same fuel: glucose. So if people eat lots of sugar, they can make both their cancers and/or fungal infections grow. Cancer and fungi play well together. In summary, cancer and fungi most often co-exist together, so at our clinic, we treat them simultaneously, because fungal infections often kill people much faster than cancer.

Anti-Coagulant Therapy

We utilize anti-coagulant therapy such as subcutaneous heparin, and enzyme products such as Nattokinase, Serrapeptase, and Lumbrokinase to thin patients' blood and break down debris and fibrin. Thick blood doesn't flow well through capillaries, and when blood flow to tissues is blocked, the body sends a signal to the brain to create more blood vessels, which cancer patients don't need because more blood vessels means more cancer growth. This signaling protein that does this is called vascular endothelial growth factor (VEGF). It's produced as a result of cellular hypoxia (oxygen deprivation) and stimulates the growth of new blood vessels. Heparin has a two-fold benefit: in addition to breaking up fibrin and thinning the blood, it also stops VEGF production.

Inhibiting the MDR-1 Pump

Years of genetic testing have taught us that the majority of cancer cells develop the ability to defensively pump out and eliminate threats, including toxins such as chemotherapy, using what is called the MDR-1 pump. This pumping mechanism is over-expressed in most cancers, and so must be addressed. If it isn't, then no treatment, conventional or naturopathic, will be effective.

We use natural substances as well as conventional drugs such as Celebrex (an anti-inflammatory drug) to inhibit this pump. Anti-inflammatory drugs are also helpful in blocking the Cox-2 inflammatory pathways, which is important because inflammation creates an ideal environment for cancer to thrive in.

Dendritic Cell Vaccines and Stem Cell Therapies

There are certain out-of-clinic, or outpatient, treatments that we sometimes recommend to our patients which enhance what we do, such as stem cell therapy and dendritic cell vaccines. Dendrites are immune system cells that, when presented with a cancer cell antigen, "spread the word" to the rest of the immune cells. It's as if they put up a "wanted" poster so that everyone (the other immune cells) knows what the bad guy (the cancer) looks like. So dendritic cell vaccines improve the body's ability to recognize cancer. We don't do these vaccines at our clinic, but we can refer our patients to people who do.

Another out-of-clinic treatment that we sometimes recommend is stem cell therapy. Stem cell therapies are expensive and not all patients can afford them, but we have seen some impressive results when they are used together with a small amount of well-placed chemotherapy and CyberKnife, a therapy which delivers high doses of radiation to tumors with extreme accuracy. This latter therapy requires a trip to our sister clinic in Seoul, Korea.

Dietary Recommendations

We generally recommend that our patients avoid grains and night-shade vegetables (tomatoes, potatoes, chili peppers, eggplant, tobacco, and paprika) because they cause inflammation. We also encourage them to consume low-glycemic foods, because this helps to starve their cancer and fungi, which thrive on sugar. Low-glycemic foods are also essential for bringing the body's blood sugar levels back to normal, and for reducing inflammation, which is the body's greatest enemy. A low-glycemic diet void of the aforementioned foods is the best possible anti-inflammatory diet.

Furthermore, we recommend that our patients take aloe vera extracts, which contain a type of "communicatory sugar" that's essential for maintaining effective cellular communications in the body. Mushroom extracts also work well for this purpose: Shitake, Maitake, Ganoderma and Reishi, to name a few. In China, mushrooms are always part of patients' cancer regimens. We recom-recommend green drinks that contain lots of phytochemicals, and smoothies with coconut milk, predigested rice bran extract (to stabilize blood sugar), and lots of botanical extracts like ashwagandha and milk thistle, to regulate cortisol production in the body, among other purposes. Substances that support the immune system such as colostrum, Saccharomyces boulardii, and pharmaceutical grade probiotics are also a standard part of our protocols.

Detoxification

We routinely recommend that our patients do coffee enemas every morning. Enemas stimulate the release of bile from the gall bladder and the excretion of waste from the lower bowels. We also recommend that they do colonics, whenever these are available. In addition, we prescribe very high amounts of pancreatic enzymes to help stop inflammation, break down circulating immune complexes in the blood, and inhibit the formation of fibrin, which contributes to thick blood and angiogenesis.

Balancing the Hormones and Neurotransmitters

Balancing the body's hormones is essential, no matter the disease condition. We give our patients pharmaceutical and botanical aromatase inhibitors, which block the synthesis of estrogen and thereby lower estrogen levels and slow cancer growth. We also prescribe bio-identical progesterone to some to prevent estrogen dominance. Additionally, we give them 5-alpha reductase inhibitors (5-alpha reductase is an enzyme involved in steroid metabolism) to lower levels of dihydrotestosterone (DHT). Lowering the body's levels of estrogen and DHT is important because both hormones encourage the growth of certain cancers. We use adaptogenic herbs, phosphatidyl-serine, and DHEA to bring down elevated cortisol levels and enhance energy production.

We assess our patients' brain biochemistry and normalize it with the proper amino acids, which are the building blocks of neuro-transmitters. Hormone and neurotransmitter levels have everything to do with patients' mood and attitude. As we like to say, "attitude determines altitude!" A happy patient tends to get well more quickly than a sad, stressed, and depressed patient.

Treatment Outcomes

Overall, we have observed an improvement rate of about 70 percent at our clinic. This doesn't necessarily mean that our patients no longer have cancer. What it means is that they either go into total remission, or have symptomatic improvement and a better quality of life, diminished pain, and a disease process that has stabilized, instead of progressed.

Some of our patients recover completely. We have patients who have fully recovered from end stage breast, lung, liver, brain, and prostate cancers, and who are still alive ten to twelve years following their treatments with us. We also have plenty of patients whose tumors have either stopped growing or shrunken to some degree, and who have been stable for many years. These people, even though they still have tumors, feel fine. Sometimes, their tumors are just scar tissue. We find that most people seem to be fine living for a long time with a lump in their bodies, as long as that lump isn't harming them. Increasing our patients' length and quality of life is our main priority.

Still, it's important to note that we also see many people who don't make a full recovery. The more conventional treatment that they have received, the harder it is for them to get well. Our treatment outcomes depend substantially upon this factor. Furthermore, people who have very advanced cancers are more difficult cases. We tend to take impossible cases, which many other clinics refuse, because it doesn't make a clinic's success statistics look very good when their patients don't survive, and it's also very stressful to work with such patients—but we take on this challenge. When you start with patients who are near death and have already failed every conventional treatment, saving even twenty percent of them (which we do) is heroic. Our consciences are more important to us than our statistics, which is why we accept such patients.

Our typical patients, if they haven't already been in hospice, are on their way there by the time they come to see us. Most of them have only weeks or months to live and are usually on morphine or codeine (strong narcotic drugs) for pain. Our goal for these people, first and foremost, is to improve their quality of life. This means helping to alleviate their pain and increasing their energy and cognition. We are mostly very successful in this area, and are also generally able to significantly extend their lifespan. For many of the terminally ill, we are even able to double or triple it.

Often, cancer patients die not from cancer, but from malnourishment or infections that are totally ignored by mainstream oncology. Many patients are in agonizing pain not because of their cancers, but because of an infection or, more commonly, constipation due to morphine or other pain medications.

In all cases, we treat our patients as if they were going to live, instead of expecting them to die. Conventional oncology treats advanced stage patients in a palliative manner, which means "keeping them comfortable" by giving them OxyContin (oxycodone) and morphine. We have never been successful in remitting our patients' cancers without getting them off these drugs. Opiate drugs are terribly immune-suppressive. Ironically, cancer itself isn't generally painful unless it's encroaching upon major blood vessels or is in the bone. We are generally very successful at alleviating our patients' pain with other methods, and are often able to get them off the painkillers that they were taking when they first came to our clinic.

Finally, patients' physical condition helps us to determine which treatments to use and enables us to predict the outcomes that may be attained with those treatments. If their kidneys are compromised, for example, then we may have to work on healing those before we can work on their cancers. If they are diabetic, we have to treat their diabetes first, because high blood sugar causes hormonal imbalances in the body and allows cancer to thrive.

Factors That Influence Healing

Emotional wellbeing is critical for healing. We have an incredible pastoral counselor on staff at our clinic named Marco who helps our patients with this aspect of their healing. We have seen many who were mean, angry, and miserable, go into his office and come out smiling, happy, and content. He's truly a tremendous blessing to them.

Over the years, we have noticed an amazing correlation between the incidence of cancer and emotional and/or physical trauma; for example, the death of a loved one, a divorce, or just outright, inescapable stress. Grief, depression, and anxiety have all been scientifically proven to cause immune suppression. Hans Selye (1907-1982) was a scientist who understood this. He developed the General Adaptation Syndrome model in 1936, which demonstrates, in three phases, the effects that stress has upon the body. He theorized that stress is a major cause of disease and proved that chronic stress causes long-term chemical changes to the body. He also observed that the body would respond to any external biological source of stress with a predictable biological pattern in an attempt to restore its internal homeostasis. The General Adaptation Syndrome and the classic "fight or flight" response, which he also described, have been studied extensively in medicine.

We can't tell you the number of times that we have had a breast cancer patient report a lump in her breast within two years of getting a divorce or losing a child. Fortunately, our pastoral counselor, Marco, has given us many tools to help these patients. Without his emotional support, we would be much less effective in our work.

We are a Christ-centered clinic and staff that treat patients of all religious backgrounds. We are a staff of "huggers." Like it or not, if you come to our clinic, you will be hugged and told that we love you! We have had so many patients say that out greatest asset is our clinical environment, but some patients might be uncomfortable if they don't like to be "loved on."

Lack of sleep, which many cancer patients struggle with, can affect recovery. So we do everything possible to help our patients get a good night's sleep. Sometimes, we can accomplish this by weaning them off their medications, especially pain killers. Such medications cause anxiety and constipation, and if patients are constipated, they won't be able to sleep, due to toxicity. We prescribe natural transdermal sleep aids like melatonin, including our own topical formula, as well as valerian, passion flower, 5-HTP, and pharmaceutical drugs like Lunesta and Ambien. Basically, we will do whatever it takes to get them to sleep.

Roadblocks to Healing

Lack of forgiveness toward oneself or others is one of the greatest roadblocks to healing. Our pastoral counselors try to help our patients reframe their problems, and provide them with solutions, so that they can let go of their anger. Emotional health and physical health are inseparable.

We also have our share of patients who don't comply with our dietary and stress relief recommendations, and even some who, with a little prompting, will admit to self-destructive behaviors. Such behaviors can also block healing. If patients are drinking, smoking, and abusing drugs during their treatments, this obviously won't help them in their recovery.

What More People Should Know About Cancer Treatments

The truth! If people knew, from the time of their diagnoses, about the types of treatments that are available, and the outcomes that result from conventional and holistic therapies, there would be fewer people dying prematurely. When deciding upon which treatments to pursue, people should always get a second and third opinion from other doctors, especially holistically-oriented doctors. They should never make fear-based decisions, but instead, get the facts about different treatments, take their time making decisions, and do their homework. They should never accept a death sentence just because someone in a white coat tells them that they only have "X" number of days to live. Very few oncologists know much about healing; they just know about treatments, which isn't the same thing! Many treatment options are available in holistic medicine, the least effective of which generally produces better outcomes than the "standard of care" in conventional medicine.

Our Greatest Challenge as Practitioners Who Treat Cancer

Our greatest challenge in treating cancer patients usually has to do with their lack of trust in the medical profession. Patients are skeptical about seeing us, after having spent their life savings going down the "standard of care" road, only to find themselves now dead broke and nearly dead! They have already spent so much emotional and pain "capital," to end up where they are at, so they don't have much left to give. Their vital force and will to live are so low that we have to "drag them out of the gutter" so to speak, to get them to believe that they can get well.

Patients should pursue the holistic approach first, not last. They can always do conventional therapy if the holistic approach by itself isn't successful. If they do it the other way around, it makes the clinician's job and their recovery so much more difficult.

Dangerous and Ineffective Cancer Treatments

Although I abhor them both, I would do chemotherapy over standard radiation any day. Ask anyone within 500 miles of Chernobyl in the former Soviet Union, and they will tell you the same thing.

In November 2004, *Swiss Medical Weekly* published findings by workers at the Clinical Institute of Radiation Medicine and Endocrinology Research in Minsk, Belarus (70 percent of the fallout from Chernobyl happened in neighboring Belarus), which showed that cancer rates rose by 40 percent in that area between 1990 and 2000. The nuclear catastrophe happened in April, 1986. Most of the cases of metastatic bone cancer that we have seen at our clinic in Mexico have resulted from previous radiation treatments that our patients received. We have successfully treated many post-mastectomy breast cancers only to have them recur in the plural lining of the lung or the rib cage. Sometimes, a totally new primary lung cancer even appears, and all of these recurrences are due to previous radiation which patients received.

The damage that the body incurs as a result of radiation is nearly impossible to heal. The damage to the oral mucosa (mucous membranes of the mouth) after radiation treatments for the throat or mouth cancers is unimaginable. The chronic yeast infections and burning pain that occur as a result of radiation are almost more than some people can endure.

This isn't necessarily the case with the well-orchestrated Cyber-Knife therapy, however, which was mentioned earlier in this chapter. Under the right circumstances, and especially when used in conjunction with stem cell therapy and dendritic cell vaccines, CyberKnife can stimulate a local immune response. However, unless it's combined with the latter two therapies, it's generally of little benefit to patients.

We aren't opposed to the use of well-thought out chemotherapy, if chemo sensitivity testing is done on the patient, the right chemotherapy agent is used in low or divided doses, and it's followed up with an MGIK drip. The MGIK drip is a restorative therapy that we use at our clinic which contains magnesium, glucose, insulin, Vitamin-C, and potassium. When chemotherapy is done this way, most people do fine. It's the unbridled, "We're going to treat this cancer with the big guns" kind of chemotherapy that ends up being dangerous to patients. The damage and gene mutations that chemotherapy causes can be dramatically minimized by simply giving patients some IV Vitamin C along with antioxidants the day after they receive treatments.

Conversely, on the naturopathic side, patients should guard against "holistic nonsense," such as relying solely upon 120 ounces of carrot juice daily and a few homeopathic remedies to get well. While not harmful to the body, people with cancer may be left with a false sense of security about the effectiveness of such approaches, and in the process of trying to get well may be burning valuable daylight. Cancer is no walk in the park; we must be wise and employ a bigger arsenal against it.

It's important for doctors to look at their patients' genetics, financial resources, age, medical history, emotional stability, and family support when helping them to decide upon a treatment regimen. I have seen many patients who didn't want to do any standard (conventional) therapy but who ended up caving in to the demands of their closest family members. Unfortunately, it was only after these family members witnessed the devastating effects that the "standard of care" had upon their loved ones that they repented for scolding Mom or Dad for being so stupid in their desire for a different type of care! By this time, however, it may be too late. Therefore, patients must be strong in their decision to not do conventional care, right from the start, and in the face of pressure from family and friends.

Inexpensive, but Effective, Cancer Treatments

There are some inexpensive, but rather heroic, cancer treatments that people who are short on funds can use. Haelan 951 is one such treatment. This is a super nutritious, fermented soybean protein beverage that contains a substance called Genistein, as well as numerous isoflavone compounds that have been found to have anti-estrogenic and immune-stimulating properties. Haelan 951 inhibits the formation of new tumor blood vessels and is thought to stop uncontrolled cell growth, most likely by inhibiting the activity of growth factors in the body that regulate cell division and cell survival.

...nnatech are great, too. Scien-
...polysaccharides have strong
...operties.

...al agents such as Sporanox
...l part of any cancer treat-
...are often found in people
..., can even masquerade as

Also, people who are fighting cancer or autoimmune diseases should talk to their physicians about low-dose naltrexone, which is another standard part of our treatment regimens. More information can be found on the Internet at: www.lowdosenaltrexone.org. This one compound, by itself, is more powerful and effective for treating cancer than almost anything in the conventional treatment arsenal.

Coffee enemas and gallbladder liver flushes give people with cancer a "big bang for the buck" in that they provide tremendous detoxification benefits to the body at a low cost. See the "Liver Flush" instructions on our website: www.hopewellness.com, for more information.

Another heroic botanical is Oleander soup. This recipe is truly amazing for many patients. We have seen stage four cancer patients who failed all treatments and who were at death's door recover with this simple soup. Instructions for making it are also on our website.

Finally, we recommend that every cancer patient get the book, *The Road to Health*, which can be purchased at www.hopewellness.com. This book was written by Laura Schroeder and me (Steve Hines). It contains information on a gut-healing, anti-inflammatory, and anti-fungal diet, which has profound healing benefits for those with cancer.

How Family and Friends Can Support Their Loved Ones with Cancer

To the friends and family of those with cancer: Remember, it's not your life at stake here. Please don't force your fearful, uninformed opinions on others. Get informed about effective cancer treatments, and try to be encouraging.

To the forceful and heavy-handed: Forever is a long time to feel guilty over the loss of your loved one!

Final Words

We go to every cancer conference and read every book and scientific study that we can get our hands on. We pick the brains of everyone who will let us, but we still sometimes fail in our treatments. After reasonably assessing a patient's case, if we feel that we aren't progressing with treatments in a positive manner, we are more than happy to refer that person to another practitioner or clinic that may have a better chance of saving the patient's life. We can't be everything to everyone. We do, however, try to be as much as we can for as many as we can.

None of us has a guarantee of tomorrow, so we advise our patients to live every moment of every day as though there were no tomorrow.

Other Recommended Books/Websites

We enjoy the "Moss report" by Ralph W. Moss, PhD: www.cancerdecisions.com.

Other great websites for general information on cancer include: www.curezone.com and www.cancertutor.com.

Contact Information
Elio Martin Rivera Celaya, MD and Steven Hines

Hope Wellness Center
Treatment Facility
Calle Trigo #3319
Fraccionamiento Valle Verde, D.
Ciudad Acuña, Coahuila, Mexico

For more information, contact our United States location:
Hope Wellness Center
2118 W. Beauregard Avenue
San Angelo, Texas 76901
Phone: (325) 947-5266
Fax: (325) 223-2853
eFax: (866) 716-4945
Email: info@hopewellnesscenter.com

Author's note: This interview was conducted with Steven Hines and Dr. Rivera.

•CHAPTER 7•

Martin Dayton, MD, DO
SUNNY ISLES BEACH, FL

Biography

Martin Dayton, MD, DO, is licensed and Board Certified as an osteopathic physician and surgeon by the state of Florida. He received his DO degree from Still University (Kirksville College of Osteopathic Medicine) in 1970, as well as an MD degree from Ross University in 1983. He also studied electrical acupuncture from 1974-77, at the Ryodoraku Institute of North America.

He is currently the medical director at Dayton Medical Center, in Sunny Isles Beach, Florida. His clinical experience includes emergency and intensive care medicine, as well as family and nutritional medicine. He is also a clinician, author, researcher, lecturer, and teacher.

Dr. Dayton has received certification by all of the following organizations: the American Board of Clinical Metal Toxicology, the Ryodoraku Institute of America (in electro-acupuncture), and the former American Board of Homeopathy and Certifying Board for Clinical Nutrition.

He is a past fellow of the American Academy of Family Practice (1983-2003) and the International College of Applied Nutrition (1981). His past teaching positions include: Assistant Clinical Professor of Family Medicine at Nova Southeastern University; Clinical Assistant Professor of Family Medicine at the College of Osteopathic Medicine of the Pacific; Adjunct Clinical Assistant Professor at New York College of Osteopathic Medicine; Preceptor at the University of Miami, and Preceptor at the University of Pittsburgh.

Approximately twenty percent of Dr. Dayton's patients are cancer patients. He has been treating cancer with Insulin Potentiation Therapy (IPT) since 2001, and has been using homeopathy and heavy metal chelation therapies since the 1970s. He combines medical concepts found in both Eastern and Western medicine. The Eastern concept of medicine has to do with balancing the body. The Western concept of medicine has to do with destroying what doesn't belong in the body. Dr. Dayton has found that combining these two branches of medicine, carefully and prudently, produces the best outcomes for patients.

Dr. Dayton's professional and certifying board affiliations, both past and present, include the following:

- American Academy for Anti-aging Medicine (A4M)
- IAACN, International American Associations of Clinical Nutritionists (past President/Chairman of the board)
- American College of Emergency Physicians, charter member (circa 1972-1976)
- IBOMF, International Oxidative Medical Association
- ABOM, American Academy Board of Oxidative Medicine (1998-2001 Board Member)
- CNCB, Clinical Nutrition Certification Board
- Life Extension Foundation, Advisory Board Member (present)
- American Board of Clinical Metal Toxicology (present Board member)
- National Center of Homeopathy (circa 1983-2000)
- ACAM, American College for Advancement in Medicine (1980-present, past Board Member)

- AMA, American Medical Association (1979-2005)
- AOA, American Osteopathic Association (1970-present)
- FOMA, Florida Osteopathic Medical Association (1970-present)
- AAFP, American Academy of Family Practice, Fellow (1980-2003)
- APMA, American Preventive Medical Association
- American International Associations of Cytobiology
- Arizona Association for Homeopathic and Integrative Medicine
- International College for Integrative Medicine, Board Advisor
- CNCB, Clinical Nutrition Certification Board, Scientific Council member (circa 1996-2003)
- ABCT, American Board of Clinical Metal Toxicology
- American Holistic Medical Association (1980-circa 2000)
- FAMA, Florida Academy for Advancement in Medicine, President (circa 1995-1997)
- American Society of Teachers in Family Medicine (Circa 1981-84)
- ACOFP, American College of Osteopathic Family Physicians (circa 1985-1988)
- ACOPMS, American College of Pain Management and Sclerotherapy (circa1998-2002)
- International Association of Cytobiological Therapies (1999-2003)
- Arizona Association for Homeopathic and Integrative Medicine Association (circa 1990 - 2002)
- ICIM, International College for Integrative Medicine, Board Advisor (circa 2000)
- Ryodoraku Institute of North America, PhD Candidate in Electrical Acupuncture (1974)
- Society for the Advancement of Healing Arts, President (1980-1983)
- Aslan Institute, Medical Director (1994-1995)

What Cancer Is and What Causes It

Cancer is characterized by the excessive and uncontrolled growth of abnormal cells. These cells deviate from the anatomical and organizational features of normal and benign cells and take on bizarre appearances and maladaptive physiology. They proliferate and spread throughout the body through local tissue invasion, or via the blood and lymph, causing the potential destruction of organs and bodily functions.

Cancer is caused by many things. In general, it's caused by the interaction of the body's genes within their environment. Our chromosomes are like banks of genetic switches. Certain switches are turned on, while others are turned off, to elicit specific behaviors in the body. Genetic switches are influenced by heredity as well as environmental toxins and radiation. Deficiencies and excesses of nutrients, hormones, emotions, and many other factors, such as viruses, also play a role in genetic behavior.

Cancer cells have common characteristics which distinguish them from benign cells. For instance, the ability to self-destruct, which is found in benign cells, is impaired in cancer cells. As such, cancer cells don't contribute to the welfare of the body. Normal cells self-destruct so that new, vibrant cells can take their place. This process is called apoptosis, or programmed cell death. Cancer cells, instead of self-destructing, produce more dysfunctional cancer cells, eventually producing tumors and metastases. Many therapies target the induction of apoptosis, or programmed cell death, in cancer cells.

Cancer cells are also different from normal cells because they create energy for function, propagation, and repair by metabolizing sugar without oxygen, while normal cells rely upon the metabolism of sugar with oxygen for the production of their energy.

Cancer cells use various strategies to survive at the expense of normal cells, one of which is immune system evasion. Accordingly, targeted therapies for cancer are intended to exploit the differences between malignant and benign cells, in order to improve immune recognition, and cripple the energy producing pathways that cancer uses.

Diagnostic and Testing Procedures

When patients first come to my clinic, I try to gather as much pertinent information as I can about them, including specific information about their cancer tissue. The more I know about my patients, the more I am able to determine what treatments they need. My initial evaluation involves taking a diagnostic history, doing a physical examination, and reviewing patients' medical records, including their pathology and treatment reports. I then discuss their case and treatment options with them and their family members. After that, we may do more testing.

We do blood, hair, urine, electro-dermal and biofeedback testing, the latter of which uses acupuncture points on the body to measure the functioning of the body's systems and organs.

If cancer cells are found to be circulating in the patient's blood, we use blood tests to determine what anti-cancer agents those cancer cells will be sensitive to. We order tests from a laboratory in Germany called BioFocus (www.biofocus.de) and another in Greece called Research Genetic Cancer Centre, LTD. We send our patients' blood samples out of the country because we don't have labs that do this type of testing in the United States. These labs look at the genetic (and therefore, metabolic) characteristics of cancer cells, and their sensitivity to various anti-cancer agents, including the natural substances and drugs that cancer cells are most likely to respond to. In addition, the tests can help us determine what synergistic substances may be used to enhance the effects of other substances.

The tests are far from perfect, though, because they can only ascertain the characteristics of the cancer cells that are circulating in the blood. They don't necessarily tell us the characteristics of cancer in other parts of the body. Cancer cells aren't homogenous. Even within the same tumor, they can have different characteristics, and therefore, can be sensitive to different treatment agents.

I also select anti-cancer agents based on the standard pathology diagnosis, which is based upon the characteristics of the cancer tissue, such as bodily location, microscopic appearance, and other laboratory findings. Testing labs here in the United States can help to determine which cancer agents may be most therapeutic based on this pathology. Rational Therapeutics (www.rational-t.com) is one such lab, which examines small clusters of cancer cells and takes a snapshot of the cancer's behavior in response to different drugs and combinations of drugs. By analyzing tumor responses in the laboratory, RT can identify which chemotherapy drug or combination of drugs will induce programmed cell death, and which ones will not. The general overall estimate of positive predictive accuracy (the measure of what drugs will work) from this type of testing is 77 percent, and the negative predictive accuracy (the measure of what drugs won't work) is 87.9 percent, but the reliability of the testing varies and depends upon the tissues that are tested. Weisenthal Cancer Group (www.weisenthalcancer.com) is another lab that determines which drugs cancer cells will best respond to, based on their pathology.

In order to do this type of testing, both Rational Therapeutics and Weisenthal generally require cells that come directly from the patient's tumor (except in the case of blood cancers like leukemia), and most patients, by the time they come to see me, have already been through surgery and/or usually are in a more advanced state of cancer, which means that we can't take a biopsy of their tumors for testing.

We want to avoid prescribing ineffective therapies. The following is an excerpt from Pharmacogenomics, a book published in 2001: "Chemotherapy drugs selected empirically and based on the results of clinical trials, using limited patient specific data (tumor size, site, and metastasis) induce positive responses (in patients) only 30 percent of the time." We need to do better than that when selecting treatments for our patients, which is why we do more extensive testing than many other clinics.

After we do the aforementioned blood tests, in addition to perhaps a pathology test (if we are able to obtain a sample of the patient's tumor), we end up with several treatment options. We do electro-dermal biofeedback testing to help us evaluate those options. This type of testing is done at our clinic, and provides further insight about the agents that might be most effective or most problematic for our patients. Devices that can be used for this type of testing include the EDS 2000 and the Asyra, as well as others. The Asyra evaluates the body and its general needs using sophisticated computer programs that electromagnetically analyze bodily energy patterns via hand-held electrodes.

Electrodermal testing may also involve placing different anti-cancer substances, such as herbs, homeopathic medication, and chemotherapeutic drugs, "in circuit" with the patient and a testing device. The substances are typically placed on a metal plate which is electromagnetically connected to the testing device and the patient. For example, if a patient has a tumor in the left lung, an electrode is placed on an acupuncture point on the hand corresponding to the left lung (according to principles of Chinese medicine). If a positive change is measured, then that particular substance may be helpful for treating that patient's lung cancer.

When treating cancer patients, I prefer to use substances that are both anti-cancer and not likely to harm the rest of the body. So when testing substances, I also put them in circuit with acupuncture points that correspond to other parts of the body—the kidneys, liver, etc. to determine the likelihood that they will cause undesirable side effects to those parts of the body. By testing more than one substance at a time, I can obtain information about which substances work together well in the body.

Patients may have a lot of metastases, and different tumors that are sensitive to different agents. We need to determine how our treatment choices will affect the overall body as well as all of the tumors that are present. A chemotherapy agent that tests well for one tumor may not test well for another. Electrodermal testing can alert us to the potential need to change therapeutic strategies. Electrodermal biofeedback testing is also useful for monitoring patients' progress, because the results that we get from this testing are immediate. And because its cost isn't high, it can be done frequently.

None of the testing modalities that we use provides a perfect perspective on what patients need: not blood tests, not empirical knowledge, (e.g., tumor type and diagnosis), nor any other test.

Viewing all of the information as a collective "mosaic" of knowledge is the best way to determine what combination of treatments is likely to be the most appropriate; the whole picture is greater than the sum of its parts.

Additionally, we test our patients for substances that they might need to treat other problems in their bodies, such as heavy metal poisoning and other types of toxicity. We also do organic acid urine tests, which give us an idea of how much their bodily functions are impaired. We often look at how they react to different foods, to determine whether they have allergies and sensitivities. We also look for infections, because often, people with cancer have active Candida, viruses, and other pathogens that are causing them problems. We do tests to determine their genetic weaknesses and then try to support them in whatever fashion is appropriate. Our goal during treatment is to reduce the body's overall stress load so that the immune system can better fight the cancer. We treat for toxicities either before or after their cancer treatments, depending on what's most practical for our patients.

Treatment Approach

Our overall treatment approach is to create an environment in the patient's body which is conducive to health and not disease. We treat the cancerous tissue, but we also treat the rest of the person. We base our therapies upon our patients' preferences and needs, their ability to do certain treatments, and the options that are available to them based on testing, financial resources, and other factors. We also look at the cost, or risk, of different treatments, versus their benefits.

Our treatment approach can be broken down into three components: treating deficiencies in the body, eliminating its toxicities, and improving cell signaling (both inter- and intra-cellular communication). These are described below.

1. Toxicity is caused by an excess of harmful substances or processes that prevent optimal function and repair of the body: for example, mercury poisoning, or toxic thoughts.

2. Deficiencies have to do with what the body is lacking (in a variety of areas): for example, nutrients such as Vitamin C or D. It may also be associated with psycho-emotional factors, such as patients not having enough nurturing in their lives.

3. Defects in inter and intra-cellular communication may involve photons, chemicals called cytokines, or hormones (hormones are produced in one area of body and travel throughout it to regulate different functions, such as metabolism). Signaling defects also encompass nerve impulses that conduct information from one area of the body to another through the nervous system.

Basically, we concern ourselves with anything that impacts the body and attempt to establish a harmonic state within it which leaves patients in a condition that's more conducive to health. We also look for infections that need to be treated, as well as substances that need to be removed from the body and nutrients that need to be added to it. We need to pay attention to the body's excretory and other vital functions in order to help the immune system to perform better. Vitamins and phytonutrients are some of the substances that we commonly use to support these vital functions.

The following sections describe in greater detail some of the treatments that we use to address the aforementioned areas.

IPT-Insulin Potentiation Therapy

Author's note: IPT is described in Chapter Five, as well as in other chapters throughout this book. Therefore, the basics of how it works won't be repeated here.

We use IPT in our clinic for the treatment of cancer. IPT can be used to deliver both natural substances and chemotherapy drugs to cancer cells. We generally use chemotherapeutic drugs for this procedure, but we also use natural substances. We may include dimethyl sulfoxide (DMSO) in the IVs, which helps the drugs to penetrate the cells better.

I sometimes recommend full-dose chemotherapy to patients with certain types of cancers, and will refer them to an oncologist, who has more experience in full-dose chemotherapy than I do. It is of utmost importance that I recommend treatments that are in my patients' best interest, even if it means that I must refer them elsewhere.

We sometimes use conventional medicine, but overall, and more often than not, we prefer natural, less toxic approaches to treatment. For example, patients with pancreatic cancer respond poorly to conventional treatments, so we would be inclined to use more natural therapies for them. But sometimes we use chemotherapy in an IPT format for pancreatic cancer, as well, in order to get the best of both (medical) worlds.

Some time ago, a study was done in which researchers tracked two groups of patients with pancreatic cancer. One group was treated with conventional chemotherapy, and the other was treated with a macrobiotic diet. At the end of the year, most of the patients that had been on the macrobiotic diet were still alive. Hardly any of the patients who had done chemotherapy were still alive. While natural treatments may be more effective for certain types of cancers, they are not for all types. For instance, testicular cancer is almost always curable by conventional means (ie: chemotherapy) and therefore such therapy should be the treatment of choice for patients with this type of cancer.

Natural Substances to Poison Glycolysis and Prevent Angiogenesis

One anti-cancer strategy that we use involves the poisoning of glycolysis, which is the metabolic pathway that cancers use to create energy and which metabolizes sugar without oxygen. Various products on the market are useful for poisoning this pathway, including wheat germ extract, which is found in products such as Avemar, and substances which come from tangerines and blueberries, which are found in products such as Salvestrol. We sometimes use these as part of our IPT treatments. What's interesting is that we can poison these pathways without harming the metabolic pathways of normal cells. So feeding cancer things that selectively suppress this particular energy pathway can be helpful for destroying the cancer, and is one of the strategies that we use when treating our patients.

Preventing angiogenesis (or tumor blood vessel creation) is another component of our anti-tumor protocol. Bindweed, bovine cartilage, sea cucumber, curcumin, and soy are some effective agents that we use to do this. Copper chelation is used to reduce copper levels in the body so that tumor blood vessels don't have enough copper to grow.

Melatonin

Melatonin has been shown to have anti-cancer properties. It also appears to be statistically safer, more effective, and much less expensive than chemotherapy drugs for treating certain types of cancer. For instance, a drug called erlotinib (Tarceva®) is commonly used to treat lung, and sometimes, pancreatic cancers, but melatonin has proven to have greater beneficial effects upon these cancers than erlotinib.

Some time ago, a series of studies was done by oncologists in Italy, in which the benefits of melatonin were assessed on patients with non-small cell lung cancers. In one study, researchers gave ten milligrams of melatonin daily to patients who had non-small cell lung cancers and who had stopped their chemotherapy regimens due to their failure to respond to them. They were compared with similar patients who didn't receive melatonin. A year later, 26 percent of the patients who had taken melatonin were still alive. None of those that had done chemotherapy without melatonin were alive. In another study, a group of patients was given chemotherapy along with twenty milligrams of melatonin, while another group of similar patients was given only chemotherapy. After one year, 44 percent of the patients in the melatonin group were still alive, compared to 19 percent in the group that didn't take the melatonin. This represents a twofold increase in the survival rate of patients who took melatonin! In yet another study, patients with glioblastoma, a type of brain cancer, were given either radiation and melatonin, or radiation alone. Twenty-three percent of the patients who took the melatonin were alive after one year, while none of those who received radiation without melatonin were still alive.

Oncologists don't usually recommend melatonin to their patients. You would think that they would, given that many studies have been published which attest to its effectiveness. Instead, they recommend drugs like Tarceva, which is an antineoplastic medication that inhibits epidermal growth factor receptors in cancer. Research shows that melatonin also inhibits this receptor, and has other beneficial effects upon cancer, as well. Studies of patients with certain types of cancer demonstrate that those who have failed chemotherapy but who take melatonin have a 26 percent survival rate after one year, compared to 10 percent of those who just take Tarceva. Furthermore, Tarceva may cost more than $4,000 per month, while twenty milligrams of melatonin cost only $11 per month. That's medical politics for you.

Other Anti-Cancer Nutrients

We administer high doses of Vitamin C to our patients, sometimes concurrently with Vitamin K. When given at high doses together in an IV, both of these vitamins have strong anti-cancer properties. We also use resveratrol, delta-tocopherols, and sometimes bicarbonate. Of all the natural forms of Vitamin E, delta-tocopherols have the greatest effect upon cancer. We also give our patients Vitamin D, which has anti-cancerous properties, but it's important to dose Vitamin D properly, as the wrong doses can be immunosuppressive. All of these substances function in various ways to disadvantage cancer cells. Resveratrol is an example of a substance that influences cancer cells via its cell signaling effects.

Using Pharmaceutical Drugs Off-Label: Viagra, Naltrexone and Persantine

Using some pharmaceutical drugs off-label (for purposes other than what their label indicates) can also be useful for treating cancer. For example, some phosphordiesterase inhibitor drugs, such as Viagra (sildenafil), reverse tumor suppression mechanisms, which means that they unmask cancer cells so that the immune system can more easily attack them. This effect has been proven in studies on mice and humans. Additionally, if Viagra is used in conjunction with Adriamycin (a chemotherapy drug), it helps to reduce negative side effects that Adriamycin causes to the heart. So Viagra seems to be helpful for treating certain cancers in a variety of ways and can be used in conjunction with chemotherapy.

Low-dose naltrexone is another powerful anti-cancer drug. When given in a full 50 mg dose, it suppresses endorphin activity, but when given in small doses, it has the opposite effect. It has been used to treat a variety of cancers with favorable clinical results. I gave low-dose naltrexone to one of my 80 plus-year-old patients who had developed B-cell lymphoma. This patient had failed to respond to various treatments, and was in hospice. He didn't want to regularly come to my office, take a lot of medicine, or spend a lot of money, so I gave him a prescription for naltrexone, which he took on a nightly basis. Six weeks later, he was out of hospice— ballroom dancing! I provide this example because he had such a dramatic response to the medication, and was one of the few patients that I treated with only low-dose naltrexone and nothing else. So his case provides insight into how effective this treatment can be.

Persantine (dipyridamole) is a drug that augments the activity of various chemotherapeutic agents, including Etoposide and Methotrexate, and has also proven to be helpful for treating melanoma. Basically, it helps to unmask cancer cells so that the immune system can more easily recognize them. Cancer cells have ways of hiding from the immune system, or suppressing it, and this is one substance that helps it to recognize them.

Immune Support

Stimulating the immune system is important if people are to effectively heal from cancer. We often recommend Beta-1, 3-D glucans to our patients, which give the most "bang for the buck" by providing the greatest benefit at the lowest price. We also recommend various mushroom products, shark liver oil, and many other substances that stimulate white blood cell production. There are also other naturally occurring substances that aren't commercially available which we put together and use for this purpose.

Detoxification

At our clinic, every patient's detoxification protocol is different. Unlike the field of oncology, where everyone follows the same protocol, integrative doctors like me tailor treatments to the individual patient. So detoxification means different things for different people. For example, we may recommend coffee enemas to some of our patients, and saunas to others. Saunas may be appropriate for some, but they aren't helpful if patients are debilitated. We may also recommend substances to support the body's excretory organs (those which are responsible for processing toxins). Silymarin (milk thistle) and alpha-lipoic acid are two that we use for the liver. We may recommend herbal formulas, like Triphala, which is also used for gastrointestinal detoxification. We may prescribe probiotics, which replace healthy bacteria within the intestinal tract, as well as substances which contain fiber, because these help to carry toxic substances out of the body. Additionally, we may recommend foods that contain high amounts of sulfur, such as asparagus, eggs, and garlic because sulfur aids in detoxification.

For heavy metal chelation, we use everything from pharmaceutical medications such as DMSA and DMPS to natural substances like zeolite. I may or may not recommend heavy metal detoxification to patients who are doing chemotherapy. We don't tend to recommend it to those that are weak and doing chemotherapy, but it depends upon patients' overall condition. When treating cancer, there are no hard and fast rules. Doctors must take into account their patients' overall integrity and response to treatment, and tailor treatments to the individual. For example, if patients are strongly mercury-toxic, and their overall condition isn't bad, then I may not treat their cancers until they get the mercury (dental amalgams) out of their teeth, because mercury weakens the immune system.

Dietary Recommendations

Like other aspects of treatment, my patients' diets are individualized. I usually refer people to the nutritionist at our clinic, who spends time with them and reviews their dietary issues. Generally, I recommend that people with cancer avoid red meats and sugars and instead consume high quality, alkaline foods. Juicing fruits and vegetables is also beneficial. I also recommend that they do electrodermal and chemical tests to determine what their food allergies are, so that their immune systems aren't focusing on allergens when they should be focusing on cancer.

Strategies for Emotional Healing

The Importance of Awareness, Spontaneity and Intimacy

Sometimes, we take an inventory of our patients' emotional condition, to see what can be done to improve their emotional and psychological well-being, since this is intertwined with their physical health. If patients are feeling suppressed, then their immune function will be down. If they are feeling empowered, then their immune function will be good. A Canadian-born psychiatrist named Eric Berne wrote a book called *The Games People Play* (1964), in which he indicated that there are three things that people need in order to be psychologically healthy (after their physical needs are met). Those three things are awareness; that is, being able to appreciate one's surroundings; spontaneity, the "spice of life;" and intimacy, the sharing of one's self. This doctor believed that if people were deficient in any one of these three areas, then they wouldn't be as happy as they could be.

Some psychologists think that disease is the body's way of express-ing that the person doesn't want to participate in society and that cancer is the ultimate socially acceptable way of not participating. So after taking an inventory to find out what needs to be added and eliminated from our patients' lives, we may need to help them to change the conditions in their lives which have made them not want to participate in life anymore, and create new conditions which would favor them wanting to participate.

Healing Regret, Resentment and Self-Righteousness

We also look for emotional roadblocks to healing in our patients, and help them to remove these, so that their other treatments will be more effective. In particular, there are three health-robbing attitudes that I observe and attempt to address in my patients. I call these "the three R's": regret, resentment, and righteousness (or rather, self-righteousness).

When events don't unfold in life as people think they should, they may be living with feelings of regret or resentment, and theoretical-ly, these feelings can be associated with the development of chronic degenerative diseases. So dealing with these emotions is important. Two ways that people can do this are by forgiving others or rationa-lizing past events. Whatever they can do to make the past okay is helpful for their healing process. People who live with regrets must realize that they can't change the past, and so must instead change their perspective, such as by forgiving those who hurt them, or rationalizing past events so that they are now okay with whatever happened.

Also, having an attitude of self-righteousness can block healing, because people who are self-righteous tend to go around thinking that they are right all of the time and that everyone else is wrong. Such people may find themselves living in a world that appears to be very hostile towards them—a world that, in their eyes, is full of wrong. Because of this, they are angry, and their feelings of anger are counter-productive to their healing.

There are various ways to heal such attitudes. Group therapy, self-help books, counseling, and tapping on various acupuncture or other historically effective points on the body through techniques such as Emotional Freedom Technique (EFT), are some ways to do this. EFT (www.emofree.com), for example, reprograms the sub-conscious mind through the use of affirmations and touch. Another approach is neuro-linguistic programming, which is a therapeutic technique that's used to detect and reprogram unconscious patterns of thought and behavior, in order to alter psychological responses.

Using Energetic Devices and Homeopathy to Release Emotional Trauma

There are many ways to de-stress the body and heal emotional trauma, and everyone's needs are different. Some people go to counselors, while others may practice Qi Gong, which is a Chinese form of healing that happens via the manipulation of energies. I usually go through different treatment options with my patients to help them determine what they most need. I use energetic devices that, at least in theory, can release emotional trauma from the cells. I also use homeopathy, which has proven to be effective for releasing emotional trauma.

Scientific evidence is proving that the body's cells hold memories, although not in epic pictures like the conscious mind. Theoretically, if you put the right signals into the body, those memories can be unlocked. There are various devices that produce an energetic, homeopathic-like resonance which can unlock the memories. The Asyra is one such device, although specific medical claims can't be made about this (or any other device that hasn't been approved by the FDA). Other methods and devices exist which may alter the body's energetic patterns and thereby promote healing, as well.

I have used homeopathy on my patients for over 25 years and I believe that it heals, both emotionally and physically. To provide a modern analogy of how it works, suppose that you have a remote control device on your car key which unlocks your car door. If the remote control button on the key is pressed, and the battery and the receiving device on the car are working, and an effective signal is emitted and received, the car door lock will either close or open, provided that the car door mechanism is in good shape and there is enough power coming from the battery. Just as the car door lock is programmed to open and close, we are programmed for self-healing. So theoretically, if the right energetic signal is put into the right person, and that signal is received by the body, it can initiate a process of self-healing. The goal of homeopathy is to initiate a cascade of events in the body using the person's own power (or energy). It's based upon the body's ability to self-heal.

Treatment Outcomes

The later the stage of cancer that patients are in, the more difficult it is to treat them. Fortunately, we have patients with late stage cancers who have survived for years past their initial diagnoses. Recently, we had a patient who came to us with breast cancer and metastases masses in her lungs. She decided that she didn't want to receive chemotherapy, radiation, or surgery. Instead, she spent ten thousand dollars on treatments for her teeth, and her family wasn't happy because she was 95 years old! We also treated her five days a week for three months. We gave her herbs and high dose Vitamin C, and did detoxification treatments on her, as well. No detectable cancer remained in her body after we completed those treatments. She died at age 99, but not from cancer. Our treatments appeared to help her, but more importantly, she had a great attitude, which probably put her over the top so that she could overcome her cancer. She also repaired her bad teeth prior to initiating cancer treatments, which may have been significantly helpful. You wouldn't think that a 95 year-old lady could survive all these treatments and go into remission. It's interesting how things like this occur.

Then there are people who seem to do everything right, but who go downhill anyway. It's sometimes difficult to predict who is going to do well, although I think attitude has a lot to do with it. People who are angry and who refuse to stop being angry, have the worst prognoses. Those who seem to be grateful for life and who want to share with others, seem to do better. In any case, people with metastatic disease, even the angry ones, do better if they utilize a holistic approach to healing.

Roadblocks to Healing

Unresolved emotional problems can be a roadblock to healing. We try to do everything that we can to keep our patients' spirits up, so that they are able to follow our treatment program. It's important that they reduce as many negative influences upon their lives as possible. When their insurance companies don't pay for their treatments, for instance, this can be a major source of stress for them. Some insurance companies cover IPT treatments and some of our tests, but not all of them do.

Also, when patients don't understand their treatment options, this can be a block to their healing. Oncologists use vague words with their patients when referring to the outcomes that they can expect from different treatments. For example, they will often say, "the tumor will respond to this treatment." People think "response" means remission. But it can also mean that their tumors will grow less quickly, partially shrink, or disappear, as a result of treatment. Reducing the tumor's size may or may not have any relevance to how long patients live. So it's important for them to understand what their treatment options are.

Finally, it's really dangerous when doctors give their patients death sentences, and tell them how long they have left to live. The power of suggestion can really screw up the immune system, especially when doctors say, "There's nothing else that can be done for you." They forget to add that very important phrase, "...by me!"

Low-Cost Treatment Solutions

For patients that don't have a lot of money for treatments, low-dose naltrexone can be helpful. I had a patient with B-cell lymphoma who came into my office yesterday who was told that she had a year and a half to live. She was no longer responding to conventional medication, so I sat down with her, and told her about the older patient that I had treated who had been in hospice, but who had gotten well with low-dose naltrexone. I also told her about another woman who had refused conventional treatments at the Mayo clinic and to whom I had also prescribed naltrexone. This other woman, like my current patient, also had B-cell lymphoma. After a few years on naltrexone, she called the other B-cell lymphoma patients that she had met at the Mayo clinic a few years prior, only to discover that they had all died. She was still alive and working, thanks to the low-dose naltrexone, but she still had her tumors. Unfortunately, after awhile, she ran out of naltrexone and for some unknown reason didn't call me for a refill. Three months later, she was back in my office in a wheelchair. A lymphoma had grown in her spine, so she went to a hospital to receive radiation.

There are people who don't have a lot of money for treatments and who will volunteer to participate in clinical trials, because some of the costs of treatment are covered under such trials. I have seen some people "hit home runs" with these clinical trial treatments, but unfortunately, most aren't aimed at making patients better. Rather, they are only done to test patient response and tolerance to new treatments. People don't usually do very well on them, but they may be an alternative for those who don't have a lot of money for treatments.

How Family and Friends Can Support Their Loved Ones with Cancer

One of the best things that family and friends of the sick can do is create intimacy with their loved ones and provide reasons for them to "hang out" instead of "check out." Helping them to experience pleasurable things in life, assisting them with a proper diet, getting them to where they need to go in a timely fashion, providing them with loving guidance in other areas, and creating an atmosphere which motivates them to want to hang around, are beneficial for their healing.

Recommended Books and Websites

Studying the National Cancer Institute website (www.cancer.gov) can provide helpful insights into "in vogue" cancer treatments in conventional medicine. It can also give outcome-based results on conventional treatments for different types of cancers. I recommend this site because people with cancer should start treatments with their eyes wide open and with a strong knowledge of their options.

Cancer websites that advocate conventional medicine don't recognize the benefits of holistic alternative and complementary medicine, though, even though many studies have been published which support such care. For example, the benefits of taking anti-oxidants, along with chemotherapy, is well-supported by published research, but most oncologists don't advocate their use. Patients should be aware of this when researching treatments.

Burton Goldberg, one of the world's foremost experts in alternative medicine, has a patient advocacy site, www.burtongoldberg.com, which contains a lot of information for people with cancer. Another website, www.cancertutor.com, offers a "smorgasbord" of alternative cancer treatment ideas. Patients should have a competent coach to help them navigate the options presented on such sites.

Last Words

Life and health are too dear to be left to chance alone. Take charge of them for the sake of those you love, including yourself. Love and accept yourself.

Strive to supply what is needed for your physical and emotional well-being and remove anything that may impair it. Embrace goals that make life rewarding. Experience the joys of life in the form of intimacy, spontaneity, and appreciation of the beauty in the world that surrounds you. Do these things and you will enjoy stellar and prolonged survival during your time on earth.

Contact Information
Martin Dayton, MD, DO

18600 Collins Avenue
Sunny Isles Beach, Florida 33160
Telephone: (305) 931-8484
Fax: (305) 936-1849
E-mail: drdayton@daytonmedical.com
www.daytonmedical.com

•CHAPTER 8•

Robert Eslinger, DO, HMD
RENO, NV

Biography

Robert Eslinger, DO, HMD, or Dr. Bob, as those in his practice fondly call him, finished his formal medical training in 1978. He has been in clinical practice for over thirty years. He is certified in Family Practice, Osteopathic Manipulation and Homeopathy. In November, 2008, he was appointed by the governor of Nevada to sit on the Board of Homeopathic Medical Examiners for the state of Nevada; a board that supervises not just homeopathic practice, but all of alternative medicine. Dr. Eslinger currently practices at the Reno Integrative Medical Center in Reno, NV.

For thirteen years prior to coming to Reno, Dr. Eslinger was the Medical Director of Cascade Medical Center in Cascade, Idaho. Before concentrating in the area of alternative/integrative medicine, Dr. Eslinger developed a broad background in traditional medical disciplines. His work involved everything from being stationed on a remote Indian reservation in the Public Health Service to establishing a private practice and spending years working in clinics and emergency rooms. He has been on a lifelong quest to find the treatments that work best for his patients. He has many hours of training in homeopathic and alternative medicine and is a compassionate physician who takes time to listen to his patients' needs. He brings an abundance of life and professional experience to his practice.

He presently focuses on a specialty known as biological medicine, which combines older and more natural traditional treatments with modern technology and uses therapeutic measures to strengthen and balance the body. The primary goal of biological medicine is to support or restore the body's systems to promote maximum self-healing. It involves methods of diagnosis and therapy that are guided by the principles of maintenance and furtherance of the human bio-system and its regulatory mechanisms. Biological medicine is holistic because it's based upon the supposition that the body is a matrix of interconnectedness; physical, mental, emotional, and spiritual.

What Cancer Is and What Causes It

I don't believe that cancer is some alien life form that invades the body with the sole purpose of trying to kill it. The body has infinite wisdom, which sometimes surpasses our conscious minds, but things can run "amok" in it at times. So in many ways, cancers are really just adaptations to different stressors that people experience in their lives, either early on or within approximately two years prior to their developing a tumor. So cancer is driven by the subconscious mind, and it's the body's attempt to adapt to something. Of course, it can also be triggered by various toxins, genetic abnormalities, and infectious organisms.

I don't accept any theory 100 percent, but in my experience of treating cancer patients, I have witnessed what Douglas Brodie, MD (the founder of this clinic and a renowned cancer treatment physician) calls "cancer personalities." There are basically two kinds of personalities that he observed to be preponderant in those with cancer. In over half a century of medical practice, Dr. Brodie saw that cancer tended to happen either to people who had long-suppressed bitterness and anger deep within themselves, or to those who were martyrs—the kind of people who would do things for everyone but themselves.

Another doctor, Ryke Geerd Hamer, MD, who was an oncologist from Germany and the head of the main chemotherapy program in Munich in the 1980s, had a son who was shot and killed. Dr. Hamer subsequently developed testicular cancer, which caused him to wonder if there was a connection between his son's death and the development of his cancer, because he had never been sick a day in his life. So he started asking his cancer patients questions, and learned that the vast majority of them had specific stressors—conflict shocks, he called them—which were blows to their psychological, mental, and emotional wellbeing, and which had happened to them within two years prior to their diagnoses. His findings were so specific that he was able to develop a map which correlated particular types of cancer with specific stressors.

For example, he believed that a particular type of lung cancer called adenocarcinoma resulted from people experiencing a threat to their lives. He thought that this death threat triggered the subconscious mind to want to grow more lung tissue to help to prevent death in the future, because breathing is the most basal reflex in the body. Humans have a strong drive to breathe, and if something impinges on that, then Dr. Hamer believed that the subconscious mind would trigger more lung tissue to grow in order to avoid strangulation; hence, the cancer.

I have observed a strong correlation between specific emotional traumas and the development of specific cancers in many of my patients. Once, I was explaining to a liver cancer patient the connection between the body, mind and psyche, and Dr. Hamer's theories. I said to him, "Take pancreatic cancer, for example. Dr. Hamer believes that pancreatic cancer develops from conflicts surrounding family inheritances, or frustrated entitlements." And the man almost fell out of his chair, He said, "My sister just died of pancreatic cancer!" Then he proceeded to tell me that his mother had died, and that he wanted to keep his mom's wedding ring, and had told his sister that he wanted the wedding ring but that she could have their mother's engagement rings. She said to him, "No I want both rings!" and she fought him, even up until a court battle, which she lost. Six months later, she developed pancreatic cancer.

I notice that these kinds of specific associations happen often. I'm not ready to say that cancer is caused purely by psychological factors, but they play a large role in its development. What is interesting about Dr. Hamer's work is that if you ask any oncologist where cancer most commonly spreads to in the body, from any other organ and no matter the cancer, they will always say that it's the lungs. Lung metastases are the most common type of metastases. So Dr. Hamer would say that lung metastases are due to doctors delivering cancer diagnoses to their patients, which causes immediate death fright in the patients and in turn triggers tumor growth in their lungs. These little associations have made me wonder. Another interesting theory of Dr. Hamer's is that cancer doesn't spread through the blood. Instead, every new location where it shows up in the body is an entirely new cancer.

Strategies for Mind-Body Healing

Because of the associations that I have observed between specific traumas and the different types of cancer in people, my nurses and I talk to our patients about what kind of stressors were going on their lives roughly two years prior to their diagnoses, because this information can provide us with clues about how to heal them on a mind-body level. It's important to bring their subconscious minds into the treatment process, because the subconscious mind is what runs the body and controls all of its automatic processes.

I do a therapy called Psych-K in my office, which uses bio-kinesiology, or muscle testing, along with affirmations, to communicate directly with the subconscious mind, in order to alter its beliefs. By testing my patients' muscle responses to different questions, I can ask their subconscious minds if they really want to heal. And nine times out of ten, even if on a conscious level they want to heal, the initial answer of their subconscious to this question is "no." I must then explain to them that if we don't address the underlying subconscious drive that's causing them to want to remain ill, then none of my therapies will be effective for them. This is one reason why I believe that cancer has such a terrible cure rate. People have all these subconscious motivations for illness that don't often get addressed, especially in Western medicine.

Ninety-nine percent of my patients with cancer are in sympathetic overdrive, which means that their bodies are in a state of "fight or flight," or high arousal, and they are scared to death. I tell them that the worst thing that they can do is declare war on their tumors. There's no activity that creates as much of a sympathetic response in the body as war, and if patients have the mentality that they are in a war, then their bodies' fight or flight response becomes activated, and their immune and digestive systems shut down. This is because the functioning of the immune and digestive systems is considered to be non-essential for the body's immediate survival when it's behaving as though it were in a war. It's not a big deal if the body is in a state of sympathetic dominance for a few days, but when it's for a few years, it's a big problem.

Frequently, the onset of people's symptoms occurs when some major stressor in their lives finally gets removed. It's amazing how many people get sick when they go on vacation. So I teach my patients the importance of strengthening and stimulating the parasympathetic nervous system (which is opposite to the "fight or flight" system and is what gets stimulated during relaxation and meditation). This in turn strengthens and stimulates the digestive and immune systems.

We use specific mental healing exercises to accomplish parasympathetic dominance in our patients, including CDs that use different sound technologies to synchronize and stimulate neural development in the two hemispheres of the brain. The left side of the brain in most people is scientific and analytical, and the right side is artistic; it's the side that looks at the sunset and smells the flowers.

In our daily lives, rarely do we activate both hemispheres simultaneously, but whenever we do, the parasympathetic system gets strongly activated. One of the things that we use to activate the parasympathetic branch of the autonomic nervous system is a CD called *Insight*. It uses sound technology to coordinate communication between both sides of the brain. It does this by causing both hemispheres to vibrate simultaneously and at the same frequency. This ultimately brings patients into a state where optimal healing can take place.

Getting to subconscious lies that can block healing is also important. I often have discussions with my patients about the circumstances of their pasts, because it gives me insights into their diagnoses. For example, I might ask them what their childhood and relationship with their parents was like, because the answers to this question can provide me with important information about their self-image and what might be blocking their healing. I find that the most common belief associated with a poor self-image, and which blocks healing, is that people aren't worthy to heal. And if they don't feel worthy of wellness, then they won't heal.

We then use Psych-K to de-program those harmful beliefs from the mind and re-program healthier ones into it. This is accomplished through the use of affirmations, body postures, and muscle testing. First, we develop affirmations for our patients to recite, which serve to replace the lies that they believe. Then we put them into a certain posture (crossing their hands and legs, for instance), according to kinesiology techniques (muscle testing). We want to find out what the most empowering position is for them to be in, then we ask them to start repeating the affirmations for two or three minutes. Then we retest them, and nine times out of ten, we find that their harmful subconscious beliefs have been reversed. The patient's specific posture, combined with the affirmations are what re-program the subconscious mind. People use body language to communicate subconsciously with other people, and when used with affirmations, it can also be a useful tool for communicating with the deepest part of ourselves.

Most of the people that I test are astonished when they discover that their subconscious minds are telling their bodies that they don't want to heal. "What do you mean I don't want to heal? Of course I do!" they will say. And I will tell them, "Well you do, but your subconscious doesn't."

I find that if my patients can work for awhile synchronizing the hemispheres of their brains with an *Insight CD* or something similar, followed by Psych-K, then even those who haven't been responding well to treatments seem to turn around.

The other tool that we use for emotional healing is called Heart Math, which is a biofeedback tool. A recent issue of the medical journal "Alternative Therapies," discusses the benefits of putting the body into a state of what is called "coherence," which is what Heart Math does. Coherence, on a very basic level, refers to order, harmony, and stability in the body's physiology. Researchers are finding that the heart is much more than just a pump; it releases various neurotransmitters, and sends impulses to the brain to direct its thought activities. So the old Egyptian idea that the brain is really in the heart wasn't so crazy, after all.

Sometimes, when nurses take their patients' pulses and measure their heart rate for 60 seconds, the number that they get (called the pulse rate) can be misleading. In reality, heart rate varies from beat to beat, and if the body is in a state of incoherence, it varies radically; it's up and down and all over the place, especially if the person is in a state of sympathetic (or "fight or flight") dominance. When the body is put into a state of coherence, the parasympathetic system becomes dominant and heart function normalizes. In coherence, the heart's beats are of the same strength, and its rhythm is steady. Also, endorphins get released from the brain, which is important, because endorphins stimulate the immune system. A whole cascade of beneficial effects results from putting the body into state of coherence, or parasympathetic dominance.

In Heart Math therapy, patients focus on a series of flashing lights and control their respiration as a meter measures their pulse rate. As they do this, they picture themselves breathing through the heart, as they project thoughts of love and compassion and all that is associated with positive emotion, into it. As a result, their hearts flip into coherence and they are put into a state whereby they are able to start eliciting their subconscious minds as an ally.

I think that addressing the trauma in the subconscious mind is an important area of healing that's being missed in medicine and cancer treatments today. Of course, psychologists deal with it, but they want people to go back and relive all of the traumas in their lives, and I don't know how helpful that really is. In addition to that, they only deal with the mind. I believe that the best healing comes from addressing the body (with physical treatments) as well as the mind (with non-physical treatments).

So these three things: Heart Math, Psych-K, and the *Insight CD* are what we use to address our patients' healing on a mind-body level.

In addition to these therapies, we also do a variety of biochemical treatments to treat our patients' cancers. There is a time and place for everything from pharmaceutical medication to herbs and foot baths, and only fully trained doctors of integrative medicine can understand what remedies to give their patients, how much, and when. Also, the only way that physicians can practice true integrative medicine is by receiving a lot of training and experience in both conventional and alternative medicine so that they can decide which therapeutics to apply to their patients. At Reno Integrative Medical Center, we have accomplished such training.

Cancer Treatment Approach

My primary treatment approach has six components, which are discussed in the following sections.

CHAPTER 8: Robert Eslinger, DO, HMD

Boosting Immune Function

The first of the treatment components involves boosting my patients' immune system function with IV vitamins and mineral formulas, along with oral supplements. These formulas were developed by Doug Brodie, MD, who owned Reno Integrative Medical Center for thirty years. I worked with him for two years before he passed away. He worked here until the day he died, at age 80.

One oral product that we use is an extract of thirteen different medicinal mushrooms called "My Community-Host Defense" by Fungi Perfecti, which has been proven to boost the body's T-cell counts. T-cells are lymphocytes which are made in the thymus gland. T-cells can become what are called NK (natural killer) cells, which kill cancer cells. We also use resveratrol, oral Vitamin C, and a vitamin formula that Dr. Brodie developed called Chela-Vite, which is a potent multi-vitamin and mineral supplement.

I also use a specific line of homeopathic remedies; bacterial and fungal extracts, to positively alter the body's "terrain," or internal environment. This is important because the status of the body's terrain determines what grows in that terrain. As an analogy, if you pull all of the weeds in your garden to plant marigolds, and you load up your garden with marigold food, you create an optimal environment for marigolds to flourish. And if you plant them right, within a year or two, you will see marigolds, not weeds. A similar thing happens with the body; if you get rid of its weeds, and give it the proper food, it will heal. The homeopathic remedies that we recommend alter the body's terrain so that its organisms become more in balance with one another and with the body itself.

According to microbiologists, we have more microbes in our bodies than normal cells. We are literally walking communities of organisms. My wife doesn't like it when I jokingly say that we are "walking compost heaps." We shouldn't necessarily try to kill off all of these organisms, though, which is Western medicine's approach to healing. The western medical model basically teaches that the body is sterile inside, unless you have an infection—but nothing could be further from the truth. So rather than kill the organisms, a better approach would be to balance them in the body.

It's good for people to maintain a humble, open attitude about new knowledge, because there's so much more out there besides what we know, and we (in the medical community) are probably in kindergarten when it comes to our knowledge about healing.

Bio-Oxidative Therapies

The second component of my treatment approach involves giving patients bio-oxidative therapies, which oxygenate the body to higher than normal levels. Otto Warburg, a Nobel Prize-winning PhD and MD, discovered in the 1930s that cancer cells of all types use anaerobic metabolism to produce energy, which means that they thrive in low-level oxygen environments. In fact, oxygen is toxic to them. Normal cells have enzymes that help them to handle oxidative stress, but cancer cells don't, which is why bio-oxidative therapies can weaken or kill them.

So we do bio-oxidative treatments using different combinations of substances such as ozone and intravenous pharmaceutical grade hydrogen peroxide. For one treatment, we combine ozone with UBI (ultraviolet blood irradiation) or bio-photonic therapy, which is discussed later in this chapter.

Intravenous Vitamin C

Next, we give our patients high doses of intravenous Vitamin C, which we administer in conjunction with bio-oxidative therapies. Biochemists have proven that while Vitamin C is an antioxidant, at doses much above ten grams, it actually becomes an oxidative therapy that kills cancer cells. So we may give 75 grams (or 75,000 mg) of Vitamin C in an IV, over the course of two hours, along with the bio-oxidative therapies.

CHAPTER 8: Robert Eslinger, DO, HMD

Laetrile

The fourth component of my treatment plan involves administering laetrile, which is a naturally cytotoxic (cancer-killing) substance made from apricot pits. Dr. Brodie was involved in the "laetrile wars" which took place in the 1940s in California. During these so-called wars, medical boards would go after doctors who were using laetrile to treat their patients—because God forbid you should use a natural substance to treat people! The government actually burned the bitter almond trees in California which contained the highest concentrations of laetrile. Laetrile has a cyanide molecule in it, and the FDA claimed that it was necessary to destroy the almond trees, because cyanide is dangerous.

The fact is, though, many products contain cyanide, including some foods and medicines. It's most prevalent in a type of Vitamin B-12 called cyanocobalamin. The "cyano" part of this word refers to cyanide, but because the cyanide is bound up chemically in the vitamin, it's really harmless. As it turns out, the same thing is true of laetrile; there's a cyanide molecule that's bound up within the substance, but it's totally safe. Interestingly enough, though, by nature or God's grace, there's an enzyme that's found only inside of cancer cells, which cleaves off the cyanide molecule in laetrile. Because free cyanide is deadly poison, this means that laetrile only releases deadly poison inside of cancer cells.

Dr. Brodie was involved in the original work with laetrile, and found it to be effective, so we continue to use it on all of our patients. Doctors have been taught that laetrile is ineffective for treating cancer, but there's a lot of brainwashing that goes into doctors' training. I went through that same training myself, but somehow, I ended up thinking that we were missing something.

Insulin Potentiation Therapy

Insulin Potentiation Therapy (IPT) comprises the fifth element of our treatment approach. This therapy is also based on Otto Warburg's work, which was developed 100 years ago in Mexico, when insulin first became understood in medical science. In IPT, we first drop our patients' blood sugar levels with an intravenous dose of pharmaceutical grade insulin: the same type diabetics use, as we closely monitor their blood sugar levels. A low-normal blood sugar level is 65, but in IPT, we shoot for the mid 30s. It's commonly said that cancer loves sugar. Well, it doesn't love sugar; it requires it, more so than normal cells because of its anaerobic metabolism. In comparison to normal cells, cancer cells are like a car that gets fewer miles per gallon.

When the body's blood sugar levels are extremely low, cancer cells start starving, so they open up their cell membranes in order to grab any sugar molecules that might be in the bloodstream. At that point, we give our patients an intravenous dose of sugar, along with multiple cancer-killing compounds (including chemo drugs at one-tenth of a full dose). These agents are mixed with the sugar in a syringe, so that when the mix goes into the patient, the cancer cells suck up both the sugar and the cancer-killing agents, at a much higher concentration than they would had the patient been given normal chemotherapy. Following the IPT treatments, we give our patients IV and oral sugars to bring their blood sugar levels back to normal again.

There are some negative perspectives about IPT on the Internet. People claim, for instance, that it's dangerous to lower the body's blood sugar levels. I want to say to them, "Oh really? Dangerous compared to what? Chemotherapy? Crossing the street? Well, only if you don't know what you're doing." The majority of people who have put such reviews on the Internet have never received training in, or done, an IPT treatment. In our office, we have done over 7,500 IPT treatments since 2003, and we have never lost a single patient to this type of treatment. I challenge any conventional chemotherapy program in the country to be able to make that claim about its chemotherapy drugs.

The IPT approach uses standard chemotherapy drugs, at only one-tenth the dose of what would be used in a traditional chemotherapy regimen. When used in an IPT format, I've seen chemotherapy drugs help many people, without them suffering the typical side effects of traditional chemotherapy. They don't lose their hair, throw up, get diarrhea, and so forth. So it's still much safer than regular chemotherapy. That said, while we sometimes use chemotherapy drugs for IPT, we prefer to use combinations of natural agents such as cesium, laetrile, mistletoe, and DMSO for the IPT IV.

The mistletoe extract that we use in the IVs comes from Germany (which is far ahead of the United States in its approaches to natural healing) and has a potent anti-cancer effect. (I previously discussed laetrile, which we give our patients both intravenously and orally). We also put DMSO in their IVs, which is a solvent that enhances the cancer cell's absorption of these other cytotoxic compounds, thereby making them more effective.

Finally, every cancer patient that I have ever seen has a very acidic body, because tumors crank out acids. On an intracellular level, tumors don't like alkaline environments. So we use cesium chloride as part of our cancer-killing treatment regimens, because it creates an alkaline environment in the body that's toxic to cancer cells. Cesium chloride is one of the most alkalizing minerals found in nature.

MEAD Analysis and Balancing the Body's Meridians

The last component of our approach involves doing a MEAD analysis (MEAD stands for Meridian Energy Analysis Device). This device measures patients' energy levels in all of their acupuncture meridians and then re-balances the energy in those meridians. Nearly 80 percent of all hospitals in China use the MEAD on all of their incoming patients.

After measuring patients' energy levels with the MEAD, we do electro-acupuncture treatments to balance their energy, using electrodes and a TENS (transdermal electrical nerve stimulator) unit—rather than needles—to pump energy into the meridians that need electricity. The human body is comprised of energy, and these treatments raise its voltage, which in turn increases its immune function and cancer-fighting ability.

Other Adjunct Treatments

Ultraviolet Blood Irradiation or Biophotonic Therapy

Ultraviolet blood treatment involves extracting the patient's blood into a chamber and irradiating it so that the bacteria and viruses within it get altered or destroyed. The blood is then put back into the patient's body, and as a result, a vaccination-like effect is created in the body against these organisms. The freshly irradiated blood also provokes an immune system reaction that destroys most or all of the other pathological bacteria and viruses in the body.

The treatment functions by stimulating the red blood cells to emit a kind of light called biophotons. Biophotons destroy viruses, bacteria, and (in autoimmune diseases) activated white blood cells. In autoimmune disorders, it appears that metabolically active T-cells and other immune cells absorb much greater numbers of biophotons than ordinary immune and other types of cells. This has the effect of destroying them and slowing or stopping the autoimmune problem, because it is hyper-metabolic, or over-active T-cells, that cause autoimmune disorders.

The practice of ultraviolet blood irradiation (UBI) therapy began in the 1920s (in the United States), when a UBI device was developed for extracorporeal (outside the body) treatment of the blood. By the 1940s, UBI was being used to treat bacterial, viral, and autoimmune diseases, but in the 1950s, enthusiasm over the development of new antibiotics and vaccines caused UBI to be put on the shelf by the medical authorities, even though for certain conditions such as hepatitis, herpes, and viral pneumonia, its effects were demonstrably superior to those of drugs.

The development of multi-drug resistance to antibiotics in recent years and the search for less toxic therapies have led to a renewed interest in UBI therapy. By now, thousands or millions of patients have been successfully treated with UBI and scores of clinical trials have been conducted in Russia, Ukraine, and the former East Germany. UBI is also currently being used by some physicians in China and the United States.

UBI therapy is effective against many disorders. American medical science has made a significant mistake by ignoring years of documentation (which have included several controlled studies) which demonstrate the beneficial effects that UBI treatment has had on hundreds of thousands of patients and which has been used by reputable physicians since 1928. It's especially hard to justify this oversight, given the fact that the scientific community has been intensively seeking to identify promising new approaches to HIV treatment and related viral conditions, many of which can be effectively treated with UBI.

In addition to killing pathogens, UBI treatments inactivate toxins, increase oxygen transportation to organs, activate steroid hormones and white blood cells, dilate blood vessels, stimulate cellular and humoral immunity and fibrinolysis, decrease blood viscosity, improve microcirculation, and decrease platelet aggregation.

UBI has been successfully used to treat viral and bacterial pneumonia, polio, botulism, non-healing wounds, herpes, encephalitis, peritonitis, asthma, hepatitis, chronic fatigue, fibromyalgia, rheumatoid arthritis, and many other infectious, inflammatory, and autoimmune disorders, along with cancer.

UBI is beneficial to cancer patients not only because it increases oxygen to the tissues, but also because it strengthens and balances the immune system and is toxic to cancer cells. So far, the FDA has approved the principle that ultraviolet treatment of the blood can convey therapeutic benefit to patients. This is an important statement, as this governmental agency is usually hostile towards all therapies that aren't considered to be mainstream.

Revici Remedies

Another line of remedies which we give our cancer patients are specific selenium formulations based on the work of Emanuel Revici, MD, a New York doctor who passed away in 1998. Selenium is a beneficial micronutrient trace metal which, when taken in tiny amounts, is healthy, but when taken in large amounts, is poisonous. Dr. Revici found a way to encase the selenium molecule in lipids, or fat, in such a way that the selenium wouldn't get dissolved in the blood. He also found that specific lipids or fats concentrated in different tumors, so being the very biochemically-minded doctor that he was, he developed lipid envelopes around selenium molecules and gave these to his patients. These molecules would then selectively dissolve inside of their cancer tumors. So the treatment mechanism of selenium is similar to that of laetrile. A healthy dose of selenium is around 200 mcg (micrograms), but by encasing the mineral in certain fats, Dr. Revici was able to use it therapeutically in doses of as high as ten grams, which he administered to his patients intravenously. Although ten grams of selenium is high, his patients didn't die of selenium poisoning, but the selenium successfully dissolved their tumors.

This New York City doctor, originally from Romania, made house calls to patients in Manhattan until he was 100 years old. Every night, he would eat dinner and then go into his research lab, where he would work for most of the night. He slept three hours per night, on average. He ran his own hospital, and had so many grateful patients that they purchased the hospital and asked him to be its director. He developed a whole line of remedies to treat cancer and other conditions, most notably drug and alcohol addictions. He worked "outside the box," and ran afoul of the American Medical Association, so they blacklisted him. He had to operate under the radar, so to speak, but he still managed to keep his own hospital in New York City. The medical authorities tried to take his license away but failed. It would take hours and many pages to explain all the details of his amazing treatments. I'm working on incorporating Dr. Revici's work into mine, and am also now working with his niece, who is a biochemist in New York who runs his clinic and provides me with certain remedies for my practice.

Poly-MVA

Poly-MVA is a new supplement in the fight against cancer that we have been using at our clinic. It's a patented combination of palladium (a mineral) and alpha-lipoic acid. It also contains a combination of vitamins, minerals, and amino acids. It promotes energy production and potent antioxidant protection at the cellular level. When palladium is sequestered in alpha-lipoic acid, it's beneficial to healthy cells, but toxic to cancer cells.

Heavy Metal Chelation

We also do heavy metal testing and chelation therapies. Ninety-nine percent of all people have some heavy metal toxicity in their bodies, and these metals interfere with their immune function in one way or another.

As one treatment for heavy metal toxicity, we give our patients cracked cell chlorella to take at home, which binds metals in the bowel and gets them out of the body. Cracked cell chlorella is a type of fresh water blue-green algae. We do both IV and oral heavy metal chelation treatments at our clinic but we usually don't start these until after our patients have completed an aggressive cancer therapy protocol because these, in and of themselves, are intensive and all-consuming protocols.

Detoxification

Another important aspect of our cancer treatment involves enhancing our patients' drainage systems (or detoxification pathways) with homeopathic and herbal preparations. One that we use is a German herbal formula called Lymphonest, in addition to homeopathic remedies by Pekana, which assist with the drainage toxins through the detoxification organs. Pekana has remedies for liver, kidney, and lymphatic drainage, as well as others.

Additionally, we use a Chi machine, which also helps with detoxification. For this therapy, patients lie on the floor and place their feet into grooves on a machine. The machine then swings their feet back and forth for fifteen minutes, creating a wave-like motion which reverberates throughout the entire body and enhances lymphatic drainage. I also recommend that they purchase a mini-trampoline, because rebounding on a trampoline is the best exercise there is for stimulating lymphatic drainage, and it only costs $30-50. Just bouncing up and down on it, for five to ten minutes, enhances lymphatic circulation.

We also have a far infrared dome, which patients can climb into and sweat out toxins. Additionally, we recommend far infrared saunas, as well as steam or hot baths because sweat glands are like miniature kidneys that help the body to unload toxins. We encourage our patients to load up on good healthy liquids (water, especially), and do sweat-inducing detoxification therapies, two or three times per week.

We also encourage them to have regular bowel movements. If they are on strong pain medications, then their bowels sometimes become sluggish and they get constipated. This causes them to retain toxins which then need to be cleaned out. So we have specific remedies which we recommend for constipation.

Finally, we do standard lab tests to monitor our patients' organ function. I use several different herbal formulas to restore the functioning of the organs.

Earthing or Grounding Therapy

This ancient therapy, which has recently gained new attention, involves connecting the patient to the earth through various techniques of "grounding." By transferring electrons to the body, the earth balances its electrical system and thereby neutralizes inflammatory and dysfunctional cellular processes. Walking barefoot on the earth is the simplest way to experience the benefits of this therapy, which have been proven in several studies. Most notably,

Earthing decreases inflammation and improves immune system function, which is important for beating cancer.

Dietary Recommendations

Most people in the USA eat the SAD (Standard American Diet), which is comprised of too much animal protein, fats of the wrong kind, and too much sugar.

Until recently, we didn't provide our cancer patients with many specific dietary recommendations. However, we have always advocated a diet that includes a small, measured amount of clean, (i.e. organic) animal protein and lower amounts of carbohydrates. We now also recommend a protocol called CAAT (Controlled Amino Acid Therapy), which was developed over 40 years ago by a molecular biologist and cancer researcher named A.P. John, Sr. It involves following a very specific high protein, low carbohydrate diet, and taking a certain amino acid formula that has been proven to shut off cancer cell energy production and reproduction. It's a very exciting addition to our existing treatment plans.

Treatment Duration

We usually start our patients on what we call the "intensive" protocol, which was originally developed by Dr. Brodie. For this protocol, patients receive intravenous treatments five days a week, for three to six weeks, depending upon the severity of their diseases. They also take a variety of oral supplements. Every protocol is different though, and depends upon patients' condition, how they respond to treatments and what their lab test results are. Sometimes, we will have them stay here for an extra week or two.

After this, we monitor them on a weekly basis while they continue to get lab tests done with their primary care doctors. We generally recommend that they continue to come to our clinic three days a month, for an additional three months, during which time we also continue to do tests and IVs and monitor their progress. Then, if they are feeling well and improving, we may have them come in for a total of three days every other month, until we get a CAT or PET scan which shows that their cancers are completely gone. Then, (following the example of Dr. Brodie), I recommend that they come back to the clinic for two or three days, every six months or once a year, to get a tune-up, retested, and to receive IV treatments. They continue on oral supplements in the interim. Dr. Brodie felt that cancer was like a degenerative disease and that once patients were diagnosed with it, they would have to forever pay attention to it, whatever the length of their lives. So even if their tumors were to disappear, they would still have to pay attention to their diet, mental status, and life stressors, while continuing to take supplements. In reality, though, everybody should pay attention to these things.

Treatment Outcomes

Providing information on treatment outcomes is difficult. When most people with cancer come to us, they are already at death's door, and have already had chemotherapy and radiation treatments, so getting them into remission can be difficult. We have the best outcomes with patients who are "treatment virgins" who haven't had their immune systems destroyed by chemotherapy and radiation. Also, there's a time and place for surgery, but it's far less than what conventional oncologists would have their patients believe. Admittedly, I almost gag when I see these "race for the cure" campaigns to raise money for cancer research. I want to tell people, "Don't you realize where all that fundraiser money goes? It's for pharmaceutical companies that only want to make money— they aren't interested in developing remedies that cure people!"

We gauge treatment success according to three factors: increased length of life, improved quality of life, and of course, tumor remission. Yes, everyone wants their tumors to go away, but sometimes, people can live for years and enjoy a decent quality of life, while still having a tumor. So overall, we get very positive results within the confines of the three above-mentioned criteria, roughly 50-60 percent of the time. I wish that it was 100 percent, but we are working towards increasing that percentile. If we consider only total tumor remission, in which the tumor completely disappears, our success rate is approximately 20-30 percent.

There's a reference on our website about a study that was done in 2004 on full-dose chemotherapy, which was published in the Journal of Clinical Oncology. From 1990-2004, over 150,000 people with all types of cancer were studied, and it was found that only 2.1 percent of them were still alive after five years. All had done full dose chemotherapy. Another study revealed that roughly 30 percent of people who receive full dose chemotherapy die from their treatments, not their tumors. This is something oncologists don't ever tell their patients.

In my practice, we sometimes define increased length of life as patients surviving two years when their oncologists told them they would survive two months. I think it's criminal for doctors to tell their patients that they have only three months to live, anyway, because of the power that this suggestion brings to the subconscious mind. Sometimes, when patients come to see me, by the grace of God or our work here at the clinic, their tumors go away after they have been given a terminal diagnosis. And a year later, they will go to their oncologists, who are astonished that they are still alive, and they will say to them, "Do you want to know what helped me?" and their oncologists will often say, "No, don't tell me. Leave the office."

I have been doing IPT for seven years, and I see people who are still alive since the time that I started doing this. Sometimes, people die of other causes, too, such as heart attacks. Also, the general success terms that I describe here reflect our outcomes prior to doing Psych-K work. I believe that our survival statistics have probably increased since starting Psych-K.

There are those for whom our treatments don't work well, and in some cases, I think it's because subconsciously these people want to die. Some choose to use their cancer tumors as a way to leave a bad relationship, for example. There are all kinds of psychological issues going on in people that heretofore medicine hasn't examined in the least, which I think have a lot of bearing upon their diseases, and not just their cancers. When people come here, I tell them that if they think they will be cured as a result of getting a needle plugged into them, then they need to leave and go somewhere else, because healing is a co-participatory process, involving both the patient and practitioner. I tell them that they will get treatment homework, and that they will be graded on their homework. They have to participate in their treatments, or else those treatments will have a far lesser chance of working. People can survive for years and years with a tumor if they live well and do their homework. There is a difference between dying of cancer and dying with cancer.

Roadblocks/Challenges to Healing

It's amazing to me how I can explain all of what I just shared in this chapter to my patients, and they still won't follow my advice. I think this is self-sabotaging behavior; evidence that they don't really want to heal. The patients that tend to get well are those that are enthusiastic and do all that I ask of them, and follow all of their treatment guidelines. When I tell them to jump they say, "How high?" This is my greatest challenge as a practitioner: getting patients to understand how important it is for them to participate in their healing process.

How Family and Friends Can Support Their Loved Ones with Cancer

Family and friends can help their loved ones with cancer adhere to their treatment regimens, diet and mental exercises. They can help support them emotionally, and help them find reasons for wanting to heal. If a husband thinks that it's a nuisance to come to Reno and hang out here while his wife gets treatment, then his attitude won't help her to get better.

Risky Treatment Approaches

I don't believe that it's possible to cure cancer by just taking supplements. Some people would like to do this. There are different therapies which people with cancer can do at home but it's better for them to do them under a physician's supervision. Of course, there are therapies like the *Insight CD*, which anyone can order and use without a doctor's help. People can order natural remedies like laetrile and cesium over the Internet, maintain a good, clean, nutritious diet, and take good, quality supplements on their own. In general, though, following a doctor's protocol in a clinic, along with doing the aforementioned things, is the best approach to treatment.

Dangerous/Ineffective Treatments

Full-dose chemotherapy is by far the most dangerous type of cancer treatment.

Final Words

The most important thing that I would say to people who are seeking out cancer treatments is, "Don't just swallow everything that your oncologist tells you!" One of the biggest roadblocks to healing is people not being able to make the leap into thinking, "There must be a better way," when nobody tells them that there's a better way. There's a lot of information on the Internet. I would also say, "Don't be afraid to do the research, and don't be just another sheep going into the chemo kitchen."

Contact Information
Robert Eslinger, DO, HMD

Reno Integrative Medical Center
6110 Plumas St. Ste. B
Reno, Nevada 89519
Tel: (775) 829-1009
(800) 994-1009
Fax: (775) 829-9330
www.renointegrativemedicalcenter.com

•CHAPTER 9•

Hufeland Klinik and Nina Reis, MD
BAD MERGENTHEIM, GERMANY

Biography

Hufeland Klinik (Clinic), a small family practice, was founded by Wolfgang Woeppel, MD, and his wife Gabriele in 1985, and is still run as such today. Dr. Woeppel worked closely with Joseph Issels, MD, a German oncologist famous for his immunological approach to the treatment of cancer. In 1951, Dr. Issels was the first person to open a hospital in Germany for conventionally incurable cancer patients which specialized in comprehensive immunotherapy. A world-renowned pioneer of integrative medicine, Dr. Issels was also the first physician to integrate conventional and alternative/complementary treatments into a comprehensive treatment program. He became internationally known for his successful treatment outcomes.

Since Dr. Woeppel's death in July 2006, Gabriele Woeppel and her daughters have run Hufeland Klinik. Hufeland employs four doctors, eight nurses, three massage therapists, a psychologist, and an art therapist, as well as other health care practitioners, who all work together as a team to provide their patients with the best individualized care. They consider each patient to be unique, and seek to combine treatment methods in both conventional and biological medicine to formulate protocols that are best suited to the individual patient. (Note: German biological medicine is a field which integrates modern medical science with traditional European natural medicine and homeopathy. It also integrates philosophies from Traditional Chinese medicine and Ayurvedic medicine into its disciplines).

Nina Reis, MD, is Hufeland Klinik's senior physician. She was born in 1957 in Kytmanowo (Russia), and earned her medical degree (MD) in 1980 from the University of Altaisk in Russia, where she specialized in pediatrics and surgery. In 1999, she moved to Bad Mergentheim, Germany, with her two children. During 2000-2004, she worked in the areas of internal medicine and surgery at the Caritas hospital in Bad Mergentheim. In February, 2004, she met Wolfgang Woeppel, MD. Dr. Reis was impressed with Dr. Woeppel's way of thinking and his successful results with cancer patients, the likes of which she hadn't seen before in conventional oncology. Because she believes that healing is a holistic process and appreciated Dr. Woeppel's treatment methods, she started working with him at Hufeland Klinik in 2004.

What Cancer Is and What Causes It

We see cancer, like most chronic diseases, as the result of disharmony in the body. Its causes are multi-factorial, so the treatment approach at our clinic involves bringing the body back into balance again. Dr. Woeppel, the founder of Hufeland Klinik, believed that chronic and (especially) malignant diseases occur when the metabolism and natural resistance of an organism are negatively altered by various "causal factors." These causal factors may happen either in the womb or after birth, and include things like genetic abnormalities, microbes, dental and tonsillar foci, abnormal intestinal flora, poor diet, physical and chemical influences in the environment, and other possible factors.

These factors cause complex disorders and weaken the body's defense mechanisms, organs and systems, and especially the immune system, which is responsible for protection against disease.

In the presence of these causal factors, the body is weakened and cancer cells are able to develop easily, like seeds in well-prepared soil. Since they aren't met with any resistance, they quickly form tumors that spread out, metastasize, and further weaken the body. Therefore, cancer is simply the outward symptom of an ongoing, serious, generalized chronic disease that has already been present in the body for years. Dr. Woeppel often said, "The tumor is not the disease." So when a surgeon removes a cancer tumor, he has only eliminated one symptom of the patient's disease; he hasn't cured that patient. Whenever patients have had malignant tumors totally removed, they are at an increased risk for developing new tumors or metastases, and should therefore consider immunobiological treatments to prevent this from happening.

Cancer isn't just about the disorder of a single organ, but is instead always about the expression of a comprehensive disorder of the whole person's body and soul. Therefore, holistic therapy must address the individual causes which led to cancer in the first place.

Our Holistic Approach to Healing

Holistic therapy stimulates and supports the body's self-healing powers. Our clinic's main aim is to discover the best treatment strategy for each one of our patients and then convey that strategy to them. In this process, we strive to integrate conventional medicine with holistic, biological medicine, in order to discover which proven methods of treatment to apply to each patient.

The so-called "spontaneous remissions" that happen in some people seem to indicate that the body's natural healing power is able to cure even fatal diseases, and that holistic therapy is worthwhile, even for people with advanced cancers. So our biological immunotherapy treatments are suitable for malignant diseases (including brain tumors, M. Hodgkin's and non-Hodgkin's lymphomas), even if patients have metastases and have been diagnosed by conventional medicine as incurable. Our treatments still offer them a chance at wellness. For cases of severe illness, we combine our natural biological treatments with mild conventional treatments because the combination of both can provide better results than if one or the other type of treatment is used alone. Otherwise, our treatments are predominantly biological (natural) and are designed to rebuild the body's immune system. They are based on Dr. Josef Issels' work.

Treatment Protocol

Our treatment protocol consists of the following:

1. **Basic biological treatments to detoxify and regenerate the body.** These involve stimulating the detoxification functions of the liver, kidneys, skin, and mucosa (mucosa is the moist tissue that lines some organs and body cavities throughout the body, including the digestive tract, lungs, nose and mouth) with homeopathic and herbal medicines. It also involves supplying the body with vitamins and minerals, especially intravenous infusions of high doses of Vitamin C and B-vitamins, selenium, magnesium, potassium, and trace minerals; providing enzymes to the body and controlling symbiosis, or the interactions of different organisms within the body. It includes ozone therapy (which is given twice a week), oxygen multi-step therapy, and colon hydrotherapy, as well as various physical therapies like hydrotherapy, permanent shower, lymphatic drainage, reflex zone therapy, cupping massage, and auto-hormone therapy. Some of these therapies are discussed in greater detail in the following sections. We recommend that our patients extract their root canals and other infected/problematic teeth before beginning these biological treatments.

2. **A special diet that heals the metabolism and increases its healing influence upon the body.** Nutrition at the Hufeland Klinik is predominantly based upon an ovo-lacto-vegetable diet, which basically consists of vegetables, eggs, milk and other dairy products. We recommend dairy products to our patients because they need protein and fat in order to heal. We also recommend high-quality oils such as

olive, flax, and walnut oil. We serve cooked and uncooked vegetables in their natural state. Once a week, we serve meat (lamb, beef, game, chicken, or fish). We limit our patients' meat consumption to once per week because it's difficult for people with cancer to digest meat, so we recommend dairy products instead, as these are a bit easier for the body to digest. Dairy products also cause less acidity in the body than meat. In addition, we recommend that our patients avoid sugar, which means that they should also reduce their fruit consumption, which provides the body with a natural form of sugar. Our meals are freshly prepared without artificial additives.

3. **Immunotherapy to strengthen the body's natural defense mechanisms**. This is done through the use of active fever therapy, passive hyperthermia (moderate whole body hyperthermia and local hyperthermia), thymus peptides and other organ-based products, special serums, biological response modifiers, and mistletoe.

4. **Psychological treatments to strengthen the patient's will to get healthy again.** This aspect of healing is very important. We have different treatments which address the psyche, including: therapeutic dance as a means of experiencing the body, art and clay therapy, yoga, deep relaxation, group hypnosis, visualization techniques, meditation, and intensive talk therapy. Our practitioners attempt to discover and dissolve patients' emotional or mental blocks to healing, which are often present, even when patients aren't aware of them. As a result of these therapies, patients may experience increased freedom in their beliefs and thinking patterns, and regain the courage and willingness to face life again.

5. **Carefully applying conventional treatment and specifically targeting the tumor.** When necessary, we prescribe low-dose chemotherapy, which is often given as Insulin Potentiation Therapy (IPT) or in combination with

moderate whole-body hyperthermia or local hyperthermia. We also use anti-hormone therapies and medications which prevent bone loss (bisphosphonates), prescribe pharmaceutical painkillers, and use conventional methods of diagnosis.

Our therapies don't fight against the body, but instead, harness its healing power. They don't destroy the body, but rebuild it, and in doing so, open up possibilities for healing, even in patients for whom conventional methods would normally be ineffective or even harmful. Following is a more detailed description of some of these therapies.

Immunotherapy

Immunotherapy is a key element of our integrated treatment approach, and involves activating the immune system and increasing the body's resistance to cancer. Successful immunotherapy causes tumors to stop growing or even shrink, and improves the patient's overall sense of wellbeing. It takes a great deal of knowledge and experience to successfully use immunotherapy, as the wrong use of immune stimulants can have the opposite effect upon the immune system and completely block it, thereby opening the floodgates to disease.

At our clinic, we've experienced very positive results activating our patients' immune systems with active fever therapy, moderate whole-body hyperthermia, thymus preparations and other organ-based products, plant extracts, and so-called biological response modifiers. Each of these treatments is applied on an individualized basis, depending upon the patient's level of responsiveness.

We do immune therapies after detoxifying our patients, because it's not always beneficial to stimulate the immune system if the body hasn't been regenerated or is very toxic. So our basic treatment protocol starts with detoxification, and is followed by immune-stimulating therapies.

Thymus Therapy

We also use highly purified thymus peptide extracts, which provide sustained stimulation of the body's hormonal production and immune system. The peptides cause the immune system to produce more immune cells in the bone marrow and train mature immune cells to support an active defense system in the body. This remedy helps to effectively counteract the weakening of the immune system that's caused by cancer, other infections, or conventional therapies such as chemotherapy and radiation.

Local and Moderate Whole Body Hyperthermia

Local hyperthermia involves applying concentrated therapeutic heat to a tumor. Its benefits in medicine are well-known. When heat is applied locally to a tumor, vital nutrients and oxygen are cut off from tumor cells. This results in the collapse of the tumor's vascular system and cancer cell destruction. To accomplish this, we use special electrodes that heat the tumor region of the body. We often combine local hyperthermia with other methods of cancer treatment, such as low-dose chemotherapy, anti-hormone-therapy, or high-dose mistletoe preparations.

Moderate whole body hyperthermia has different effects upon the body than local hyperthermia. We also use this type of hyperthermia at our clinic because it stimulates the immune system, and as such, is especially beneficial for patients who are not able to undergo active fever therapy because they are too weak or old. Whole-body hyperthermia is also used to boost the effects of low-dose chemotherapy. In moderate whole-body hyperthermia, we use special heating beds (called "fever tents") to bring the body's temperature to a minimum of 40 degrees Celsius (or 104 degrees Fahrenheit).

Fever Therapy

Dr. Issels and others have found active fever therapy to be particularly effective for the treatment of cancer, and this has been our experience, as well. We use it mostly to stimulate the immune system and to speed up the body's elimination of toxins. Of all the immune supportive therapies, fever therapy provides the maximum amount of immune stimulation to the body.

Unlike passive hyperthermia, where the body or tumor is heated up from the outside using different devices, active fever therapy doesn't kill tumor cells by raising the temperature of the body. Instead, it triggers a fever and a broad range of immune functions, so that the body can more effectively fight the cancer.

We induce fevers in our patients through the intravenous administration of bacterial lipopolysaccharides. (Lipopolysaccharides (LPS), also known as lipoglycans, are large molecules consisting of a lipid and a polysaccharide. They are found in the outer membrane of Gram-negative bacteria, act as endotoxins, and elicit strong immune responses). This type of treatment must be performed by an experienced doctor because serious complications can arise if the relevant contraindications are ignored.

Permanent Shower Therapy

This is a type of detoxification therapy in which patients lie in a bathtub of warm, continually running water for an hour and a half. The warm water, combined with the length of time in which they sit in the water, causes them to sweat and release toxins through their skin.

Programmed Oxygen Multi-Step Therapy (OMT)

We use Oxygen Multi-Step therapy to improve the supply of oxygen to the body, which can in turn help reduce the rate of metastases or disease recurrence in our patients. It also serves to strengthen their immune systems.

During this therapy, patients inhale oxygen for two hours, then do some form of physical activity for at least thirty minutes. Movement helps the body to absorb oxygen and improves its overall metabolism and immune function. We use oxygen in our cancer treatment protocols because it benefits the body in a multitude of ways. For instance, cancer patients are often anemic, and oxygen helps to heal them from this condition.

Ozone Therapy

In medicine, ozone should only be used in applications where it's proven to be beneficial and doesn't cause damage. Medical ozone is always a mixture of pure oxygen and pure ozone, with the percentage of oxygen always being higher. The ratio is generally 99.5 percent oxygen to only 0.5 percent ozone, depending upon its intended use. Since ozone molecules are unstable, they react immediately with the components in the blood to which they are added, so that pure oxygen is formed, along with other compounds.

Ozone has many positive and scientifically proven beneficial effects upon the body. It activates red blood cell and tissue metabolism as well as immune cells; frees the cytokines (interferons, interleukins etc.) for use by the body, and detoxifies the body by activating its antioxidants and free radical scavengers. Ozone is beneficial for cancer patients because it removes toxins and other harmful substances, including inflammatory mediators that result from cancer, from the body. Also, by optimizing the metabolism and immune system function, it aids the body in its fight against cancer.

Colon Hydrotherapy

Enemas have been used for detoxification for centuries. In the United States, coffee enemas are often used to cleanse the intestines and liver. The caffeine in the coffee increases bile flow, activating the liver so that it releases toxins. American scientists have taken this ancient form of treatment and used it as the basis for modern colon hydrotherapy (COHT), which can now be done hygienically, comfortably, and almost completely odor-free. Patients are able to lie down during treatment, which is one of the reasons why COHT is well-tolerated.

Massage Cupping

Cupping involves creating a partial vacuum inside glass cups, which are then applied to the skin to relieve areas of congestion, which are often referred to as areas of stagnation in Traditional Chinese medicine. By creating suction and negative pressure, Massage Cupping therapy is also used to soften tight muscles and tone attachments (ligaments, tendons and vessels), loosen adhesions and lift connective tissue, hydrate and increase blood flow to the body's tissues, and drain toxins by opening up lymphatic pathways. It also stimulates blood flow through the lungs.

Antioxidants

Antioxidants are substances that protect the body from damage caused by free radicals. Free radicals are aggressive and unstable molecules that result from the body's own metabolic processes, chemicals that have been taken into the body, or radiation. Under certain conditions, such as cancer or excessive exposure to environmental or other toxins, the number of free radicals in the body increases so dramatically that the normal concentration of the body's own antioxidant defenses becomes insufficient. These free radicals can then cause a lot of damage. They destroy cell membranes, genetic material, and important protein molecules in the cells. If this excessively high concentration of free radicals remains constant, a condition known as oxidative stress is created in the body. Oxidative stress plays a role in many illnesses and diseases, including cancer. It weakens the immune system, creates chronic inflammation and allergies, as well as faulty fat and sugar metabolism.

Supplying the body with an optimal amount of antioxidants can prevent oxidative stress, so our patients receive antioxidants as part of their basic treatment protocol. These can be taken orally or given intravenously. Of course, supplementation with vitamins and trace elements can't take the place of a healthy, balanced, whole foods diet, so maintaining a healthy diet is important, too.

The vitamins and trace elements that we use aren't given randomly, but rather, are prescribed in therapeutic doses that are tailored to the individual patient.

Following is some information on Vitamin E, Vitamin D-3, selenium and Vitamin C; four important antioxidants which we often give our cancer patients.

Vitamin E

Vitamin E is a fat-soluble vitamin that's found in high quantities in plant and animal fats, such as sunflower seeds, wheat germ, sunflower oil, nuts, seeds, milk, butter, and margarine. As a natural antioxidant, it stabilizes cell membranes and protects unsaturated fatty acids from oxidation by reacting with free radicals before they can destroy cell structures. Vitamin E also prevents the oxidation of other substances, such as Vitamin A. This is why germ oils with a high concentration of polyunsaturated fatty acids are also rich in Vitamin E. In animal studies, Vitamin E deficiencies have been shown to cause damage to the muscles, heart, nervous system, liver, and reproductive organs. In addition, such deficiencies have been shown to cause the destruction of blood cells, though this phenomenon has not yet been observed in healthy humans. People with chronic diseases, including cancer, need more Vitamin E than the average person.

Vitamin D-3

Vitamin D has many beneficial effects upon the body. Its influence upon calcium metabolism strengthens bones and muscles. It also has positive effects upon the immune system and cellular metabolism, and many studies have shown it to be very helpful for preventing cancer. Therefore, we recommend Vitamin D as part of our cancer prevention and treatment protocol.

Selenium

Selenium is an essential trace element that's an integral part of the enzyme glutathione peroxidase, which is involved in important metabolic processes and helps the body to detoxify by destroying free radicals. Selenium is also important for maintaining an intact immune system. We use selenium in both tablet and intravenous form as an adjunct cancer treatment for our patients, because replenishing the body's stores of selenium strengthens the immune system and prevents the recurrence of tumors. It also effectively reduces the side effects of radiation or chemotherapy, and improves the effectiveness of cytostatic drugs (which inhibit cancer cell growth and multiplication).

Vitamin C

Vitamin C is found in different concentrations in the organs, with the highest amounts being found in the liver, adrenal glands, eye lenses, brain, and immune cells. Vitamin C is involved in a variety of metabolic processes in the body. It's essential for strengthening and activating the immune, hormonal, and nervous systems, for regulating fat metabolism and detoxification, and for the formation and functioning of the bones and connective tissues. Vitamin C is an important antioxidant for the human body. It helps wounds to heal faster, plays a decisive role in inflammatory diseases and helps to counteract the negative effects of radiation exposure.

High-Dose Intravenous Vitamin C Therapy

Much research has been done since the 1990s on the beneficial immune-boosting and cytotoxic (cancer-killing) effects of intravenous Vitamin C. Medline, one of the key medical databanks, shows that there have been around 8,000 publications that have focused on Vitamin C since 1990. These studies have led to the development of high-dose Vitamin C therapy for the treatment of cancer, and increasing numbers of physicians and alternative practitioners have been using it for this purpose with excellent results. In general, IV treatments are useful because the body's need for Vitamin C can be much higher than what it can absorb via the gastrointestinal tract. Additionally, many illnesses, including cancer, reduce the intestinal lining's ability to absorb Vitamin C. As a result, sometimes a therapeutically effective level of Vitamin C can only be achieved through injections or intravenous infusions.

Auto-Hormone Therapy (AHT)

Auto-hormone therapy was developed by Erwin Schliephake, a renowned professor of physical therapy at the University of Wuerzburg, Germany. Schliephake discovered that flooding the brain with short waves (which are a certain type of electrical energy), led to measurable changes of hormone levels in the blood. In 1934, he succeeded in curing a patient of a brain tumor by using "short-wave flooding." His method was later researched and perfected. He describes the method and numerous cases of successful tumor treatment in his book, *Short-Wave Therapy: The Medical Uses of Electrical High Frequencies.*

Treatment involves flooding the vegetative centers of the interbrain with electrical waves, including the hypothalamus and pituitary gland, which are responsible for regulating hormonal balance in the body. This is done using two capacitor places (called "Schiephake electrodes"), which increase blood flow to the brain and warm its tissue. The result is apparent normalization of the endocrine system, which is often impaired by disease. Because the vegetative centers are also closely connected to the immune system, the immune system is also positively affected by AHT.

Other Natural Anti-Cancer Treatments

In addition to thymus, we use spleen and other organ serums to support the body and immune system. We use mistletoe for its cytotoxic (anti-cancer) and immune-supportive effects, as well as a homeopathic remedy called Horvi, which contains extracts made from snakes. These extracts are proteins that function as enzymes within the cancer cell. They support the regeneration of the malfunctioning cell, so that it no longer behaves like a cancer cell, but instead, a normal cell.

Additional Treatments

We do other treatments at our clinic. For instance, we give all of our cancer patients brewer's yeast, which alters tumor metabolism so that tumor cells start behaving more like normal cells. We also have a machine called the HiToP® 182, which is used to treat pain and revitalize the entire body. Other treatments include magnetic field and chromo (color) therapy, hypnotherapy, intestinal cleansing, and various physical therapies.

Conventional Therapies

Conventional treatment methods, such as surgery, chemotherapy, radiation, and hormone therapy, have been improving in recent years. When used in a carefully targeted way, their use is thoroughly justified. It's certainly wrong to reject them as a matter of principle, merely because a patient prefers to be treated with biological or natural medicine. Biological therapy must not be seen as an alternative to conventional therapy, but instead must complement all of the other conceivable and familiar forms of treatment. Conventional treatments must form the basis of any type of cancer therapy protocol, but in the majority of cases, and by itself, they are insufficient to effectively halt tumor growth. At the same time, it's important to note that conventional treatments, particularly chemotherapy, are often overvalued by many orthodox clinicians and administered too frequently when their use is inappropriate.

Conventional treatments are overused because some doctors are poorly educated and over- or underestimate the effects and side effects of treatment. They also display an uncritical acceptance of research study results that have been prematurely published. Furthermore, they lack an understanding of the value of meaningful palliative cancer therapy because they are stuck in the autistic grip of a scientifically-oriented, quantified way of thinking, and also view themselves as the only real healing doctors.

It's extremely important to apply strict diagnostic criteria when using conventional treatment methods and integrate them meaningfully and individually into the therapeutic approach. This obviously requires appropriate experience on the part of the doctor, who must be as knowledgeable about orthodox medicine as biological healing methods. As a rule, all conventional treatments negatively affect the patient's immune system. The worst of these effects is caused by radiation, which is why strict limitations must be placed on its use. On the other hand, we know that low-dose chemotherapy, when administered, for example, in an IPT (Insulin Potentiation Therapy) format, can be effective. In some circumstances, chemotherapy can even help to improve the patient's immune condition, as paradoxical as this may sound.

Treatment Procedure

When patients first come to our clinic, we take their medical history, perform a physical exam and do tests, which may include an echocardiogram, blood tests, ultrasound and lung-function check. We then usually start by giving them intravenous vitamin and detoxification infusions at least twice a week, for about three weeks. The IV's contain high doses of Vitamin C, selenium, B vitamins, magnesium, and potassium. During this time, we also do other therapies, such as ozone and oxygen, and physical therapies like magnetic field, brain light and color therapy; reflexology and electrotherapy.

We also give them injections to stimulate the immune system, which we administer at the same time as their vitamin and mineral IVs. We do hyperthermia and other strong immune-stimulating therapies only after they have received nutrient and detoxification IVs for a few weeks, but we also continue with the nutritional IVs after they start the immune therapies. We don't start them on treatments such as hyperthermia right away, because they usually need to be built up and detoxified first, especially if they have done conventional treatments prior to coming to our clinic. If utilized too early, strong immune-stimulating treatments such as hyperthermia and fever therapy can cause them to release too many toxins at the outset of their treatment program. We also want to support the liver and other detoxification organs, so that the body is better prepared to receive the immune-stimulating treatments. Throughout their entire stay at our clinic, we offer our patients various psychological therapies, such as talk therapy, meditation, art therapy, and yoga, since psychological care is a very important part of a holistic treatment program (this is discussed in further detail below).

Length of Treatment and Maintenance Program

Patients stay at our clinic for approximately six to eight weeks, and are given a maintenance therapy program to do after they leave. After six months to a year, we recommend that they come back for a follow-up treatment/visit with us.

Because our treatments are individualized, our follow-up treatments are different for every patient. We might recommend that one continue doing fever therapy at home with his or her doctor. For another, we might recommend hyperthermia or Vitamin C infusions.

Psychological/Mental Health Treatments

"You take the lead," said the soul to the body, "for 'he' won't listen to me."
"All right," replied the body, "I'll fall ill, then 'he' will have time for you."
—Author unknown

Taking care of our patients' mental and emotional health needs is an important component of our holistic therapy plan, because almost all diseases have mental causes and/or effects behind them, which our patients often don't perceive because they don't pay attention to their souls. At our clinic, we have a psychologist, an art therapist and other practitioners who work to improve our patients' mental health by teaching them yoga, meditation, and relaxation therapies, and by offering them counseling and the opportunity to paint and work with clay. Like our other treatments, our patients don't all do the same therapies. We might recommend painting therapy to one and talk therapy to another, for example. Some of these therapies are described in more detail in the following sections.

Psychotherapy

We know from experience that cancer patients are often isolated because neither relatives nor doctors are willing to talk with them openly about their diseases. It's imperative for us to be honest and open while talking with our patients about what they are going through. Only in this way is it possible for us to provide them with a way of living positively and purposefully with, and in spite of, their diseases. Doing this can also relieve their feelings of isolation.

The cause of our patients' mental stress isn't limited to cancer. It frequently has its origins in their childhoods, marriages, or occupations. Often, their needs and feelings have been inhibited and repressed to the point that their mental states have now become determined not by themselves, but instead by others. As a result, they suffer from depression, feelings of guilt or being overburdened, and despair—all elements of severe mental stress, which are often unconscious, but which have paralyzed their immune systems and caused disease.

Medical doctors like Bernie Siegel, Simonton, and many others, have impressively pointed out the connection between mental disorders and tumor development. Doctors or psychotherapists can only make suggestions to their patients about how to heal these disorders, but it's ultimately up to patients to take those suggestions and use them. Part of psychotherapy involves informing patients about what they need to do to change their lives. Support groups can be a good first contact point for this.

The purpose of mental health therapy isn't to dig up problems. We have arranged our programs in such a way that they provide our patients with simple hints and techniques that they can use which will better enable them to deal with their diseases.

Even if patients are firmly convinced that mental problems don't play a role in their diseases, we invite them to take advantage of the various range of psychotherapeutic treatments that we offer at our clinic, because they might "break new ground" in their thinking, in a way that would end up enriching their lives.

Painting Classes

Another mental health therapy that we offer is painting classes, in which our patients paint pictures and then talk about what they have painted with a therapist. Through their paintings, therapists can discern whether patients have aggression, or are experiencing emotions such as terror or shock, because their emotions are expressed through their art. We can't solve their problems, but we can help to identify them so that they can resolve them. Painting also enables patients to become far more aware and conscious of nature and the outside world. It helps them to rediscover the joy of creating art and using colors, and in doing so, alleviates their stress, helps them to abandon exaggerated pretensions, and overcome inhibitions. Being a mirror of the soul, painting also contributes to self-knowledge. Through it, patients can express their innermost selves, which is healing for the body. Additionally, no previous experience is required to do this kind of therapy. Everybody can do it. Our patients enjoy doing art therapy and are generally very happy when they leave our clinic with a package of paintings that they have created.

Clay Field Therapy

This therapy was founded and developed in 1972 by Professor Heinz Deuser, a German art therapist. Today, it's used in a variety of therapeutic settings. Clay Field Therapy is a powerful tactile medium that can profoundly evoke, structure, and transform a person's life story. All of our life experiences, especially those that involve touching and being touched, are stored in the memory of our hands. By working with clay, patients can retrace how they learned to "grasp" the world, and if they wish, rewrite the script of their relationship with it. As a material, clay also strengthens their relationship with the earth and with themselves. CFT enables them to develop more self-confidence, as it stimulates clarifying and healing processes.

Meditation

In his book, *Love, Medicine and Miracles*, author and physician Bernie Siegel, MD, describes the essence of meditation in a meaningful manner: "Someone once said, 'Praying is talking; meditating is listening.' "

Meditation can indeed help patients to forget the stress and distractions of everyday life, thereby enabling them to perceive other things: their deepest thoughts, emotions, products of their subconscious mind, the peace of pure consciousness, and spiritual concerns. There are many ways of achieving this state of mind. Some meditation teachers recommend concentrating on a symbolic sound or word (mantra) or on a single picture, the flame of a candle or a visual symbol (mandala). Others recommend concentrating on the relaxed flow of the breath or shutting oneself off from thoughts that "flicker" on the surface of the mind. In the end, all methods produce the same effect upon the person: a feeling of deep and peaceful emptiness or of being in a trance, which strengthens the mind that is now free from the usual chaos.

At our clinic, we teach our patients to do different meditation techniques, which they practice individually or in groups.

Visualization Therapy

Finally, we teach our patients how to do visualization therapy, according to a technique that was established by Carl Simonton, MD, an internationally-known oncologist. It's based upon the idea that patients' state of mind can influence their ability to survive cancer.

The technique utilizes the tremendous powers of the mind, and specifically, its faculty for visualization and imagination, to control disease. First, patients are shown what a normal healthy cell looks like and are asked to imagine a battle going on between the cancer cell and the normal cell. Next, they are asked to visualize a concrete image that represents the cancer cell, and then another image of the normal cell. Then they are asked to see the normal cell winning the battle against the cancer cell. The results from Dr. Simonton's techniques have been nothing short of extraordinary and have helped many cancer patients in their recovery.

Treatment Outcomes

We often see stage three and four patients living for many years past their original diagnoses. Many of our patients (about ten percent) follow up with us for years after they finish their treatments. We can't offer statistics regarding patient treatment outcomes, though. No doctor can guarantee that any patient will heal from a severe cancer, and neither can they provide a "success rate" for any type of cancer.

Worldwide, there is no treatment that is guaranteed to cure cancer. For this reason, it's difficult for us to say exactly how our patients will benefit from our biological treatments, but we have healed conventionally incurable cancer patients, or at least enabled them to live for many months or years past their original diagnoses.

Columbia University and other institutions have done studies on our treatment outcomes which hint at their effectiveness in different situations. For example, in a dissertation from the University of Wuerzburg, we examined 133 women with breast cancer who were treated at our clinic from 1985 until December 31, 1989. The results of that study are summarized in the following quotation, which is found on page 70 of the dissertation: "The probability of survival depends, among other things, on the early beginning of an immunobiological treatment...the mean survival of women with metastases and bad risk factors was (from the operation until death): in group I (9 patients) 81.27 months; in group II (25 patients) 53.06 months; in group III (7 patients) 58.33 months, and in group IV (92 patients) 62.33 months" (Note: the Roman numeral of each group indicates the stage of cancer that the women were in. Group IV had 92 women with generalized metastases; 82 of them had very bad prognostic factors, and yet their average survival time was 62.33 months, or just over five years). Thus, the mean length of survival of our patients with generalized metastases was much higher than the statistics that are mentioned in the scientific literature for conventional therapies. It's also important to note that many of the women in this study were still alive after the study was completed on December 31, 1989, so these data must be adjusted in a follow-up study, because some have lived for much longer periods than what is indicated here.

A study performed by the University of Freiburg, in which only patient satisfaction was measured, showed that 75 percent of our patients were very content with the therapies that we had provided them, and believed that we had improved their quality of life. At many worldwide cancer conferences, we have provided reports on many of our patients who were previously diagnosed as incurable, but who instead attained full remission and have remained in remission for many years now due to our biological therapies, which involved no full-dose chemotherapy, radiation, or surgery. These conferences included the World Congress of Spontaneous Remissions, which took place in Heidelberg in 1997, and the International Cancer Congress, which took place in 1998 at Kalithea, as well as several others, in Washington, Philadelphia, and Atlanta. Also, our rate of so-called spontaneous remissions after therapy is much higher here (about 1:600) than what is seen worldwide at most clinics (1:80,000). The results of a scientific evaluation that was done by experts at Columbia University in New York, demonstrates our extraordinary success. The results of that study, called "Cancer Outcomes at the Hufeland (complementary/alternative medicine) Klinik: A Best-Case Series Review" can be found on the Internet at: www.ncbi.nlm.nih.gov/pubmed/15911928.

If we aren't able to heal our patients' cancers with our immunobiological treatments, we can often at least stop their progression and add more years to their lives so that they feel well for a long time.

The success of our therapies doesn't usually depend upon the type of tumor that our patients have, but instead, upon their individual reactions to our immunological treatments, and, most of all, upon their will to get well again. We can't promise success, but if we weren't successful, then patients wouldn't come to our clinic from all over the world.

The first aim of our therapy is to detoxify our patients and to strengthen their bodies' defense mechanisms as well as their overall condition. We are successful about 90 percent of the time in doing this. The second aim of our therapy, and especially in patients who have been diagnosed as incurable, is to stop their tumor growth and then reduce their tumor load. The third aim of our therapy is to prolong and improve their quality of life. We are usually successful at accomplishing all of these things.

Factors That Influence Healing and Roadblocks to Healing

Patients' age, their family history of disease, environmental influences, as well as other diseases that they might have, such as diabetes or thyroid gland problems, can influence their healing. We treat their other problems as well, because many have so-called additional diagnoses like diabetes, and our therapies have a positive effect upon these types of metabolic diseases, as well.

Patients' mental outlook greatly affects their healing. Those who have accepted their diseases do better with their treatments. Those who have worked not only on their bodies, but also their minds, tend to heal better. If patients accept their diseases, and don't fight against their bodies, they tend to have better outcomes. We once had a remarkable patient with melanoma, who would say to his cancer, "If I die, then you die, too!" He would communicate with his tumor, and the tumor ended up disappearing! He had a spontaneous remission. It was a remarkable case.

When patients have allergies or other diseases that make it hard for them to do treatments, this can sometimes block their healing.

Dental problems and infections in the teeth can also compromise recovery, which is why we sometimes recommend that they extract all of their root canals and take care of other infected teeth problems, either before or after their cancer treatments. Also, because we are a private clinic and receive no funding from government or private parties, our patients usually have to pay for their treatments, so financial problems can sometimes be a roadblock to recovery. Our patients from the United States sometimes have health insurance plans that cover their treatments here. They work with the American Medical Health Alliance (AMHA, www.amhabilling.com) which helps them to get reimbursed for treatments through their insurance companies.

The Problem with Conventional Cancer Treatments

The main aim of cancer therapy shouldn't be to kill the cancer but to support the healing power of the body, and most conventional treatments these days are designed to treat the cancer, but they harm the body at the same time.

Nearly all conventional doctors attempt to use drugs to get rid of and defeat the cancer tumor, but we aim to strengthen the body so that it can defeat the cancer itself. Conventional oncologists give strong therapies to cancer patients that harm the organs in which their cancers are found, but these therapies don't end up defeating their cancers. Most of the time, full-dose chemotherapy and radiation aren't appropriate for treating cancer; they are extreme and destroy the body, and don't have the desired effect upon the patient's cancer. As previously mentioned, we do chemotherapy at our clinic, but we administer it in low doses and using different techniques, so that it has beneficial effects upon the cancer but doesn't destroy the body.

Our patients' quality of life is important; it's usually more important than how long they live. If they are living completely damaged and disabled due to harsh treatments, then they have no quality of life anymore. Nowadays, more people are aware of the many treatments that are available in conventional and alternative medicine, but most still take the "normal" (conventional medicine) path. It isn't until conventional medicine doesn't help them anymore that they start doubting it and looking for another way to get better.

Lifestyle Recommendations for Healing

People with cancer should be conscious of every day that they live, and really live life to the fullest, because every day that they are alive is precious. They should change any unhealthy habits they have, such as eating the wrong foods, and sort out what is and what isn't important to them in life.

They should also consider the treatments that they are being offered, and not do anything that destroys their bodies. They should fight their fears and consider the effects that different treatments will have upon them. Of course, when people get diagnosed with cancer, they are terrified, but they should do whatever they can to manage those fears. There's no medication in the whole world that can heal cancer. People must heal themselves. Doctors and treatments can only support the body in its power to heal itself.

How Friends and Family Can Support Their Loved Ones with Cancer

Once patients have decided upon a treatment, their families should support their treatment decisions and not insist that they do more aggressive therapies. Family members should treat them with love and warmth, and help them to feel supported, important, and cared for.

Contact Information
Hufeland Klinik and Nina Reis, MD

Hufeland Clinic for Holistic Immunotherapy
Loeffelstelzer Str. 1-3
D - 97980 Bad Mergentheim (Germany)
Phone: +49 7931/536-0
Fax number: +49-7931-536-333
www.hufeland.com

• CHAPTER 10 •

Julian Kenyon, MD, MB, ChB
LONDON, ENGLAND

Biography

Dr. Julian Kenyon is a physician of integrative medicine and Medical Director of The Dove Clinic for Integrated Medicine, which has locations in Winchester and London, England. He is Founder-Chairman of the British Medical Acupuncture Society, which was established in 1980, and Co-Founder of the Centre for the Study of Complementary Medicine in Southampton and London, where he worked for many years before starting The Dove Clinic in 2000. He is also Founder-President of the British Society for Integrated Medicine and is an established authority in the field of complementary treatment approaches for a wide range of medical conditions.

He graduated from the University of Liverpool with a Bachelor of Medicine and Surgery degree in 1970, and subsequently with a Doctor of Medicine research degree. In 1972, he was appointed a Primary Fellow of the Royal College of Surgeons, Edinburgh. Dr. Kenyon has written approximately twenty books, has had many academic papers published in peer review journals and has been granted several patents. He has a particular interest in immune function and its relationship to the development of life-threatening illnesses and chronic disease in general.

The doctors and nurses who form The Dove Clinic team are committed to a multi-disciplinary and holistic approach to health care, which means giving equal attention to the body, mind, and spirit, in a caring, peaceful, and nurturing environment. Dr. Kenyon's wife, Tanya, works with him at The Dove Clinic. She has many years of experience as a trained nurse, counselor and complementary therapist.

What Cancer Is and What Causes It

Cancer is a wound that doesn't heal. In normal wound healing, a lot of growth processes happen, but these processes stop when the wound is healed. In cancer, the growth processes don't stop, and what results is a tumor that continues to grow unchecked. Environmental factors have possibly played a role in the increased incidence of cancer over the last fifty years, but it depends upon where people live. For example, in China there's a lot of pollution and consequently, an increased incidence of a range of cancers, especially lung cancer.

To some extent, dietary changes are also related to the rapid increase in the occurrences of cancer. In England, the longest-lived population was the mid-Victorian working class (the Victorian period was from 1837-1901). This has been well-studied, and research has established that these people lived longer than we do today. Their cancer incidence was about ten percent of ours, and their cancers were mostly hereditary. The working class Victorians were mostly laborers, and the vats in which they stored their food were high in many different types of polyphenols, which are nutritional constituents of food that have anti-cancer properties. These vats also contained significant amounts of oligosaccharides, which protected the people's guts and in turn, aided in their cell-mediated immune function, which is the body's main defense against cancer. Also, they had large amounts of phytonutrients in their diets, which came from food that they grew themselves.

It's hard to know specifically what factors are causing an increase in the incidence of cancer today. On an immunological level, cancer happens when the body switches from a Th-1 dominant, cell-mediated immune function response, to one in which it produces more antibodies, which is a Th-2 response. When the body produces too much of a Th-2 response, it makes people more susceptible to allergies such as hay fever, and causes their cell-mediated immune function, which the body needs to fight cancer, to be poor. In people with cancer, there has been a movement away from a Th-1 dominated phenotype response to a Th-2 dominated phenotype response. Exposure to mycobacterium early in life can upregulate the body's cell-mediated immune response, so factors such as the environment in which children are raised can determine the strength of their cell-mediated immune response later in life. For example, children who grow up on farms, and who get cuts and scrapes, and are exposed to all types of organisms, tend to have stronger cell-mediated immune responses as adults.

Treatments

My treatment approach to cancer is fundamentally based upon trying to shift the patient's immune system from a predominantly Th-2 response to a Th-1 response. At our clinic, we are heavily involved in cancer immunotherapy, the results of which have allowed some of our patients with metastatic cancers to live for ten years or more.

Sonodynamic and Photodynamic Therapy

The most common, and by far most effective cancer-killing approaches that we use at our clinic are called sonodynamic and photodynamic therapy, both of which have produced very encouraging and positive results in our patients.

Photodynamic therapy involves giving patients light sensitive substances (usually chemical compounds called porphyrins, which are breakdown products from recycled hemoglobin, although chlorophyll derivatives are also used). These substances accumulate preferentially in cancer cells and cause the cells to auto-fluoresce. When the substances are then exposed to light of a certain wavelength, energy is created. This energy is transferred to neighboring oxygen molecules and alters their configuration in such a way that they become an aggressive chemical species that rapidly reacts with any nearby biomolecules; in this case, cancer cells, and destroys them directly or via apoptosis. Tumors tend to be hypoxic (lacking in oxygen), so in some treatment protocols, we also use ozone autohemotherapy, which is a strategy for increasing oxygen at the tumor site. It also enhances the cytotoxic effects of the photodynamic therapy.

Some versions of photodynamic therapy have a very shallow penetration of only one-half centimeter. However, we use a specialized light bed, which patients lie on, to activate the light-sensitive agents. The light bed consists of tens of thousands of light-emitting diodes in the red light and infra-red regions of the electromagnetic spectrum. In comparison with standard photodynamic treatments, these diodes produce energy that penetrates much deeper into the body, allowing us to treat many types of tumors from the surface of the body.

Photodynamic therapy has several advantages over conventional treatments such as surgery and radiotherapy (radiation): It's comparatively non-invasive, can be targeted to the tumor, and repeated doses can be given. It has no total dose limitations, unlike radiation, and the healing process results in little or no scarring. It can always be done on an outpatient basis, and it has no significant side effects.

Sonodynamic therapy is another method by which to activate the above-mentioned light sensitive substances in order to destroy tumors. Sonodynamic therapy is similar to photodynamic therapy, except that the light-sensitive substances are activated by ultrasound rather than by light (the light sensitive agent that we use is also sensitive to ultrasound frequencies). The non-thermal effects of ultrasound also create cavitations in malignant cells, thereby destroying them. The ultrasonic energy utilized by sonodynamic therapy provides deeper penetration into the body than standard photodynamic therapy.

The procedure of sonodynamic therapy is carried out using a simple therapeutic ultrasound machine with a specially-designed treatment head known as a maniple, which is applied over the affected area, along with ultrasound gel.

In our practice, patients usually do photodynamic treatments on the light bed followed by sonodynamic therapy. Sonodynamic photodynamic therapy (SPDT), or the combination of the two therapies, represents a significant advancement over earlier methods of photodynamic therapy. We can now give patients the light-sensitive substances to take orally, whereas previously, we had to administer them intravenously. This is advantageous because giving patients a light-sensitive agent orally (sublingually) allows it to accumulate more slowly at the tumor site, which means that less of that agent gets excreted through the kidneys. When given intravenously, there's an immediate, large peak of the light-sensitive substance(s) in patients' serum (blood) which leads to significantly larger amounts of the substance getting excreted through their kidneys. The agents that we use in sono- and photodynamic therapy accumulate selectively at the tumor sites and don't produce the same photosensitive side effects that occur with standard photodynamic therapy. SPDT is a whole body treatment, and doesn't require the undesirable practice of using lasers on the patient, which are used in standard photodynamic therapy. Instead, we use the light bed, which contains banks of emitting diodes which emit red light frequencies that are effective for killing cancer cells.

It should be noted that those with advanced tumors should be treated slowly to prevent their tumors from breaking down too quickly and over too short a period of time.

Treatment Procedure Using Sonodynamic Photodynamic Therapy (SPDT)

We assess our patients clinically, and then give them a photosensitive agent in the form of drops, which are absorbed under the tongue. Over the next 48-72 hours, the agent accumulates selectively in tumor sites. Following this, patients lie on the light bed, where they are exposed to appropriate light frequencies from the light-emitting diodes. The time of exposure is important, and can vary from up to twenty minutes for patients with less advanced tumors, to only a few minutes for patients who have more advanced tumors (the more advanced the tumor, the slower the treatment program). Patients do treatments on the light bed for three consecutive days. We then calculate on an ongoing clinical basis whether they need further treatments.

Anecdotally, we have had the best success using next generation SPDT with breast and prostate cancers. We have also had encouraging results with several types of brain tumors including glioblastoma multiforme. Many brain tumors have significantly regressed during photodynamic therapy. In one case of glioblastoma multiforme, the patient's tumor completely disappeared.

Additional information on sono- and photodynamic therapy, including research studies which prove its effectiveness, can be found on the following websites: www.spdt.org.uk, or www.doveclinic.com.

Beta-glucans

The innate immune system is a complex network of immune cells which includes monocytes, macrophages, neutrophils, and natural killer cells—all of which circulate throughout the body to identify and destroy foreign pathogens and damaged cells. Extensive research has proven that cancer rates are higher in people who take immunosuppressant medications and in those who have poor innate immune cell function.

Of all the natural compounds known to activate the innate immune system, the best documented and most effective are the 1-3, 1-6 beta glucans, which are generally derived from baker's yeast. Wellmune (which is sold in the United States) and Immiflex (which is sold in the United Kingdom) are two reputable products that we recommend to our patients which provide an inexpensive, effective way to stimulate the innate immune system, and thereby, the body's response to cancer.

Intravenous Vitamin C

For years, our clinic worked with the Riordan family in the United States, which did the original research on the effectiveness of high dose Vitamin C for treating cancer. Intravenous Vitamin C at very high doses has a pro-oxidant, rather than anti-oxidant effect, which means it can kill cancer cells. It does this without producing the same side effects as chemotherapy. Although published research demonstrates that high dose intravenous Vitamin C can kill cancer cells, there are currently very few studies which demonstrate how effective it is for specific cancers and various types of tumors. At our clinic, we administer Vitamin C therapy concurrently with oral supplements such as alpha-lipoic acid and quercetin, which increase the body's serum levels of Vitamin C.

Pancreatic Pro-Enzymes

Another effective approach which we have developed for treating cancer involves pro-enzymes. It's similar to pancreatic enzyme therapy, but goes one step beyond. In our study of pancreatic enzyme therapy, we realized that it wasn't the enzymes themselves that worked to stop people's cancers, but the pro-enzymes, or enzyme precursors. The pancreas secretes pro-enzymes (or zymogens) partly to prevent the enzymes from digesting proteins in the same cells in which they are synthesized. The body secretes proenzymes to keep us alive; without them, we would digest ourselves. In our practice, we worked out a treatment (suppository) using pancreatic pro-enzymes, and had remarkable results from using it on many of our cancer patients.

Our pro-enzyme treatments were so successful that we decided to spend huge amounts of money to do animal studies and cell cultures to have them formally developed. We took out a couple of patents on them and have started a pharmaceutical company in Australia, called Propanc-Pty-Ltd., which is now responsible for its research and development. There is nothing about this type of treatment on the Dove Clinic's website, since I have turned the intellectual property rights over to the Australian company, but it's one of the first, totally safe, biological remedies to ever be developed for cancer treatment.

At the moment, I can't get pro-enzymes made for use at our clinic because we don't currently have the funds available for re-development. When the clinical trials have been completed, we will be able to use pro-enzymes as part of our treatment programs again. We expect them to be out on the market in about four or five years. We could continue to make them ourselves, but we currently don't have access to all of the raw materials. We could get them made under a research banner, but then we would have to manufacture them to pharmaceutical standards, which would require millions of dollars.

I developed this treatment, along with the sonodynamic and photo-dynamic therapies, right here at our clinic in New Hampshire. We are the only major clinic in the world that has developed two new, major, effective types of treatment for cancer, both of which are completely safe, non-chemotherapeutic and non-radiotherapy approaches. We feel justly proud of that.

Dendritic Cell Therapy Vaccines

Over the past ten years, the medical community has rapidly increased its understanding of immune surveillance and its appreciation of the mechanisms by which tumors escape its notice. This has led to the development of promising new strategies against cancer, of which the most exciting and consistently successful are dendritic cell therapy vaccines.

It's clear that the immune system is capable of recognizing tumor cells. Cellular immunotherapy or dendritic cell therapy vaccines consist of giving patients cells that stimulate anti-tumor activity. The aim is to harness the body's own potent immunological weapons to destroy cancer cells.

So-called cytotoxic T-lymphocytes are one of the critical cells that are able to destroy tumor cells. Receptors on the surface of T-cells recognize proteins called tumor-associated antigens on the surface of the tumors. The process is complex, but basically, in order for the T-cell to become activated, it must recognize the tumor-associated antigen and receive a co-stimulatory signal in order to kill off a cancer cell. In the absence of this, T-cells become resistant to the cancer's antigen and the tumor continues to grow. The cellular orchestrators of this T-cell activation are antigen-presenting cells, which are the dendritic cells.

Dendritic cells possess a remarkable ability to stimulate immune response. Under the microscope, these cells are about the size of an average white blood cell and have long finger-like appendages which often divide. It's on these appendages that the tumor-associated antigen is carried and presented to T-lymphocytes. In that process, the co-stimulatory signal is provided and the T-cells recognize the particular antigen presented to them. They then go to the tumor bearing that antigen and, if all goes well, are able to kill the tumor cells.

Dendritic cells are present throughout the body but are particularly prevalent in the skin. This is why some dendritic cell therapy injections need to be given into the skin (intra-dermally) instead of under the skin (subcutaneously). This is absolutely critical and is an important reason why some dendritic cell therapy vaccines fail.

In order to make a dendritic cell therapy vaccine, a tumor-associated antigen needs to be obtained. This can come from either a biopsy of the tumor, or ideally, from tumor cells from a tumor cell line (a line of cancer cells that have been kept alive in a laboratory). Such cell lines can be kept alive for many years, and used to make an allogeneic dendritic cell vaccine.

Many hundreds of papers on dendritic cell therapy vaccines have been published in the medical literature, and more are being published all the time. Dendritic cells are being used to treat more and more types of cancer. The first vaccines were used for the treatment of melanoma, but now they are also being used to treat stage three and four kidney, prostate, brain, and bowel cancers, along with others.

It's unusual for our stage four cancer patients who include this type of therapy in their protocols to go into complete remission. Yet, we often see an increase in their median survival time, and some patients attain complete remission after following our cytotoxic tumor killing program and receiving a dendritic vaccine. This is gratifying for us to witness, especially since our patients have experienced no significant side effects from the use of such vaccines. Also, it's important to note that most clinical trials with dendritic vaccines have been done on patients with advanced disease who have some degree of immune suppression from their cancers and/or as a result of conventional treatment, particularly chemotherapy.

In the future, it's likely that all patients with cancer, after having received tumor-killing therapies, such as surgery, radiotherapy (radiation), and chemotherapy, will go on to receive dendritic cell therapy vaccines to improve their immune function, because prospective studies have demonstrated a high recurrence of cancer (approximately 50 percent) in those with low cell-mediated immune function. This situation commonly happens following chemotherapy, which significantly depresses immune function.

Finally, it's important to note that stimulating the immune system with just any old agent is crude and ineffective. Dendritic vaccines work because the immune system is taught to recognize specific tumor associated antigens, which is key to its success. Simply activating the immune system with other immune-stimulating substances may not work.

While we don't administer dendritic cell therapy vaccines at our clinic, we are heavily involved in other aspects of their use, and can recommend clinics overseas that do administer them.

Ukrain and Metronomic Low-Dose Cytophosphamide

We also use Ukrain, which consists of the herbaceous perennial plant *Chelidonium majus* (greater celandine) and Thiotepa, which is a very old chemotherapy medication. In Ukrain, Chelidonium binds with Thiotepa to make it less toxic. Ukrain is useful for treating a variety of late-stage cancers, as well as patients who have previously had chemotherapy, because it's typically well tolerated. Several published studies demonstrate its benefits for treating cancer. For instance, in killing tumor cells, it also upregulates cytotoxic (or cancer-killing) activity in the tumor microenvironment, which helps to reduce tumor mass. This is very important because there's a great deal of evidence which shows that surviving cancer is based mostly upon an adequate amount of cytotoxic T-cell activity within the tumor microenvironment.

At the same time, these cytotoxic T-cells tend to be down-regulated by other immune cells called T-regulator cells, which means that it's also important to lower the number of T-regulator cells that are affecting the cancer-killing T-cells. To do this, we use a very low dose of a chemotherapy agent called cytophosphamide: about 1/20th of the dose that would be given in full-dose chemotherapy. This treatment lowers the number of T-regulator cells that prevent the cytotoxic T-cells from being fully effective.

Sono- and photodynamic therapy also cause T-cells to get upregulated in the tumor microenvironment. As previously mentioned, such upregulation is associated with an increase in the median survival of the patient. So the more tumor-killing T-cells (or CD8 cytotoxic T-cells) that there are in the tumor microenvironment, the longer the patient is likely to live. Clearly, these cells help to reduce tumor mass and increase patient survival.

Cancer is a complex illness, and it's important for doctors to give their patients several therapies at once. Doing just one type of treatment is an antiquated approach that doesn't yield good results.

The Use of Bindweed Root for Stopping Angiogenesis

As part of our protocols, we also use herbal extracts that have strong evidence for stopping angiogenesis (tumor blood vessel growth), such as VascuStatin, which is made by Allergy Research Group in the United States. This is a low molecular weight extract of bindweed root which, like intravenous Vitamin C, was also discovered by the Riordan family in Kansas. A lady with ovarian cancer visited the Riordan family and was taking an herb that was given to her by the American Indians in Kansas, which was keeping her alive. The Riordans analyzed it and discovered the effective component that it contained for treating cancer. The results of their research have since been widely published. Bindweed root is a remedy that really works for stopping angiogenesis.

Detoxification

We may use intravenous Vitamin C to eliminate the toxicity that builds up in our patients who have received chemotherapy treatments prior to coming to our clinics. We also use other detoxification treatments that are based on Traditional Chinese Medicine (TCM). I spent a lot of time in China in the 1970s, and wrote about twenty books on a range of subjects, including TCM and complementary medicine. I brought TCM to the UK, because I found that it works. It's a simple approach that's targeted to specific organ systems in the body.

We measure our patients' organ function using various unconventional energetic devices. The one that we most commonly use is a spin-off from a Russian space program device, which measures the body's magnetic vector potential. (Author's note: The subject of magnetic vector potential is beyond the scope of this book; therefore, how it works won't be described here). We then prescribe TCM treatments based on these measurements. This device can also provide clues about the type and range of treatments that we need to give our patients.

We also recommend that our patients do far-infrared saunas at home, which are very effective for detoxification. Liver cleanses can also be important, and some of our patients do these at home, too. Research papers published in the early part of the last century have also shown coffee enemas to have beneficial effects upon the liver. I don't know if they work, but some people believe that they are helpful.

Treating Hormonal Imbalances

In conventional medicine, breast cancer patients are normally prescribed the drug Tamoxifen to block the negative effects of estrogen upon their cancer cells. At our clinic, we give them indole-3 carbinole instead, which is a phytochemical that occurs naturally in cruciferous vegetables, and which has a similar effect upon estrogen.

Balancing other hormones in the body doesn't seem to influence cancer. There is medical evidence which shows that stimulating thyroid hormones also stimulates cancer growth. Similarly, suppressing the thyroid with anti-thyroid medications slows tumor growth. We don't prescribe any thyroid medications to our cancer patients.

Dietary Recommendations

The diet that we recommend to our cancer patients is based on scientific evidence that proves its effectiveness. It involves little or no dairy and red meat, and limits protein intake to 25 grams per day. The basic idea is to push the patient's body towards an alkaline state; to a pH level of seven or above. At this level, enzymes in the body work best and tumor cells die off, because tumor cells tend to grow more rapidly in acidic environments with a pH of six or below. In general, sugars, animal protein, dairy products, and certain grains are acid-forming foods. Fruits, vegetables, beans, pulses (legumes), fresh herbs, ginger, and turmeric are all examples of alkaline-forming.

Therefore, we encourage our patients to prepare neutral or alkaline meals for themselves. For example, if they eat fish, which is acid-forming, they should balance it with lots of vegetables, which are alkaline-forming. Also, no more than 25 percent of their meals should be protein, while 75 percent should be vegetables. We therefore advise them to have no more than one meal per day that's based on animal protein. Their other meals should be based on vegetables, fruits, beans, pulses (legumes), lentils, nuts, seeds, tofu, and nutritious grains such as quinoa.

More specifically, we encourage them to have liberal amounts of all of the following: whole grains, brown rice, barley, oats, millet, rye, wheat, corn and quinoa; vegetables (preferably organic), fruits, legumes, peas, lentils, beans and seeds (particularly sesame, sunflower and pumpkin), as well as nuts and filtered water. Foods that can be eaten in moderate amounts include: eggs and fish; preferably deep sea oily fish such as salmon, tuna, mackerel, herring, sardines, and pilchards; white meat, poultry (preferably organic), and soy proteins such as tofu. Finally, foods and substances that they should avoid or consume in low quantities include: tobacco, alcohol, tea, coffee, and other caffeinated drinks; chemical preservatives, processed foods, sugar, saturated fat, hydrogenated margarine, and red, smoked, or cured meats.

Consuming organic vegetables is important because they have a higher vitamin and mineral content than non-organic ones. They also contain significantly higher amounts of isoflavones, which are cancer-protective substances naturally produced by plants to resist attack by pests or fungi. Additionally, the kind of fiber that's found in whole fruits and vegetables is very important for the digestive system and also absorbs toxins from the body. People with cancer should avoid fruit and vegetable juices, however, as these drinks lack necessary fiber and are comparatively high in sugar content.

Organically-grown chicken and turkey is also preferable to non-organic poultry, because they have lower levels of fat, additives, and growth-promoting hormones, the latter of which are given to birds to accelerate their growth. Eating turkey is moderately important because it's the only meat that contains tryptophan, which is important for increasing T-cell activity and thereby, cell-mediated immunity—the body's principal defense against cancer. Occasionally, small amounts of red meat are acceptable, as long as the meat is organic or has been farmed to a good standard.

Consuming oily fish, such as those previously mentioned, is also beneficial because they contain high levels of Omega-3 fatty acids, particularly eicosapentaenoic acid. Several studies demonstrate that high levels of Omega-3 fatty acids, particularly eicosapentaenoic acid, are helpful for fighting disease because they reduce inflammation. Non-oily fish such as cod and haddock are excellent sources of protein, but they contain much lower levels of Omega-3 fatty acids.

People with cancer should avoid milk and dairy products not only because they're acidic, but also because they have high levels of estrogenic factors. This is particularly important for those that have estrogen-dependent cancers such as breast cancer or in some cases, ovarian cancer. Also, milk and dairy products are high in insulin-like growth factor number 1 and epidermal growth factor. These are important factors that encourage cancer tumor growth. Current scientific evidence reveals epidermal growth factor and their receptors to be crucial for the development of cancer stem cells, so it seems sensible that people with cancer should do everything possible to reduce any epidermal growth factors in their diets, including those which come from milk and dairy products. Many other foods contain calcium; nuts and seeds, beans, pulses (legumes), lentils, green leafy vegetables, tofu, and sardines (canned). As long as patients are consuming adequate amounts of these foods, reducing their dairy intake shouldn't result in calcium deficiencies.

Finally, sugar significantly affects cell metabolism and changes the internal environment of the body, so when patients can reduce their intake of refined sugar, it makes their bodies less conducive to tumor growth. Avoiding sugar is also effective for helping the body to starve the tumor. Specifically, the refined sugars that are found in cakes, biscuits (crackers), cookies, sweets, processed foods, and sweet drinks should be avoided. Fructose sugars that are found in fruits and vegetables are less harmful. People with cancer should aim for an intake of six to seven portions of whole fruits and vegetables daily.

The diet that's described here and on our website is a worthy, evidence-based approach, in comparison to Gerson-diet approaches. (For the Gerson diet to work, patients must do it all day long, every day, which isn't feasible for some. It works occasionally, but I have been involved in this type of medicine for years and I have never been that impressed with it).

Testing Procedures and Dark Field Microscopy

My initial visit with patients lasts an hour, and involves looking at their blood in a live state under a dark field microscope which provides an inexpensive, broad view of what's going on in the body. To do this, we take a tiny drop of blood from their fingertips and using the microscope, magnify it up to nearly 10,000 times. Patients, as well as the therapist or doctor doing the test, can see the blood cells on video and watch the blood, and contaminants in the blood, interact in real time. From these pictures, we can come to several important conclusions regarding patients' immune system status and then make treatment recommendations for them.

This blood test tells us a lot about what's going on in the body. For instance, we can obtain qualitative information about the condition of red cell membranes, the activity levels of certain white blood cells, and the quality and quantity of the blood's plasma elements. We can also look at the way the blood coagulates and dries. Certain characteristics of the blood can indicate to us whether patients have free radical damage, oxidative stress, metal toxicity, and/or digestive problems. We can also gather fundamental information related to their nutritional status, immune function, oxygen levels, toxin load, lipid levels, and heterogeneous plaque formation.

By initially screening their blood in this way, we are able to identify more specifically the areas requiring treatment. We may, for example, need to improve their nutritional status and immune function, or reduce their yeast and bacterial load. If necessary, we may do further investigations. For instance, if they have a high lipid load, we will explore their family history and dietary and lifestyle habits, and send their blood samples to a laboratory for further analysis of their lipid profile ratios.

It isn't possible to diagnose any specific disease state with live blood analysis alone; further examination and investigation are required. However, it's a good fundamental screening tool that's patient-friendly, interactive, and educational. By adjusting our patients' treatment programs to 'normalize' the appearance of their blood, we can assist them with achieving optimal health and well-being. Used in this way, live blood analysis is also a valuable clinical tool for monitoring progress.

Following the live blood analysis, we check the status of our patients' organ systems with the aforementioned Russian space program device. Then we might follow up with some conventional blood tests. We then tell our patients what treatments we can offer them, based on these results. They can then make an informed choice about whether they will do all, part, or none of what we recommend. Our treatment approach isn't like what's typically seen in conventional medicine, where treatments are done without the patient's involvement or collaboration; patient discretion is involved. We work together with them.

Other Considerations in Treatment

The specific protocol that I develop for my patients depends upon a lot of factors, such as how many co-morbid conditions they suffer from, the stage of their cancer, and the type of tumors that they have, but it's difficult to describe all of the considerations without writing an entire book. Basically, we look at all of the contributing factors to disease and base our treatments upon the individual patient's needs. For example, we can't use sonodynamic or photo-dynamic therapy on patients who have very advanced cancers, because their tumors have caused too much destruction in their bodies and they can't cope with the treatment. Treatments for such people would need to be more palliative. Pro-enzymes, on the other hand, work extremely well for any patient at any stage of disease. If we could find the raw materials to make those again we could use them at our clinic, but for now we have to wait for Propanc-PTY to manufacture them.

Maintenance Treatment Program

Our initial intensive treatment course lasts two to five weeks, three days per week, depending upon the types of tumors that patients have. Following their initial treatment regimen, they generally come back to our clinic once every several months, for at least five years, to receive maintenance treatments. During this time, we also do relevant blood tests and measure their organ and other functions through the equipment that I previously described. We decide what their ongoing prescription will be, based on the results that we get from these tests.

The maintenance program that we recommend includes strategies that support Th-1 cell-mediated immunity, such as: beta glucans, high doses of Vitamin D, and a range of nutritional supplements such as quercetin. We might also use oral TCM supplements which support organ function. These include collections of herbal and nutritional preparations, and sometimes, bovine organ extracts. We use a wide range of remedies, mostly herbs, to treat all of the organs. While certain vitamins and minerals can be helpful, most people don't seem to realize that when you give the body a bunch of vitamins and minerals, the cancer uses those, too, just like the rest of the body. Patients can take them, but they will have no significant negative effects upon their tumors.

Treatment Outcomes

Ninety-five percent of our patients come to us after they have had chemotherapy and radiotherapy (radiation), and are at the end stages of disease. We are able to bring some of them into remission, and have many testimonials of people who have been alive for ten years since being given a terminal diagnosis. These testimonials can be found on our website, in the paper that we published on sonodynamic and photodynamic therapy. Most of our patients follow up with us after they complete their treatments. We have been able to keep track of about 80 percent of our patients, for years down the road.

I have been using sonodynamic therapy for five years, which is longer than any other practitioner, anywhere else in the world, because we developed it. Since using this therapy on our patients, our treatment outcomes have literally increased by 50 percent; we have had massively improved results, even with sarcomas. Truly, the results have been extraordinary.

That said, while conventional medicine can offer statistics on its success with different types of treatments, including chemotherapy, radiation, and surgery, we don't have statistics on the results of treatments for our early stage cancer patients. We haven't been able to complete the same level of research.

Some people insist on doing our treatments before trying conventional medicine, and we accept these patients on an informed consent basis. In the end, some do well and some don't. There are no guarantees with cancer. No one treatment works 100 percent of the time.

Lifestyle Recommendations for Healing

My lifestyle recommendations for healing vary from patient to patient. In general, it's important for people with cancer to reduce their daily stress levels, whether the stress that they suffer from is emotional, job, or relationship related. One basic intervention that we recommend for dealing with stress is Mindfulness-Based Cognitive Therapy (MBCT).

Mindfulness is the Buddhist concept of allowing yourself to be completely aware of the present moment while treating yourself and your surroundings in a gentle and compassionate way. More than just a nice idea, the practice of mindfulness can bring about opportunities for happiness and re-engaging with life, ourselves, and the people around us.

MBCT combines mindfulness and the practice of meditation with the principles of cognitive behavioral therapy, which provides the skills for applying the art of mindfulness to everyday life. The course at our clinic involves a two-hour weekly class over an eight week period, and also provides patients with the opportunity to practice mindfulness meditation at home with the help of guided CDs.

In MBCT, patients focus on the present moment, instead of on the past and what might have been, or on the future and on what might be. Focusing on the past or the future wastes energy; it's important that people learn how to focus on the here and now. So we do a lot of MBCT in our practice, which is usually very effective for our patients. Our research has taught us that the psychotherapeutic approach, which involves patients talking to a counselor about mothers, fathers, and deep instincts, is mostly a waste of time.

Roadblocks to Healing

Our treatments aren't funded by insurance or any national health service, so when patients can't pay for them, this can be a block to their healing. Also, if patients have some strange fixed idea about our treatments and think that only conventional medicine can cure them, then our treatments won't help. They are wasting their time and money. If they believe that "getting blasted" with chemotherapy is going to help them, then they should be doing that instead.

Inexpensive Cancer Treatments

If people can't afford treatments at a clinic, doing treatments at home to stimulate immune function can be helpful. The most important thing that they can do is take a high-dose beta-glucan product such as Wellmune, along with other beta-glucans, at three times the regular dose. People with cancer should take beta-glucans for life, even if that means for 30 or 40 years. I also recommend high doses of fatty acids that are high in EPA, because these are anti-inflammatory, and cancer is stimulated by inflammation. Any chronic inflammatory problem in the body can eventually lead to cancer. In fact, inflammation in any part of the body is the main, or primary, condition that leads to cancer.

Patients who treat themselves at home should realize, though, that treating cancer requires a complex, multi-faceted approach. The problem with conventional oncologists is that they are too single-minded in their approach to treatment, and that doesn't work for a complex illness like cancer.

How Family and Friends Can Support Their Loved Ones with Cancer

Family and friends should do MCBT, along with their loved ones who have cancer. Also, they should try to get them to accept where they are in their healing journey. For instance, a quarter of our patients are dying, and those who accept death have a much better quality of life than those who refuse to accept where they are at. Even though we have some ten-year survivors of metastatic disease, these diseases are technically incurable. So we might say to such patients, "Look, we can't cure you, but we might be able to do this and that (to extend your life and reduce your symptoms). If you can accept where you are at, you will do much better." And being able to adopt such an attitude basically reflects a mindfulness approach to living.

Final Words

I hope that what has been written here about our treatments opens the minds of people who are suffering from metastatic cancers, and incites them to consider other approaches, particularly those involving immunotherapy.

Contact Information
Julian Kenyon, MD, MB, ChB

Medical Director, The Dove Clinic for Integrated Medicine
Winchester & London, United Kingdom
www.doveclinic.com

To learn more about sono- and photodynamic therapy, visit:
www.spdt.org.uk.

Information on our other treatments can be found on our website:
www.doveclinic.com.

•CHAPTER 11•

Constantine A. Kotsanis, MD
GRAPEVINE, TEXAS

Biography

Dr. Kotsanis is Board Certified in Otolaryngology (Head and Neck Surgery). He completed his residency at Loyola University of Chicago in 1983. He is a member of the American Academy of Otolaryngic Allergy. He is licensed to practice medicine in Texas, Illinois, and North Carolina, and is licensed by the Arizona State Board of Homeopathic Medicine.

Additionally, Dr. Kotsanis is a certified clinical nutritionist and is also certified in Auditory Enhancement Therapy and IPTLD (Insulin Potentiation Targeted Low-Dose Chemotherapy, which is also referred to as IPT). He's a certified instructor of IPTLD and has been teaching physicians about IPTLD/IPT for cancer treatment since 2002. Additionally, he serves as Assistant Clinical Professor at the University of Texas Southwestern Medical School and is a founding member of Defeat Autism Now! (DAN).

Dr. Kotsanis has been treating cancer since 2001 and has been in practice since 1983. His specialties include integrative cancer therapy, allergies, Chronic Fatigue Syndrome, autism spectrum disorder, anti-aging medicine, nutrition, and stem cell therapy research. He treats patients based on their individual physical, metabolic, and biochemical makeup.

He's an avid researcher, and educates physicians and patients alike on different treatments for cancer and other diseases. His mission is to change the way healthcare is delivered to the world, one person at a time. About 30 percent of his patients are cancer patients. He treats the most difficult cases of chronic disease, including late-stage cancers. His practice consists of people who have failed traditional oncology treatments, people who cannot tolerate traditional approaches to medicine, and those who refuse to do traditional (conventional) therapies.

What Causes Cancer

Cancer results from changes in the body's epigenetic expression, which gets altered because of the environment we live in today (Epigenetics is the study of changes in gene expression which are caused by mechanisms other than changes in the underlying DNA sequence). If I had to pick a name for cancer it would be called the "Post-Industrial Revolution Civilization Disease." Our genes don't change that much, but the expression of our DNA can, as a result of the environment we live in. Arthur Kornberg, a biochemist who won a Nobel Prize in 1959 in Medicine (together with Dr. Severo Ochoa of New York University) for his discovery of the mechanisms involved in the biological synthesis of DNA (ribonucleic acid and deoxyribonucleic acid), demonstrated how such changes in DNA expression can cause cancer. Physical, spiritual, and emotional stressors alter DNA and cause cancer, so we address all of these in our patients.

Poor nutrition is one important environmental factor which causes epigenetic changes in the body. As an advanced western society, our nutrition has gone downhill because of industrialization and commerce. We also eat too much food, which equates to too many pounds on our bodies. Additionally, we have too many chemicals, pesticides, hormones, and antibiotics in our food supply. Eating isn't a nutritional experience; it's a social event, which means that we don't eat foods that are good for us. Yet to stay healthy, we need to be mindful of what we eat, and the amount of calories that we consume. Studies have shown that the fewer calories people eat, the longer they live and the less disease they have. So eating toxic food, and lots of it, contributes to cancer development.

Emotional trauma is another major contributing factor to cancer development. The number one cause of emotional trauma is other people, especially people that we know, such as family, friends and co-workers who push us over the edge!

Finally, and most importantly, epigenetic changes result when the immune system malfunctions or breaks down. As the immune system breaks down, opportunistic infections set in and a never-ending vicious cycle of infection and toxicity gets initiated. So while cancer has hundreds of causes and contributing factors, if I could narrow it down to one thing, I would say that it happens because the immune system has been poisoned by bad food, emotional trauma, toxins, and infections.

In human physiology, basic systems need to be intact in order for a person to be healthy, and one of these is the gut. Whatever goes on in the gut affects the brain and the immune system. Seventy percent of the immune system is physically housed in the gut. There are one hundred trillion microflora here, and each has its own specific function. There is beneficial flora (bacteria), which are the "good guys" which digest foods and produce vitamins. These "good guys" also support the immune system and direct its activities. Then there is flora that I like to call the "recycler" bacteria, which are there to "take out the garbage." As an analogy, suppose that in a city of 100,000, there are five or ten garbage men. That would be a good thing. But what if 95,000 of those citizens were garbage men? It would mean that something was wrong with that city, right? So when 95 percent of the gut flora is comprised of garbage men, they are no longer garbage men, but pathogens. That's what pathogenic flora is. The pathogens then become the drivers of the immune system and they take it straight into the ditch.

As another analogy, think of the immune system as an 18-wheeler carrying fruits and vegetables, and the driver of the 18-wheeler as the healthy flora. The good guys take the 18-wheeler to the mitochondria to create good energy, which is needed by the body. But in order for that energy to be good and arrive at the right place, the back of the truck has to be filled with healthy, organic food, and the driver must be a good guy (healthy flora). In this example, the back of the truck is filled up with the foods that people consume as a part of their diets. If the truck is filled with undesirable food, this promotes pathogenic growth. These pathogens then become the drivers that take this trash into the mitochondria. Since the mitochondria are always looking for quick energy, they will accept this junk for energy, but it's like putting kerosene into a car!

So when pathogens become great in number, they populate and inflame the gut, which in turn throws off the immune system and other systems of the body. It's in this environment that cancer has the opportunity to develop. In my opinion, the normal, beneficial flora in the gut should be considered an organ. That is how important, and vast, they are.

Treatment Approach

My initial visit with new patients lasts two or three hours. I will sometimes even spend an hour or two talking to them on the phone after my office closes. We (my staff and I) follow them closely. I have three cancer care managers—one of whom has been with me for over eighteen years—who help with this. We love our work, and are a phenomenal team that works well together. We don't even look at treating cancer patients as work, actually. It's our passion! I talk to my patients anytime they want, and they can call me anytime, day or night. They have my office, home, and cell phone numbers. I work seven days a week, but again, it's not work; it's my life.

To be legal and ethical, I require that my patients have a primary care physician (in addition to me), and that they see an oncologist, to get a diagnosis and learn about their treatment options, before they do treatments at my clinic. I do this because cancer is a conundrum of a disease and people with cancer need a lot of help from many people in the medical field. Conventional medicine has some beneficial things to offer, and I want people to know about all of their available treatment options. Also, primary care physicians can take care of routine matters for my patients, such as tests, and their services are usually covered by insurance, whereas a lot of what we do at my clinic isn't.

Once patients' oncologists have given them advice about the treatments that they think they should do, those patients can then come to me for a second opinion. Then they, and they alone—not their families—can decide what type of treatment they want to do, having understood the pros and cons of the different treatments that are out there.

What we do here, above all, is support people's immune systems so their bodies can fight the cancer. Our main goal is to improve their longevity and quality of life and minimize their treatment complications from any radiation and chemotherapy that they may also be doing. We treat them with nutrition, herbal and homeopathic remedies, psychological interventions, and IPTLD (Insulin Potentiation Targeted Low Dose Therapy), along with a spectrum of other approaches. These are discussed in the following sections.

We accept all of the following for treatment:

1. Patients who prefer IPTLD as their primary anti-cancer therapy and who have refused traditional oncology treatments

2. Patients who have failed traditional oncology treatments

3. Patients who can't tolerate traditional oncology treatments

In all cases, we work closely with our patients' primary physicians and oncologists.

Summary of Our Cancer Treatment Program

We offer a comprehensive program involving both drugs and natural remedies, and this seems to be the most effective and complete treatment approach. We find that targeted low-dose chemotherapy gets rid of most of our early to mid-stage patients' cancer cells within six weeks, but it all depends upon the person and the cancer. In addition, we do therapies to lessen the body's overall toxic burden, because when we do that, then everything else, including the immune system and our IPTLD treatments, work better.

Seven Components to Healing: An Integrative Treatment Process

My treatment program consists of seven important components. Some of these are discussed more in-depth in the sections that follow. In general, the more of my program that patients can do, the greater are their chances for recovery and a better life. The components of this program are:

1. To de-bulk the tumor through oncological, traditional or alternative therapies.

2. To destroy other infections and infectious vectors, or causes of infection, in the body.

3. To de-agglutinate the blood cells, which involves thinning and cleaning up circulating immune complexes in the blood, so that red blood cells don't stick together and the tissues receive more oxygen and nutrients.

4. To increase energy at the cellular level and increase mitochondrial energy production.

5. To support the body's overall functioning with a multi-faceted approach that includes: nutritional

recommendations, hormone balancing, alkalinizing and botanical therapies, enzyme therapy, and detoxification.

6. To heal emotional trauma, build and re-build relationships.

7. To encourage patients to develop a spiritual life, through meditation, prayer, and forgiveness.

IPTLD/IPT—Insulin Potentiation Targeted Low Dose Therapy

IPT/IPTLD is one of the main therapies that we do at our clinic. IPT was developed in the 1940s by a Mexican doctor named Donato Perez Garcia, MD (who's also referred to as Dr. Donato). He did a study on cancer patients at his clinics in Mexico and Texas, and observed that most of them obtained very good results with IPT. (Note: IPT/IPTLD is described in further detail in other chapters of this book).

I once visited Dr. Donato's office in Mexico, and was amazed to find three generations of physicians working there. They also had thousands of patient charts! When I asked him how many of his stage one and two patients did well with IPT treatments, he replied that over 90 percent had extremely good results. Fifty percent of his stage three patients did fairly well; meaning, they went into remission. For his stage four patients, he primarily expected to extend their lives and alleviate their symptoms. However, a very small number of his stage four patients also went into remission.

Because IPT involves administering much lower doses of chemo-therapy than what's typically given in conventional medicine, patients experience less nausea, vomiting and hair loss, and fewer complications and major side effects than if they had done full-dose chemotherapy.

Practitioners all have their biases. I'm not sure that one type of treatment is better than another. By itself, IPT isn't superior to regular chemotherapy, and regular chemotherapy isn't superior to IPT. What matters is treating the whole person. Practitioners can't say that one type of therapy is better than another, because they must take into account all of the factors involved in healing. In our practice, we do a total revamping of the emotional and physical body, part of which involves choosing the correct therapies for each of our patients. This process is complicated but necessary.

Nutrient Supplementation

Our nutritional treatments are based on the work of A. Kornberg, an American biochemist who has made some phenomenal discoveries. For instance, he demonstrated that twenty basic amino acids are required to duplicate a DNA chain. Cancer cells require twenty essential amino acids to replicate, and if they don't have all of these, they can't do that. He discovered that it was possible to manipulate the DNA polymerase of cancer cells by putting people on a diet that didn't contain all twenty of the amino acids, and that if they followed this diet, their cancer cells would die; this clever invention won him the Nobel Prize.

According to Kornberg, people with cancer should avoid sugar and animal protein so the cancer can't get all of the amino acids that it needs to replicate. Instead, he recommends a diet of plant-based foods and herbs. Practitioners who have recommended this diet to their patients claim to get good results from it and we recommend it to some of our patients. While I (Dr. Kotsanis) follow it myself, I don't recommend it to all of my patients, because not all of them are able to follow it and/or they may have different dietary needs. So I customize my patients' diets and make recommendations that will most benefit their immune systems and promote healing. In addition to being a medical doctor, I'm a certified clinical nutritionist, which better enables me to help my patients in this aspect of their recovery. I also have a network of clinical nutritionists and dietitians that I work with and to whom I sometimes refer my patients for further help.

We're currently in the process of writing a cookbook, tentatively entitled *Free Food,* which is for people with special dietary requirements. It will contain recipes that are casein, gluten, sugar, and dairy-free, as well as vegetarian. It will be published around May-June, 2011.

We also give our patients generous amounts of Vitamins A and D, which studies have demonstrated to be beneficial for strengthening the immune system. Other remedies that we prescribe include beta-glucans, which improve neutrophil counts (neutrophils are a type of immune cell involved in fighting cancer), the herb artemisinin, IP-6 (inositol hexaphosphate, which is an anti-oxidant), and curcumin. All of these boost the immune system and increase NK (natural killer) cell activity. Vitamin D-3 and Vitamin A are essential for all of my cancer patients, as well as for people who don't have cancer.

Beyond this, I supplement nutrients, including minerals and anti-oxidants, according to what my patients need. We also administer Vitamins C and K intravenously, because they have cytotoxic effects upon cancer cells when given in high doses. I also recommend alkalinizing agents, such as wheat grass, asparagus (best when juiced), and Essiac tea.

Botanical Therapies

It's important to treat cancer patients for other infections that are weighing down their immune systems, so that their bodies can better fight cancer. The best way to control or eliminate parasitic, viral, and fungal infections is with the use of botanical remedies; the naturopathic approach is the best for treating any type of chronic infection. We use herbs such as catechu, black walnut, cloves, and wormwood, in combination with ionic minerals, to control infections in our patients with cancer.

Enzyme Therapy

Cancer patients have increased blood agglutination (red blood cell clumping). Blood agglutination promotes infections, low oxygen in the tissues, and cancer growth. A key component of all of our cancer treatments is supplemental enzymes such as amylase, lipase, protease, and bromelain, which break up blood cell clumps and thin the blood. This approach is known as "Kelly's Protocol." I find that patients who do enzyme therapy have better treatment outcomes.

Detoxification

We prescribe our patients substances for various detoxification purposes: everything from citrus pectin to DMSA (Dimercaptosuccinic acid) and EDTA (Ethylenediaminetetraacetic acid). We have a wide spectrum of heavy metal chelating agents at our clinic. Patients do some of our detoxification procedures at our clinic; others they do at home. Since all cancer patients have higher-than-average levels of toxicity, all of them are placed on some type of detoxification protocol. Detoxification must always be done under the strict supervision of a physician.

Treating Infected Teeth

We encourage our patients to address their infected teeth, if they have any. Clearing out infections in the mouth decreases the immune system's burden. Cancer must be fought on multiple fronts, because the battle occurs on multiple fronts. If patients are battling infections in their mouths and cancer in their colons, for instance, then they are fighting disease on two fronts, because the health of the mouth has a direct impact on the immune system and rest of the body.

Correcting Hormonal Imbalances

We correct our patients' hormones if they are out of balance. We test their thyroid and adrenal gland function, as well as their Vitamin D levels, using blood and saliva tests. If we find, for instance, that they don't have enough cortisol, then we may give them supplemental hydrocortisone. If their cortisol levels are too high, then we will give them herbs to lower those levels. Most people with cancer also suffer from hypothyroidism. For this, we often prescribe

Armour thyroid, which is natural thyroid hormone made from animal (pig) thyroid glands.

Dietary Recommendations

I recommend a healthy, toxin-free, low-calorie, organic food diet to my patients. Americans eat too many calories, and that has to stop if they want to avoid cancer. The amount of calories that people need depends upon their work and daily activities, but most can survive on 1,200-1,500 per day. Proper food combining is also important. For example, when people drink while they eat, their digestive enzymes get diluted, so they don't end up receiving the necessary concentration of digestive enzymes to properly metabolize their food. Ideally, people should drink before they eat a meal, and wait two hours after eating before they drink again. This makes the digestive enzymes and the body's overall digestion more efficient. When food is fully digested, nothing remains in the small intestine for pathogens to feast on. Pathogens will have a picnic whenever undigested food enters the small intestine. The byproduct of this is bloating and inflammation in the body. Mixing acidic and alkaline foods also interferes with the body's ability to produce proper digestive enzymes, which again, leaves pathogens with plenty of undigested food for a picnic.

I also individualize my patients' diets. The majority of my cancer patients are acidic with acidic cancers, so I may prescribe them alkaline water, in addition to an alkaline diet, to help alkalinize their bodies. I also encourage them to measure their pH levels at home by doing a saliva pH test, which is more accurate than a urine pH test. Ideally, I like to see people attain a body pH level of 7.4 or above, because at a pH of 7.0, cancers stop growing, and at 7.4, they begin to die.

Healing Emotional Trauma

Cancer begins in the body anywhere from two to ten years prior to its expression, and is usually initiated by an ugly emotional event. When people come into my office, I sometimes say to them, "Who are you mad at?" because I believe that they wouldn't have cancer if they weren't mad at someone. Everyone with cancer is angry at someone else, because cancer is usually initiated by a traumatic event (which produces anger), along with a garbage lifestyle.

We offer our patients therapies to heal their emotional traumas. We have psychologists, psychiatrists, and other mental health practitioners who collaborate with us on this. Psychiatrists prescribe medication for depression, which is necessary for some cancer patients.

I will also spend about 30-45 minutes in an office visit teaching my patients how to do meditation, which I consider to be a critical practice, because the brain is a powerful tool that influences healing. Meditation can be helpful, regardless of people's religion and who they believe in—whether Jesus, Moses, Buddha, or Mohammad, or even if they are agnostic. It's important for them to obtain peace in their hearts and minds and ask God to come in and help them deal with their diseases.

One of the meditation exercises that I recommend and which I have developed over the years, involves meditating before eating, three or four times per day, as well as every time people are mad about something. I teach this practice to all of my patients. I also ask their family members to participate in the exercise, so that they won't end up making fun of them and saying things like, "Come on, you need chemotherapy, vitamins, etc...not this meditation stuff!" Yes, patients need biochemical treatments, but they need spiritual therapy, too, which in my opinion, is really the main thing that influences the course of disease.

We also put our patients into the same room with their family and/or friends to discuss their treatment, and to get them all on the same page, as sometimes, they have differing opinions about which treatments are best. Patients who are mentally competent, however, ultimately need to make the decision about which treatments they should do. Their families shouldn't decide for them.

Lifestyle Recommendations for Healing

First, I would say to those who want to prevent cancer or heal from it: change your garbage lifestyle! Stop smoking, drinking, using recreational drugs, and eating fast foods. Smell the flowers, exercise, and go to church. Stop and be appreciative of your family and your surroundings. Stop watching violent movies and watch funny ones instead. When you spend time with people, elevate them. Don't tell them how bad things are. (Everyone is a grouch these days!). One of the biggest causes of cancer is other people. Some people bust others' chops all day long, and say things like, "You're no good. You're a failure." As kids, people used to hear their parents say things like, "I'm going to stick you in the closet and the boogeyman is going to get you" and then their teachers or others would say, "I'm going to flunk you" or "your boyfriend isn't going to love you." We preach hate! We need to stop preaching hate and stop trying to keep up with the Joneses'. Health is inversely proportional to the amount of wealth that you are trying to create. Not everyone is destined to be Linus Pauling or Michael Jordan. Time is a gift. Society promotes celebrities, football players, actors, and politicians, and we try to copy these guys, and it makes us sick!

Low-Cost Treatments

If our patients don't want to do IPT or can't afford these treatments, we also have a cancer program which consists of all natural therapies. It includes the use of botanicals, Essiac tea, and substances for pH control. We also recommend teas, coffee enemas, and meditation, among other low-cost treatments for patients who don't have much money.

Treatments to Prevent Cancer

We have nutritional cancer-prevention programs, which we recommend that patients come to see us for while they are still healthy, because the most ideal time for people to visit us is before their cancers even start. A famous study done by Tsunco Kobayashi, MD, in Japan, demonstrates how nutrition can prevent cancer. He has a nutritional program for people who want to prevent cancer, but there are requirements for entrance into this program. Participants must be cancer- free, and have a sibling, parent, or child with cancer. Nobody who has participated in his studies has ever gotten cancer, which demonstrates the power of nutrition to heal cancer. For more information on Kobayashi's research study, visit Gary Gordon, MD's, website: www.gordonresearch.com, which contains information on a wide range of health subjects, including cancer.

Factors That Influence Healing and Roadblocks to Healing

The most important factor affecting patients' healing is their ability to comply with a treatment regimen. Second in importance is their willingness to change their lifestyles. For instance, they may need to change their profession, or the city that they live in. If they are in an ugly situation and have a spouse that beats them up, then they need to get a divorce! Of course, the type and stage of cancer that patients have also impacts their ability to heal.

Interference of family members is the next greatest hindrance to healing. For instance, when they give negative feedback to the cancer patient, and say things like, "If you don't do this therapy, you're going to die," the patient's healing is blocked. I'm convinced that the number one cause of chronic illness is other humans. The third roadblock to healing is not having enough money to pay for treatments.

Conventional Versus Alternative Medicine

About fifteen years ago, I saw an article which stated that, when it comes to medical treatments, 29 percent of American people will do whatever treatment the government or FDA recommends. Another fifteen to twenty percent will do exactly the opposite of what the government says (some just out of spite). Then there are people in the middle, who waver but who are open to using either alternative or conventional medicine. In my clinical experience, patients choose treatments based on their personal belief systems, lifestyles, or financial abilities. In the end, we must take responsibility for ourselves and our bodies if we want to be healthy. Somehow, the United States government has convinced us that they will take care of us from cradle to grave, but this is a scary thought indeed! Ultimately, our treatment decisions should be based on the efficacy of different treatments, not the belief system behind them or any other factor.

Treatment Outcomes

No doctor has any solid statistics regarding the effectiveness of IPT or any other treatment that we do, although currently, our clinic is performing an FDA-funded, Quality of Life study to ascertain the efficacy of our treatments. This five-year study started in 2010.

I have seen our treatments completely reverse stage four cancers on rare occasion. Furthermore, we've never had to hospitalize anyone. We do all of our treatments on an outpatient basis, because IPT and our other treatments are a gentler approach to cancer treatment. (Metronomic chemotherapy is also an approach that has fewer complications for patients).

While I have seen total reversals of cancer in a few patients who have stage three and four cancers, whenever patients reach these stages, my goal is mostly to improve their quality of life. And how well this happens depends upon the person, not the type of cancer that they have. We do see many patients leading normal lives as a result of our treatments though, and participating in activities such as playing golf, going on vacation, and enjoying friends and spouses. Over 90 percent of our patients say that they are satisfied with their experiences at our clinic. Most are really happy to be here, because we lay everything out on the table for them, and treat them with kindness and love.

I have had a couple of patients with stage four cancers who were told that nothing could be done for them, and they have so far lived for a year or two past their original diagnoses. For instance, a woman who came to see us in February 2009, had had a double mastectomy, and undergone chemotherapy and radiation, but these treatments didn't work well for her. Her conventional doctors told her that they had done all that they could for her. So she came to me, with stage four cancer and metastases everywhere. We treated her, and her blood tests have been good and her CT scan results have been negative for over a year now. This is exciting news. Is she cured? I don't know, but she's working full time, going to church, traveling, and enjoying her husband and kids.

The chances for long-term survival increase if patients exercise, comply with their treatment regimens, and become loving and kind people (if they weren't before). The fourteenth century physician Paracelsus said, "There are no incurable diseases, just incurable people."

Practitioner Challenges of Treating Cancer

As a practitioner, my greatest challenge in treating cancer is dealing with medical authorities who do business a certain way and step on doctors' toes if they don't like what they do. That said, and in all fairness to the opposition, the Quality of Life study that the FDA has approved for me would have never happened two or three years ago. This year, mainstream physicians have also been referring their patients to me, which is unusual. They are more comfortable doing this now than they were in prior years. So I think we've turned a corner when it comes to making people aware of other effective cancer treatments. We are still looking for politicians to get involved, though. To step up to the plate and allow natural remedies to be a part of FDA-approved treatment regimens. I'm in favor of naturopathy, homeopathy, acupuncture, and allopathic medicine all co-existing and being accepted as part of Western medicine, and I'm dreaming of the day when all of us (practitioners) can work together under one roof. It seems as if this is a real possibility and could happen at some point in the future.

Government and commercial opposition (pharmaceutical companies) is the greatest challenge of treating cancer patients. The next greatest challenge is patients not wanting to change their lifestyles. The majority of people with cancer would be content to go through a drive-thru window, and say, "Give me an IV, don't ask me questions, and I won't ask you questions, either," then leave the drive-thru and live their lives as they please, and yet expecting to get well. Most of them would rather die than change their lifestyles and do what I tell them. They understand that they could die, but they still say, "Well, if I can't eat whatever I want and have my inappropriate medications and the booze that I drank before, then I don't want to live, anyway."

Last Words

The most important thing that people with cancer can do is become informed about their treatment options. In the Bible, when God went to King Solomon and asked him what he wanted, and told him that he could have anything in the world, Solomon chose wisdom. Information is the most powerful thing on the planet, so patients should know their treatment options. The second most important thing cancer patients should do is feed their bodies with natural, organic foods. Thirdly, they should have a complete understanding of their diseases. I'm a Board Certified surgeon, and I know what the "other side" knows about conventional cancer treatments. If we (doctors) cut out our patients' tumors with surgery, we still can't say that they are cured, because cancer is like diabetes. Once you have diabetes, you have it for the rest of your life, and you must manage it, with pills and insulin. Cancer is a chronic disease, too, it's just more advanced; the last stage of a chronic disease. So once people have cancer, even if their doctors pronounce them cured, they must continue on a treatment regimen for the rest of their lives. Patients must arm themselves with this kind of information.

It's like this: if you take a beautiful crystal ball and drop it, and it cracks into two pieces, and you put it back together with crazy glue, nobody ever knows that is has been broken. People with cancer are like broken crystal balls that have been put back together with glue, and they need to take care of themselves. Once they get a chronic disease, that disease must be "babysat." It's also similar to a car that has been in a wreck and requires more ongoing maintenance than the one that has never been in a wreck. It's not enough to have a negative CT scan and blood test results. If people go back to the old lifestyle habits which caused their cancers in the first place, then those cancers will come back. They must be vigilant and find competent practitioners who will care for them for the rest of their lives. They should have doctors who will check up on them no less than twice a year. Those are my recommendations. I tell people: "Don't give in! Continue on a regimen, and be happy! Don't forget to be happy, love, and forgive, above all."

Recommended Reading

The following is comprehensive site which describes IPT and provides a list of practitioners who use IPT: www.IPTforcancer.com.

Last year, some doctors, including me, got together and wrote a book which gives an overview of IPT. The book is called, *A Gentler, Kinder Cancer Treatment*. It can be found on Amazon.com. All proceeds go to the Best Answer for Cancer Foundation.

Contact Information
Constantine Kotsanis, MD

2020 W. State Highway 114 Suite 260
Grapevine TX 76051
www.kotsanisinstitute.com
Info@kotsanisinstitute.com
Phone: (817) 380-4992 (local)
Phone: (800) 302-9740 (toll free)
Fax: (817) 442-4040

•CHAPTER 12•

Joe Brown, NMD
TEMPE, ARIZONA

Biography

Dr. Joe Brown graduated from the Southwest College of Naturopathic Medicine & Health Sciences in Tempe, Arizona, in July 2005. He was President of his class for a year and a half before becoming President of the Student Government Association (SGA), where he also served on numerous committees and participated in the development of the Council on Naturopathic Medical Education (CNME) and Higher Learning Commission (HLC). He is a member of the Oncology Association of Naturopathic Physicians (OncANP), the American Association of Naturopathic Physicians (AANP), and Naturopathic Public Awareness Campaign (NPAC). He has also spoken at numerous open house events and taught classes at the Southwest College of Naturopathic Medicine, Arizona State University, and Rio Salado College. As well, he has been the keynote speaker on alternative cancer therapies at various breast health awareness events, which are held yearly at Del E. Webb Banner Hospital in Sun City, Arizona.

Dr. Brown is an expert in immunotherapy and naturopathic therapies for cancer and other chronic diseases. His approach is integrative, and he believes that it's important to see cancer patients as people who need to be treated in a holistic manner. His naturopathic therapies may be utilized to complement a conventional treatment protocol, or used as standalone therapies, for those who don't want to undergo chemotherapy, surgery, or radiation.

Dr. Brown has more to offer to his patients than just knowledge and expertise in integrative oncology; he offers them his personal experience of having battled cancer. In 1998, Dr. Brown was diagnosed with stage three/four melanoma. After receiving extensive therapy in conventional medicine, he was told that his prognosis was grim, and that he only had three or four weeks to live. Through the use of naturopathic and integrative medicine, he was able to overcome that prognosis. Today, he has been in remission for over fourteen years. Dr. Joe Brown's full cancer story can be viewed on the Internet at: www.youtube.com/watch?v=4c8BeNpgyvs.

Dr. Brown chose to go to a naturopathic medical school instead of conventional medical school because when he had cancer, it was naturopathic treatments that saved his life, and he believed that he would be able to effectively help more people if he had a naturopathic background rather than a conventional medical background. Conventional medicine most often utilizes only pharmaceutical drugs to treat patients, and these drugs, by themselves, are rarely adequate for treating cancer.

Although not required as part of his training, during his third and fourth years in medical school, Dr. Brown took it upon himself to work clinical rotations in hospitals, emergency rooms, and hematology, oncology and radiation clinics. Here, he worked with some of the country's top oncologists and saw cancer patients on a daily basis, learning the best of conventional medicine. This experience, along with his education in naturopathic medicine, has equipped Dr. Brown to offer his patients knowledge of both conventional and naturopathic cancer treatments.

Additionally, because of the time that Dr. Brown spent in a conventional oncology environment, he has been able to build relationships with many oncologists and clinics. These relationships allow him to help his patients more effectively, and not only because he can refer them to a good oncologist if they need one. His work and collaboration with these clinics has provided him with a deeper understanding of conventional medicine and how to better help patients who are simultaneously undergoing oncology treatments.

Dr. Brown's quest and passion to make a difference in others' lives led him to open his own clinic in Tempe, Arizona in 2006, where all of his patients, even those who are simultaneously treated with chemotherapy and/or radiation, can receive a variety of naturopathic therapies. He formulates his protocols to be compatible with his patients' oncology treatments, so they don't have to worry about potential treatment interactions and can receive the best of both worlds.

Dr. Brown has received numerous awards for his work, including the Princeton's Top Doctors award in 2008 and 2009, Good Morning America's Spirit award in 2008, and the Hero Award on 104.7 FM Radio Phoenix, AZ. He was also named among the 2008 Who's Who of Physicians. Additionally, he is a senior advisory board member for Valley of the Sun Wellness Institute (VSWI), a nonprofit organization designed to help people get free medical care.

Dr. Brown donates much of his time to the Melonhead Foundation, an organization that helps families that have children with cancer. He also donates his time and clinical services throughout the year to various people and causes, and frequently lectures around the United States on different topics, including dendritic T-cell and immune system stimulation, and lifestyle choices that lead to cancer. He also actively shares his own battle with cancer and how he overcame it. Recently, he has been asked to continue lecturing at Del E. Webb Hospital Cancer Center in Sun City, Arizona and Rio Salado College in Phoenix, Arizona, due to the overwhelmingly high attendance at his previous lectures. Dr. Joe Brown is the only naturopath who has ever been asked to lecture at a Banner hospital (a non-profit hospital, of which there are seventeen in the United States) on cancer and other medical topics.

My Personal Experience with Cancer and How It Has Affected How I Treat Patients

I was once a cancer patient who had no idea what to do after conventional medicine failed me. When I had cancer, like nearly every patient who calls my office, I was frightened. Because I have suffered the trials of cancer firsthand, I can relate to my patients' suffering. A lot of people come to me because they know that I have already walked in their shoes.

After conventional medicine failed me, I experimented with different therapies to figure out what would heal me. I tried everything under the sun: I did acupuncture and juicing regimens, and I called clinics everywhere, trying everything that they had to offer. I spent many months researching what to do and what not to do. When I finally figured out a protocol that worked, I realized that there were no clinics in the United States that were collectively doing all of these treatments. So when I opened my clinic, I wanted to make sure that we could offer all of these same therapies to our patients under one roof. I also wanted to have connections with oncologists so that I would be able to tell my patients which specialist to see if they needed radiation or chemotherapy, because even though conventional medicine failed me, there are times when it's appropriate. I wanted to have everything figured out for my patients, so that when they came to my clinic, I could simply say, "Here, call this number. I have personally worked with this oncologist for years. He's my friend and colleague, and his treatments, along with mine, are the best choice for you." I have found that being able to do these things makes such a difference for my patients. Hundreds of them have said things like, "Thanks so much for creating a ten-page protocol for me. You told me exactly what supplements to take. You have relationships with oncologists that other doctors don't have. You have hotels and shuttles arranged for my visit. You have the whole picture laid out for me, and it has made such a difference."

My personal experience with cancer has made me passionate about helping others. I spend more time than the average doctor with my patients. When they come in for an initial consultation, I try to arrange for them to spend two minutes in the waiting room and then two to four hours with me in the visit, instead of spending two hours waiting for me and then two minutes in the visit. Most doctors are too busy for this long of a consultation, because they are dealing with insurance companies and seeing fifty patients a day. It's not that doctors don't care about their patients—they are just too busy to spend much time with them due to the way the medical system is set up in the United States. Fortunately, I have found a way to run my practice so that my patients can spend ample time with me and get the proper care that they deserve and need.

It's important for me to fully listen to my patients and connect with them, not only on a professional level, but also on a personal, mental, and emotional level. I want to be available to them. My main office line is actually my cell phone (we have back office land lines as well) because I always want my patients to be able to get in touch with me if they need anything. When I was going through my own cancer treatments, I had seizures and convulsions, and my family and I couldn't get in touch with doctors or nurses in moments when I desperately needed them. So in my own practice, I decided to make myself available to my patients, so that they would be able to reach me anytime during the day or night, seven days a week, including holidays. When people go through cancer, it's serious, and they feel more at ease if they know that their doctors are available. If my patients have a problem and they call me, I am often able to meet them at my office, sometimes saving them a trip to the emergency room where they would have spent hours waiting to see an on-call physician. My patients come first!

I help my patients in other ways, too. Because many of our patients (30-40 percent) fly in from other states and countries, I have established contracts with many hotels and casinos in town. When people call my office, we can offer them information on the best places to stay, as well as set them up at hotels with suites that cost less than a full-priced standard hotel room. We also have a contract with a shuttle company that picks people up from the airport and takes them to and from their appointments free of charge. My patients tell me that these things make all the difference for them and their families. Because in reality, it's not just the patients that are suffering; it's their families, too. The whole family is crying, stressed, and concerned, and I have discovered that the more "little things" I can do for my patients and their families, to support them and help plan their treatments, the better the experience for everyone involved.

Additionally, my staff and I often work weekends, because we have patients who are only able to do therapies on the weekend, and we also have many out-of-state or out-of-country patients who fly in to see us. We accommodate their travel itineraries, which don't always allow for them to get treatment during the week.

How Naturopathy Benefits Patients

At any given time, we may have 50 percent of our patients doing both conventional and naturopathic therapies, and another 50 percent doing just naturopathic therapies. Not all choose to receive conventional treatments from an oncologist. A large percentage of them have already done conventional treatments including surgery, chemotherapy, and radiation, and have come to our clinic because conventional medicine failed them, and they are looking for a last-ditch effort to save their lives. Fortunately, over the past several years, more people have been choosing to do natural cancer therapies first. Increasingly, patients will say to me, "I got diagnosed last week, and I heard about you and want to start therapy with you before I meet with my oncologist." It's important to get the word out, and let people know that there are other options besides chemotherapy and radiation.

Treatment outcomes are radically different between patients that do only chemotherapy and radiation, and those that combine these treatments with naturopathic medicine. In fact, many oncologists now refer their patients to my office because they notice that their patients fare much better with their conventional treatments when they do them in conjunction with naturopathic medicine. People that do only conventional treatments look and feel terrible: they have low red blood cell counts, are anemic, and suffer from neutropenia (low white blood cell counts, which play a key role in fighting cancer). They also have elevated liver enzymes and low platelet counts, which usually stops them at some point from continuing their chemotherapy.

People who do naturopathic therapies along with conventional treatments can usually avoid these types of problems. Because naturopathic medicine provides them with the nutrients that they need to fight disease, they feel better and have a greater ability to tolerate treatments. Also, the color of their skin remains good, and most importantly, their ability to fight the cancer increases dramatically.

What Cancer Is and What Causes It

Everybody has cancer cells turning over in their bodies every single day, but whether or not they actually get cancer boils down to one factor: the strength of their immune systems, and what they are doing correctly and incorrectly. My patients get sick of me talking about the immune system all the time, but by the time they leave here, and after having received two months of treatment, they understand the importance of keeping their immune systems strong. And if they are able to do that with diet, exercise, supplements and nutrition, the chances of them getting sick from cancer or another disease down the road becomes slim.

The body is amazing; it's set up to heal itself if given the proper nutrition. In the United States, the role of diet is being greatly overlooked in the fight against disease. I recommend that every one of my patients see a documentary called *Food, Inc.,* because it demonstrates some of the bad things that are happening to our food supply. It shows, for instance, how our food is laden with hormones, antibiotics, herbicides, and pesticides, all of which destroy the body and drastically affect health. It also discusses how our foods have been genetically modified, which I believe is part of why people are becoming sick now, more than ever, and our cancer rates have sky-rocketed.

Modifications in the food supply have also caused many hormonal imbalances in people, and those imbalances can also contribute to cancer development. Soy, for example, has been put into many products, so people are eating soy in practically everything, and soy increases the body's production of estrogen. Women already tend to have excessive amounts of estrogen, which is due, most likely, to all of the xenoestrogens in the environment, which come from industrial compounds and pollutants. These also have estrogenic effects upon the body. Consuming soy exacerbates the problem. Women with high levels of estrogen are more prone to breast and ovarian cancer.

Xenoestrogens are found in many consumer products, as well. Plastic water bottles are one source. The plastic from bottles leaches into the water and then people consume it. Also, most bottled water is acidic, and acidity contributes to the development of disease. Studies have shown that plastics are directly linked to the development of breast cancer.

Emotional stress also plays a role in cancer development. During my patients' initial visits, I give them a therapy sheet. One suggestion on the sheet is: "I want you to find something every single day that brings you back to the calm from the storm. Don't think about cancer and treatments. For two or three hours a day, relax. Do something that takes your mind off of disease—find the calm within the storm." I think this is important for healing.

In summary, cancer is caused by many things, including poor immune system function, environmental toxicity, emotional stress, and a poor diet. Ultimately, a strong immune system is what matters most in preventing and beating cancer, and all of the aforementioned factors affect immune function.

Treatment Approach

My therapy program consists of three components. The first is a complete, ten-page diet protocol which outlines the foods that patients should and shouldn't eat. The diet is tailored specifically to people with cancer. Its main goal is to alkalinize the body and remove substances which cause cancer cells to grow. The second part of my program involves giving my patients pharmaceutical-grade nutritional supplements that feed the body antioxidants, vitamins, and amino acids, and increase white blood cell activity. The third, and most important, component involves administering intravenous and injectable substances to the body to boost immune system function. The main reason why people come to my clinic is to do these high-dose intravenous therapies and injections.

Depending upon their specific needs, my patients may receive therapy for anywhere from a few days to six to eight weeks, for three to five days per week. The duration and timing of these therapies depends upon factors such as patients' schedules and those of their conventional doctors, other treatments that they do outside of our office, their lab test results, and whether or not they are also receiving chemotherapy and/or radiation.

Dietary Recommendations

As previously mentioned, part of my diet manual for patients contains a list of foods that they should avoid. These include table sugar, salt, dairy products, wheat, and red meat. The manual also contains a list of alkaline foods that I encourage them to eat, as well as a variety of different juicing protocols and alkalinizing agents, such as alkaline water ionizers.

Consuming alkaline foods is important because many studies show that cancer cells feed on sugar and have a hard time surviving in an alkaline environment. Many cancer books discuss the importance of an alkaline diet. We drink alkaline water at our clinic and provide our patients with alkaline water that has a pH of 9.5. The higher we can push our patients' pH to bring it into an alkaline state, the better. The premise behind my therapy plan is that if I can increase my patients' white blood cell counts, boost their immune systems, and put them on an alkaline diet, then their white blood cells and immune systems will be able to overcome and effectively fight their diseases.

Finally, my diet protocol also includes information on organic labels that are put on fruits and vegetables in the grocery store. These are to help patients identify the right types of foods to eat so that they know whether they are purchasing healthy, true organic foods, without pesticides, herbicides, and other harmful additives.

Pharmaceutical-Grade Supplements

I also prescribe my patients a regimen of pharmaceutical-grade quality supplements (which can only be purchased by health care practitioners) to which they must strictly adhere. I often recommend that they take nine or ten different oral supplements, in addition to the nutrients that they receive intravenously. These supplements are used to boost immune function, alkalinize the body, cleanse the liver and colon, and provide additional nutritional support. The combination of supplements may include vitamins, minerals, herbs, amino acids, and mushroom formulas (the latter of which are used to boost white blood cell counts). Some of the pharmaceutical grade supplements that I prescribe are products that I have manufactured for my patients and are made specifically for people with cancer.

Immune-Boosting IVs

The immune-boosting intravenous substances that we use depend upon what each patient needs. My average patient receives five or six different intravenous preparations daily, which may include all of the following:

a. high-dose vitamins

b. minerals

c. anti-inflammatory substances

d. amino acids

e. herbal and homeopathic remedies

f. hydrogen peroxide

g. other immune-boosting therapeutic elements

All of these treatments are designed to super-saturate the body with nutritional substances that increase white blood cell counts and boost immunity. They are also designed to eliminate toxins from the body, which also improves immune function.

Follow-Up and Maintenance Treatments

When patients see that their scans and blood tests are normal for the first time, they tend to think, *I'm cured, so why do I need to continue doing therapy?* However, just because we get a clear scan back, doesn't mean that patients are done with their therapies. It just means that they are moving in the right direction. PET, CT, and MRI scans are fairly accurate, but they can still only pick up certain sized images, which means that some cancer cells may still be present in the body and are simply not being detected by the scans.

I once had a patient with late stage colon cancer whose scans came back normal. Because of this, he believed that he was done with his treatments and that he didn't need to come back for maintenance therapy. He didn't follow up with me or his oncologist after receiving the results of his first PET scan and so quit his treatment protocol. He went back to his old, unhealthy diet. Unfortunately, somewhere in his body, he still had microscopic cancer cells that the tests didn't pick up; those cancer cells spread and now he has widespread metastatic disease.

The term "remission" means that there is no more cancer that doctors can find in the body. Here in the United States, doctors aren't allowed to use the term "cancer free" with their patients. I haven't had cancer for over fourteen years, and would say that I am cancer free, but I can't legally say that to patients. I have to tell them that I'm in remission, due to the legalities involved in saying "cancer free."

Once my patients are considered to be in remission, I usually put them on a maintenance regimen for a few months and then carefully monitor them over the next couple of years. I do periodic scans and follow up from time to time with their oncologists. They get PET and CT scans and blood work done every few months for a while, and eventually get tested less often.

I try to make sure that my patients understand that the maintenance care that I provide is of utmost importance. Such care might involve them coming to my clinic twice a month for nutritional IVs or lab tests, or so that I can talk with them about their progress. I always follow up with my patients for months, even years, after they complete their therapies.

While patients are receiving their initial IV's at my clinic, I teach them about preventative care, maintenance, nutritional, and other supplemental therapies that they should continue to do for the rest of their lives, after they have completed their therapy with me. If they attain remission, it's important that they not return to the same lifestyle that caused them to get cancer in the first place.

Anyone who sees me quickly realizes that I am a very hands-on type of doctor. I do more frequent physical exams and lab tests than the average doctor. I often call my patients after they complete their therapies, and will even go to their houses to see how they are doing on a particular day.

Expected Treatment Outcomes for People with Late-Stage Cancers

Treatment outcomes vary for people who have terminal cancers. Again, most people don't visit a naturopath until they have a stage three or four cancer and conventional medicine has failed them, or they are in hospice. In all the years that I have been studying and practicing medicine, I have only seen a handful of people come to my clinic with stage one or two cancers, because most don't know about the benefits of naturopathic medicine when they are first diagnosed. Their choice of treatment is, by default, usually based on the standard American healthcare system. After patients go to their primary care physicians, they are referred to oncologists who participate in their insurance plans. It's as if they are led down this "dot to dot" path, according to their insurance plan, and when that path doesn't work, they show up at my door, two years later. By the time they get to me, they are usually in a later stage of disease. This is one major problem with our health care system: patients don't know the treatment options that are available to them, and if they do, their insurance plans don't pay for many of those treatments. I spend a lot of my free time lecturing and trying to spread the word that chemotherapy and radiation aren't the only types of cancer treatment available in medicine.

Despite these challenges, and even if patients are in the later stages of disease, I am often able to significantly extend the length and quality of their lives. I never know how well they are going to do, though, because I'm not God. I just try to do my best, with the understanding that God has given me. The bottom line is that people tend to do better if they pursue naturopathic therapy, and the sooner they do so, the better. Naturopathic treatments reduce their symptoms and pain; increase their lifespan, or both.

Everyone responds differently to therapy, though. For instance, about two years ago, I saw two breast cancer patients who were in a similar condition and stage of disease. I put them on the exact same regimen. One began to respond to the therapies within four to five weeks, but the other needed a few months to reach the same point in her healing. People respond differently to my therapies because everyone has a unique biochemical make-up.

Factors That Affect Treatment Outcomes

If patients have low white blood cell counts, and/or nutrient deficiencies, if their hemoglobin and hematocrit levels are low, and if they are so severely anemic that they need a blood transfusion, this can negatively affect their treatment outcome, as will their failure to comply with a treatment regimen. Sometimes, it's the small things, when taken collectively, that make the biggest difference. But if I could narrow it down to just one thing that affects treatment outcomes, more than anything, it would be the timing of patients' treatments. The sooner that people can get to my clinic following a cancer diagnosis, the better off that they will be! If they wait until the very end (after having failed conventional treatments), as most do—simply because they don't know that other options are available to them—then their chances for a full recovery are lessened. The sooner that they get the right information, and get started on good naturopathic treatments, the more likely they are to have a favorable outcome. Knowledge is power.

Roadblocks to Healing

The biggest roadblock to healing from cancer is the conventional medical system and the fact that insurance and pharmaceutical companies in the United States have limited people's access to alternative health care. Sometimes chemotherapy, radiation, and surgery are the most effective cancer treatments, but not always, and oncologists have been taught that these are the only and best ways to treat cancer. Sometimes, these therapies are the worst thing for patients. For example, even conventional research shows that giving stage four patients chemotherapy won't improve their long-term survival or prognoses because they are already immune-compromised. Yet in our society, doctors often give late-stage cancer patients chemotherapy, because it's the only treatment that conventional medicine has to offer.

In conventional medical school, students are taught that as doctors, they are supposed to figure out what their patients' symptoms are, treat those symptoms with a drug, and then see them periodically for follow-up visits. I know a lot of conventional medical doctors who believe in nutritional supplementation, the importance of a healthy diet, and other alternative approaches to healing, but who will not recommend such treatments to their patients out of fear of punishment by the American Medical Association (AMA) and associated governmental organizations. One oncologist in my area, who works with about six to eight other oncologists, has been practicing oncology for twenty-five or thirty years. He's a very smart doctor, but when patients go to see him, he tells them that all of the "naturopathic stuff" is garbage. He tells them that it won't affect their healing and that they shouldn't waste their time with it. What he doesn't say is that he is a vegetarian, takes pharmaceutical-grade supplements, and even receives intravenous nutrition from my clinic. Why won't he be honest with them? The answer is simple: because he could lose his medical license! Some conventional doctors will "come out of the box" a little by referring their patients to my office, but they won't make specific nutritional recommendations to their patients because they will get ostracized by other MDs, and possibly get in trouble with the AMA.

My Biggest Challenge as a Practitioner

My biggest challenge as a practitioner is making people with cancer aware of the fact that there are other, sometimes better, options for treating their diseases besides chemotherapy and radiation. Another challenge is getting naturopathic medicine integrated into mainstream medicine. In the United States, the medical system is set up such that primary care physicians only refer their patients to specialists who are covered under their patients' insurance plans. These are never doctors of naturopathy. One of my goals is to get naturopaths completely integrated into the medical and insurance systems. I also want my name, phone number, and website to be located in places where people with cancer can readily access them. I want it to be as easy for people with cancer to find me as it is for them to find a McDonald's sign. This isn't for my personal gain, but so that if someone gets cancer they can just look up and say, "There's Doctor Joe!" I want it to be that easy for them to find me. I want them to know who I am, because if they are desperately seeking help, like I once was, it will be easier if they know where to go for that help.

Problems with the Conventional Medical System and Conventional Cancer Treatments

Chemotherapy, while at times appropriate, can be dangerous, because it weakens the immune system, lowers hemoglobin levels, and causes anemia, neutropenia, and other harmful side effects. It makes no sense for patients to do chemotherapy when they are so fatigued and weak that they become more at risk of dying from their chemotherapy than from their cancers, but I often see doctors administering chemotherapy to patients in that condition.

For instance, not too long ago, I had a patient from Washington who was doing well until his oncologist had him do another round of chemotherapy. Two days following his treatment, he ended up in the hospital for a blood transfusion because the treatment was so harsh that it almost killed him. He then asked my opinion about whether he should do another round of chemotherapy, because he didn't want another transfusion, and I advised him to speak with his oncologist. Fortunately, his oncologist told him that he was wary about giving him another round of therapy. Some patients may be forced to pull the plug on their chemotherapy because it can weaken them to the point of death. It is, after all, comprised of toxic chemicals, and people can only tolerate so much of it.

In a perfect world, patients would get a chemotherapy sensitivity test when they are first diagnosed with cancer, to determine their cancers' sensitivity to specific drugs. In the real world, however, it's as if doctors are more or less saying to their patients: "You have breast cancer. We're going to give you this drug, because it's the standard. If it doesn't work, then we'll try another. If that doesn't work, then we'll try a third."

The problem is, if patients have metastatic cancer (which is most of them), doctors can't just surgically take a piece of their tumors and test them to discover which chemotherapy drugs they would best respond to, because surgery is contraindicated in people with metastatic disease. Doctors could end up spreading their patients' cancers in the process. Instead, they end up going from one drug to the next, starting with the one that seems to work best for a majority. Also, after a surgeon removes a tumor (before the patient starts chemotherapy or radiation), there are still usually some cancer cells that are left behind. But after the patient has had surgery, it's too late to do chemotherapy testing, because the tumor from which a sample could have been taken has already been removed and disposed of. So ideally, patients should get their surgeons to take a sample of their tumors to be sent off to a lab for chemo sensitivity testing, immediately following surgery.

Also, too many patients are being funneled into doctors' offices on a daily basis, and doctors don't have the time to adequately care for them. Doctors have to see increasingly more patients because insurance companies aren't paying them enough for the time and treatments that they provide. So they cram more and more patients into the short slots of time that they have available for patient visits, which means that they don't spend enough time with each patient. Their offices are getting so jam-packed, that some literally end up seeing over one hundred cancer patients a day! And no matter how smart they are, if they are seeing one hundred patients daily, they are going to get behind on their work. It creates a situation where patients may have to wait two to four hours just to see their doctor for two minutes. Their visit with the oncologist mostly consists of the oncologist quickly looking at their lab results, writing a prescription and saying to them, "See you in six months." And because oncologists can only spend two minutes with their patients, they miss things in their patients' profiles. Some of my good friends are among the best oncologists in the country, and while they are some of the smartest people I know, the truth is, they are so overworked that they can't keep up with all of their patients' needs.

Some radiation and chemotherapy oncologists have told me that it makes them sad that they have to treat their patients in this manner. Some have said that they can't stand their work and that if they had to do it all over again, they wouldn't go into medicine at all. But they went to school for ten to fifteen years, and have hundreds of thousands of dollars of debt to pay off from medical school, so they can't just stop practicing medicine. Sadly, they are also 100 percent controlled by drug companies. From the time that they enter medical school until graduation, they are taught that drugs are the answer to everything. And because conventional medicine has such poor outcomes with many types of cancers, this doesn't make their lives any easier. What's more, they aren't allowed to prescribe much else, because the laws which govern the practice of medicine have been influenced, in great measure, by drug lobbyists. Much of what happens in medicine is pharmaceutically-driven.

When I was in my third year of medical school, I worked rotations with the chief oncologist of a hospital. His office was huge, and during the first three weeks that I was there, there was no place for me to sit, because he always had pharmaceutical representatives lined up outside of his door, waiting to come in and show him their latest products, and to give him free tote bags or tickets to dinner or a show. His office was full of gifts from pharmaceutical representatives. The influence of drug companies and the way that insurance companies are set up have created tremendous problems for patient care in the United States.

What Patients Can Do if They Can't Afford Treatments

The therapies at my office aren't cheap, and I am one of few doctors in the United States who uses them on a regular basis. It costs me a lot of money to purchase some of the materials that I use in my practice, because only a handful of companies manufacture them, so these companies can charge more for them. These high costs are then passed down to my patients. Sadly, most people who see me have already been to their primary care physicians and oncologists and have spent a lot of money, which is unfortunate. The fact that insurance companies don't cover much of what I do doesn't help patients, either. That said, money shouldn't be a reason for people to not call my office, because I always do what I can to help others and adapt our protocol to those who can't afford all of our therapies. I was once in a situation where paying for therapy was difficult, so I understand the financial challenges that patients go through. I want people to understand that my protocols aren't an "all or nothing" deal. If they call me directly, I will work with them to get them going on some therapies that will benefit them and which they can afford.

Most people who come to my clinic don't have a lot of money, and can only do some of the recommended therapies; perhaps only six or eight of ten. I allow them to do whatever therapies they can afford, and sometimes, just doing a few of them is sufficient. For instance, I once had a patient with ovarian cancer who was given four to six months to live. She has now been alive for nearly nine years. This lady didn't have a lot of money for therapies, so she only did two out of the ten that I recommended to her, and she is still here, nine years later. As a general rule, though, the more therapies that my patients can do, the better off they are likely to be. But just because they can't afford all of what we offer here, doesn't mean that they should just turn around, leave my clinic, and be sad. I will try to find ways to help them. Switching insurance companies can sometimes be helpful. Cigna offers the best insurance coverage, by far, for naturopathic therapies. It pays for 70 percent of what we do at our clinic. If an IV costs one hundred dollars, a person with Cigna insurance will usually only pay thirty dollars for that IV. I have also heard of an insurance company in Colorado that covers 100 percent of naturopathic doctor services, but I don't know its name.

How Friends and Family Can Support Their Loved Ones with Cancer

While patients are doing their IV therapies, I often speak to their friends or family members who have accompanied them to their appointments, and offer them words of wisdom about how to best support them. Families and friends don't always know what they are doing wrong and what they are doing right in these situations. Since I have suffered through cancer personally and worked with patients for years now, I feel that I can give them a few helpful pointers.

For instance, when I was going through cancer, my mom was my biggest support. Her approach to helping me was direct and to the point. She said, "We're going to do these treatments. You are going to get better, and that's just the way it's going to be. We're going to do this and not look back. So let's go!" There was no other alternative in her mind, and her positive attitude was something that I needed at the time.

What wasn't helpful to me was when a friend of mine "disappeared" after my diagnosis. Later, after I was well, he said to me, "I'm sorry that I wasn't there for you. I didn't know what to say or do or how to support you. It was easier to not be there." That was his way of dealing with my situation, but it would have been better for me if he had tried to support me somehow. If friends or family are unsure of what do, the best thing that they can do is simply ask their loved ones what they need.

I offer these types of insights to the friends and families of those with cancer. I want to do as much as I can for my patients, because I don't want them to have to go through what I went through when I had cancer. Because emotional support is so important for patients, I also work with a couple of foundations here in Arizona which are dedicated to providing emotional support, education, and hope to people with cancer and their families.

Last Words

If you are suffering from cancer, know that there are good treatment options besides chemotherapy and radiation, such as the naturopathic care that I offer at my clinic. If you're interested in what I do, get here sooner rather than later. Don't wait until nothing works before you knock on my door or call me. I'm here to help you. I answer my phone 24 hours a day, 7 days a week, because I want to be there for you. Don't wait until the last minute when you need a miracle.

Also, understand that you aren't coming to see some naturopathic "voodoo" doctor who works with candles in his office. My approach is an intelligent, integrative one that worked for me and which has worked for others. If you need naturopathic therapy, I can help you, but if you prefer to do chemotherapy and radiation as well, I can refer you to a good oncologist. I have worked with oncologists and know many good ones; some are even my good friends. If I think that chemotherapy, radiation, or surgery is the best choice for you, I will be the first to refer you to an oncologist, so that you may receive the treatment that you need.

Many people have said that they come to my clinic because they know that I have walked in their shoes and will be able to relate to them. They also come because they have called clinics from here to Germany, and have found that I am one of the few naturopathic doctors whose true emphasis is on cancer and cancer support. I have established relationships with doctors, and not just those that are within the conventional oncology world, but with others, as well. I know dermatologists, surgeons, and physicians from many other medical specialties and my connections with them are all for one purpose—to help you to recover.

Contact Information
Joe Brown, NMD

Natural Health Medical Centers, P.L.L.C.
2055 E. Southern Ave, Suite B
Tempe, Arizona 85282
Phone: (602) 421-2613
Back phone line: (480) 456-8600

Note: Dr. Joe's back line is only answered during business hours.
www.DrJoeBrown.com (patient testimonials available on website)
Email questions to: CancerAlternatives@DrJoeBrown.com

Dr. Joe Brown's full cancer story on YouTube.com:
www.youtube.com/watch?v=4c8BeNpgyvs

Note: All opinions above are the doctor and editor's only. No comments should be taken as treatment advice for any condition without first consulting your acting physician. All people respond differently to treatments. No results are typical of any therapy. It is always recommended that you see your physician before beginning any treatment regimen. The opinions expressed herein are merely opinion and don't represent any one individual nor do they imply any therapy for any condition. These statements have not been approved by the FDA or the AMA.

• CHAPTER 13 •

Keith Scott-Mumby, MD, MB, ChB, PhD
RENO, NV

Biography

While I don't currently practice medicine as a licensed physician in the United States, I was one of the leading practitioners in the UK for over 35 years. I had several treatment centers, including one on Harley Street in Central London. Early on, word of my success in treating patients with cancer and other ailments quickly spread, and I had many thousands of patients who would come to see me from all over the world, some as far afield as New Zealand and Hong Kong. Many of these were cancer sufferers, who did extraordinarily well when I prescribed them simple lifestyle modifications: most notably a hypoallergenic diet and chemical detoxification protocol, which enabled their immune systems to better fight their cancers.

Since my time in the UK, I have become internationally recognized for my work in cancer control and immune system restoration. I have continued to advise patients worldwide on effective cancer treatments and have many who, after following my treatments, have shown no signs of declining health and who have been able to live well and for a long time with their cancers. Through my websites, blogs, and digital books, I have remained on the cutting-edge of the most effective cancer treatment breakthroughs.

I sincerely believe that cancer is a disease which doesn't deserve the fearsome reputation that has been accorded it; that most of what is horrible about cancer is the misery of brutal orthodox treatment rather than the disease itself. I have always believed that the number one cause of death is ignorance, and that if people knew more about their bodies and health issues, 95 percent of all diseases in the world would simply vanish. As a society, aging and health are within our control and we can't afford to simply submit ourselves to the so-called medical practitioners, because doctors aren't trained in health, only disease. By the time people with cancer call them for an appointment, it's often too late for effective remedies to be of benefit to them, anyway. But if the sick are willing to take charge and make changes to their lifestyles, recovery is always possible, because nature has designed the body to heal itself.

My interest in alternative medicine dates back to my time in medical school. During my first few years there, I believed in using drugs for treating cancer and other diseases, but after awhile, my perspective changed. I saw that things weren't working out as they should in conventional medicine, and that the promise of a chemical or drug to treat disease wasn't holding up. Too many people remained ill, and I observed that those who were taking drugs to be well had to take them indefinitely. If a person has to continue to take a drug in order to be well, then by definition, the drug doesn't work. If drugs work, people's health conditions should clear up and they should be able to stop their medicines at some point. My ruthless definition of a cure is: no symptoms remaining, no ongoing treatment necessary. If people have to take drugs for the rest of their lives, that's not a cure.

While in medical school, I also had a very romantic idea about what practicing medicine should look like, but in actuality, it turned out to be different than what I thought. It was very rough and unkind. So I quit my classes for three years to study natural medicine. I did end up going back to medical school after that because I wanted to be properly certified in medicine so that I could treat people's health problems. In London, doctors are required to get two degrees in medicine: a Bachelor's in Medicine and Bachelor's in Surgery. Once I became a properly trained medical doctor and surgeon in Britain, I promptly left the system again, to pursue naturopathic and alternative methods of healing. (Author's note: In some countries, such as Britain and Ireland, the qualifying degree to practice medicine isn't called a Doctor of Medicine, as in the United States. Instead, it's called the Bachelor of Science in Medicine, Bachelor of Medicine or Bachelor of Surgery, and is considered the equivalent of an MD degree in the United States system).

In my early years as a doctor, I pursued areas of medicine which were at the time considered to be radical: I learned about food allergies, environmental and chemical contamination, and other aspects of alternative medicine. Today everybody knows about this stuff, but thirty years ago, few people did, so I was called a quack. Indeed, in those times, conventional doctors referred to my knowledge about food allergies as "Mumby Jumbo!" Within ten years, however, mainstream specialist physicians were sending their wives to my clinic, and by the end of the following decade, these same specialists were showing up to see me themselves! By the end of the 1990s, the British National Health Service began ordering my treatment formulas. So I went from being considered a quack to being highly respected, in about twenty years. That's fast in medicine.

Getting into alternative medicine was the best thing that I could have done. I took more pleasure in my work and had more time to spend with my patients: on average, two hours per visit. Doctors must get to know their patients. This is the only proper way to practice medicine.

During my first years as a doctor, I was quite a pioneer in the field of alternative medicine, and I made world medical history in 1987, when a United Kingdom crime court accepted my belief that food allergies could make a person murderously violent. This came about as the result of a case in which an Irish boy tried to strangle someone and the judge assigned him to me for an evaluation, and I discovered that he had a major food allergy—to potatoes! This boy also had allergies to a couple of other foods, including beets and strawberries, which, as it turned out, were responsible for his violent behavior. His story was shown worldwide on Prime TV, and it was a big deal. He was given a conditional discharge from jail, provided he followed my diet. During that time, I was often interviewed on television, and I later discovered that the judge of this boy's case had tuned into one of my interviews and seen the types of treatments that I do.

Treatment Approach

My clinical practice in England was based upon three important components, which I called the Three Pillars of Healing. These involved nutrition, chemical clean-up (detoxification) and alternative psychology.

Pillar of Healing #1: Nutrition

My nutritional protocol for my patients was based upon a concept called nutrition by subtraction, which involves getting rid of foods in the diet that are contributing to symptoms. I found that subtracting harmful foods from my patients' diets was more important than focusing upon adding in the right ones, because most people are hurt by what they ingest, not by what they don't. So I would test them for food allergies using an inter-dermal testing technique called Miller's method. This method, otherwise known as intra-dermal neutralization therapy, was named after Joseph Miller of Alabama, who developed it. It involves either injecting food extracts under the skin or giving food extract drops under the tongue to determine food allergies. If the body doesn't react to a particular extract, it produces a small, raised bump on the skin known as a "wheal." If the body does react, the wheal that's produced takes on a characteristic appearance; it becomes white, hard and raised with a sharp edge. Also, the patient may experience symptoms similar to those normally produced by the food. The second part of the technique involves finding the specific concentration of the food allergen extract that will "turn off" symptoms, and then re-injecting that extract back into the patient. How it turns off symptoms is somewhat unknown, but it's thought to stimulate immune suppressor cells, which reduce the immune system's response to the offending allergenic food.

This test provided me with in-depth insights into my patients' physiologies. I would give them a shot of an allergen in the arm, such as wheat, and observe wheals grow rapidly on their skin in reaction to that substance. Often, they would also get symptoms as a result of the shots, and by those, I would know they were allergic to the food extracts that I had injected. Then, I would give them multiple injections of the extract, each one continually weaker than the previous one, until the opposite reaction occurred: a type of "switch off" effect that would turn off their symptoms. I would then use that dose therapeutically to treat their allergies.

I found all kinds of food allergies in my patients using this method, and constructed their diets upon the basis of the results that I got from this testing. I found that taking into consideration their specific type of cancer wasn't critical for determining an appropriate diet. Rather, it was the status of their immune system and removing anything that burdened that system, which mattered. There's no faster way to unburden the immune system than to remove inflammatory and allergenic foods from the diet. If there's one thing that I learned while in medical practice, it was the extent to which the wrong foods can destroy the body. To realize how significant food allergy reactions could be in cancer development was an eye-opener for me.

Pillar of Healing #2: Chemical Cleanup

When I started out in practice, I was one of the first doctors in the UK to mention how important it is for people to remove chemical contaminants from their environments in order to heal from cancer and other diseases. In a book that I wrote on this subject in 1986, entitled: *Allergies*: *What Everyone Should Know,* I introduced the term human canaries. (Author's note: Canaries were once regularly used in coal mining as an early warning system. Toxic gases such as carbon monoxide and methane in the mine would kill the bird before affecting the miners. Hence, the phrase "canary in a coal mine" is frequently used today to refer to a person or thing which serves as an early warning of a coming crisis). There are human canaries all around us, showing us, through their environmental illnesses, how we are being poisoned. So I came up with ways that people could eradicate chemicals from their home and work environments, as well as simple tests that they could do to detect those contaminants. One such test was called "the nose survey," which basically meant that if they could smell a chemical, then it could make them ill.

I wasn't able to do lab tests at my clinic to determine whether or not my patients were allergic to specific environmental chemicals, but if I took a careful medical history on them, they would end up telling me, either deliberately or inadvertently, what their chemical allergies were, and to what degree they were sensitive to those chemicals. For instance, if I discovered that they felt bad on Monday mornings, this meant that the chemicals that they were allergic to were coming from their office or work environments. If they felt poorly on the weekends, but fine in the office, then another set of chemicals outside of the workplace was causing them problems. I have learned a lot about medicine just by listening to my patients.

I would then tell them to throw away everything in their homes that they suspected were causing their allergies: solvents, plastics, air fresheners, household cleaners and that type of thing. If they didn't want to do this, I would tell them to put the substances into a plastic bag, seal that bag tight and put it at the back of the garage to see if they observed any changes in the way that they felt.

Women need to understand that cosmetics are lethal. Statistics have shown that the average woman absorbs around two pounds of cosmetics through her skin every year, which her liver then has to process. When I was in practice, I noticed that whenever my patients stopped using makeup, their blood test results would change for the better, and they would feel better, too—as a result of doing this one thing alone!

If my patients had high levels of liver enzymes (which indicate liver stress), and I could get those to come down through dietary and chemical clean-up recommendations, then their cancer markers would also improve. The liver is a major clean-up organ and when it's clean, the body can more effectively fight cancer. The liver gets so beat up; it's constantly getting rid of chemicals and food toxins, so anything that people with cancer can do to reduce their livers' burden will help them to heal. If they can reduce their bodies' toxic load, nature will fix their bodies.

Pillar of Healing #3: Alternative Psychology

I have spent a lot of time studying alternative psychology, which encompasses a number of highly effective techniques for healing disease that's related to trauma. Such techniques include: NLP (Neuro-Linguistic Programming), Virginia Satir's Conjoint Family Therapy, Transactional Analysis, and Robert Assagioli's Transpersonal Psychology.

A few years ago, I learned about a patented voice machine, called the Vo-Cal 360 (short for Voice Calibration), which can be used to release emotional trauma in cancer patients and thereby facilitate their healing. The Vo-Cal 360 and its more modern counterpart, the Vo-Cal II, function by detecting subconscious trauma that has been stored in the body and which is indicated through the person's voice. The results are then displayed on a computer screen as a "voice map" which reveals areas of unprocessed emotional trauma in the body and how people's relationships with different family members have impacted their DNA. Often, the disease imprints that people have in their DNA come from their grandfathers or grandmothers, which means that emotional trauma and its impact upon the DNA can be passed down from several generations.

Sophisticated software then analyzes the voice map and outputs the ideal energetic frequencies to release the trauma that has been stored in the DNA. People have experienced permanent and measurable results because of this therapy, including complete healing from different diseases.

A lady that I know of who had a brain tumor went to see Calvin Young, the developer of the Vo-Cal machine. He told her that he didn't know if the machine could help her but she wanted to try it out, anyway. She hadn't done chemotherapy or any conventional treatments. When the machine played the energetic pattern of her voice back to her, she burst into tears, and within minutes, she was wringing her hands, as pain began to course her hands and wrists. A childhood abuse memory had risen to the surface of her mind, and in it, she had been stripped and strapped to a table and abused by a bunch of adults in the forest—and that's what caused her brain tumor! But the memory had been repressed and didn't emerge until her session with this machine, when she was in her 40s. After her experience with the machine, she decided that the abuse memory had been the reason for her cancer. Sure enough, she was right, and the tumor went away.

The Vo-Cal 360 actually detects patterns in the voice, and uses those patterns to heal trauma. If people speak about their mothers, a certain audio frequency pattern emerges; if they talk about their fathers, a different audio frequency pattern appears. Just speaking about someone produces a unique voice pattern, and when these voice patterns are replayed to the person who spoke them, it encourages the psyche to push the trauma associated with that person to the surface. The energetic imprint of the trauma is present in the person's voice, so the woman with the brain tumor, for instance, carried her abuser's pattern in her voice throughout her entire life. But it wasn't until her voice pattern was played back to her that the memory of the abuse was driven to the surface of her mind.

New voice patterns emerge every time a trauma is processed, and patients keep speaking new voice patterns until their abusers' imprints don't show up in their speech anymore. Once the traumas have been processed, their voices actually sound different. Healing through the Vo-Cal 360 isn't just about recognizing specific traumas, though; it's about releasing them on an energetic level.

Traumas can be buried deep in the mind and body. I once had a patient who was doing the Gerson protocol. She came to me for nutritional IVs, and went into total remission as a result of these therapies, but she also had emotional problems, and I told her that she had to deal with those if she wanted to stay in remission. She didn't take my advice, thinking the Gerson therapy and my IV treatments to be sufficient, but the end, they weren't, and she passed away. If people with cancer don't address their emotional traumas, they leave themselves open to a recurrence of disease.

There are other ways of processing trauma, and people need to take an inventory of their personal histories to discover what they are carrying around from the past that might be contributing to their cancers. Hypnotism is another way to heal trauma in alternative psychology.

I don't have faith in just talking with a therapist. I think that if people just keep rehashing their personal stories with a therapist, over and over again for years, then it just reaffirms those stories in their minds, making them heavy, real, and difficult to leave behind. It's not good to be constantly reminded of traumatic past experiences.

Support groups can be helpful for some people. Scientific evidence has demonstrated that people with cancer who are involved in support groups have much better outcomes than those who aren't. On average, they live twice as long. People need to be with others who are sympathetic and with whom they can talk about their struggles. It's not always best, for instance, for women with breast cancer to talk about their feelings with their husbands, because they are too close to them. It may be easier for them to talk to other women who have breast cancer.

Finally, it's important for people with cancer to be able to just say "no" to things that they don't like, and "yes" to things that they do like. Many studies have been done which demonstrate the benefits of assertiveness for those with cancer. The classic cancer patient is often characterized as the obedient, submissive wife who can't assert herself and who puts everyone else's needs above her own. So it can be helpful for such people to learn to say, "No, I don't want to do that," or, "Yes, I'm going to go on holiday (vacation), so you will have to cook for yourself." Assertive behavior increases survival dramatically. Assertive people don't feel crushed and hurt by life because they feel free to express themselves, so their immune systems aren't suppressed by others' burdens.

Summary

In summary, healing is about nutrition, cleansing the body of toxins, and dealing with emotional trauma. The number one anti-cancer remedy that I know of is detoxification, and getting every-thing that's toxic to the body, out of the body. The specific protocols that I would use in my practice to accomplish this were different for each of my patients. I can't say that all people should eliminate red meat from their diets, because some things work for some people, some of the time, but not everything works for everyone 100 per-cent of the time. If the body's stressors and toxic load are reduced, then the body will heal almost anything, including deadly melano-mas and pancreatic cancers. No matter how dangerous they are.

I have also used other strategies in my practice to treat cancer. These are described in the following sections.

Homotoxicology for Detoxification

Homotoxicology involves combining several homeopathic remedies together to make a single remedy. Such remedies stimulate chemi-cal and cellular detoxification and increase cellular energy. In the 1970s and 1980s, some doctors, including me, began to realize that you can have a great detoxification program in theory, but if the cells don't have the energy to throw out their toxins, then they will remain poisoned, and that's a huge barrier to healing. The cell can't detoxify unless it has energy. Many researchers and others who write about detoxification don't realize this.

Homotoxicology remedies consist of homeopathically-potentiated minerals and herbs. There can be 10-30 different constituents in a single mixture, all of which function to support a specific organ. For instance, Hepar Composition by Heel targets the liver, and a product called Cerebrum Composition aids in brain health. Burbur is used for bowel detoxification and Populus assists with kidney function. These are very dilute, gentle homotoxicology remedies which nudge the body along in its healing and I have observed amazing results in people who have used them. There are various ways of getting toxins out of the body, and I wish more practitioners in the United States used homotoxicology because of its effectiveness. Forty percent of doctors in Germany use homotoxicology remedies, but in the United States, it's still considered to be quackery, even though it works.

Herbs are also useful for detoxification. I'm not an herbal practitioner, but there are lots of good herbs that can be used for detoxifying the body, such as schizandra, global artichoke, and milk thistle, all of which are well-known in the medical community.

Although I preferred to administer homotoxicology formulas in my practice, I believe that many herbs are in the same league as complex homeopathy or homotoxicology for their ability to detoxify the body.

Finally, I discovered that administering intravenous Vitamin C, along with two or three homeopathic mixtures, would often produce dramatic results in my cancer patients. I would watch them become invigorated after these treatments, right before my very eyes. It was wonderful to see, and the positive, evidence-based results that I witnessed in my clinic—seeing people get rejuvenated after an IV, and continually improving with each subsequent IV treatment—were more meaningful to me than the results of any double-blind, randomized trials. These are commonly used in conventional medicine to prove the so-called positive effects of certain cancer treatments, but such tests often prove nothing.

Homotoxicology for Releasing Miasms

Homotoxicology remedies are also useful for releasing miasms, which are shadows, or non-cellular energetic imprints of disease, that get passed down from one generation to the next. The classic one which the founder of homeopathy, Samuel Hahnemann, discovered was called psora, which dates back to the Black Death. (The Black Death was one of the deadliest pandemics in history, peaking in Europe in the mid 1300s. It claimed between 30-60 percent of Europe's population). Today, some people still carry the energetic imprint of psora from their ancestors, and are influenced on an energetic level by it. Sycosis is another important miasm which is linked to gonorrhea, and a third is tuberculosis, which was a major problem in the 19th and 20th centuries. These were three of the most important miasms which Hahnemann discovered and which have been carried forward from one generation to the next. These miasms continue to influence people today. People are exhausted and their immune function is low because of these miasms, so discovering and treating them can be very important. In general, tuberculosis is one of the more severe miasms that's commonly associated with cancer, but the most degenerative miasm is called luesinum (also known as syphilinum). It used to be a miasm that was associated with syphilis, and it has been with us for centuries. It was brought to America by Columbus and is characterized by tissue decay. Cancer is now a modern-day manifestation of that miasm. Other diseases, such as myotrophic lateral sclerosis (ALS) and multiple sclerosis (MS), can sometimes be traced back to this particular miasm.

Mistletoe

Ukrain, or mistletoe, is a remedy that I didn't use in my practice, but I believe that it's very useful for treating cancer. The science behind it makes sense to me and I know one doctor who has had great results using it on his cancer patients. It's a recognized form of natural chemotherapy that can keep people alive for years. When mixed with Chelidonium majus (giant celandine), it's especially powerful, because Chelidonium is one of the most potent anti-cancer herbs there is, and it has a long and honorable history of effectiveness. Furthermore, it's good for the liver, which is important, since the liver does half the job of healing the body.

How Naturopathic Treatments Benefit Those Who Do Chemotherapy

I didn't always tell my patients to avoid chemotherapy. I felt they should decide for themselves which therapies to do. I wouldn't want to do chemotherapy, personally, but I can say for certain that my therapies prevented chemotherapy from hurting my patients who also chose to do this type of treatment. During two decades of treating patients, not one of mine ever lost their hair from chemotherapy, as long as they also did my treatments. That's what alternative healing methods can do for people. I would tell my patients, "If you want to do chemotherapy, don't be scared of it. Just do something to stop it from hurting you." Everyone is scared of chemotherapy because their hair falls out, they get diarrhea, and their blood cell counts drop, but that doesn't have to happen if they take the right steps to prevent such reactions.

Patients who have done chemotherapy, along with my nutritional program, have often been able to survive terminal cancers. Of course, I lost some people, but doctors lose patients, no matter what they do. The most important thing that I could do for my chemotherapy patients was protect them from the harmful effects of their chemotherapy, mostly through intravenous infusions of 50 grams of Vitamin C, which I sometimes gave them daily, until their cancers turned around. Complex homeopathy was also useful for this purpose.

Treating Dental Problems

Treating dental problems, and not just root canals, is important for boosting immune function and therefore, for healing from cancer. Many adults with cancer have foci, which are pockets of infection in the mouth, from childhood. Dental foci are dangerous. People like to rave about how bad root canals are, but it isn't just root canals that are a problem. Tonsils can carry a certain energetic focus, much like the imprint of an old disease, which can linger in the body for years. Homeopathic remedies can address these foci. When I was in practice, tonsil problems would show up in my patients, time and time again, and I found that treating these problems also helped my patients to heal from their cancers.

Erasing the Harmful Effects of Vaccines

Childhood vaccinations are another problem which can complicate healing from cancer and are often the body's original insult that really upsets the immune system for life. The harmful effects of vaccines may not show up for 20-40 years, but homeopathic remedies can erase the effects of these, too. It's important for doctors to treat the whole person, not just the cancer, so that the person's immune system can more effectively fight the cancer. To do this, doctors must ask their patients what they were doing, ten or twenty years ago, and treat them for whatever previous insults might still be upsetting their bodies. The more that I learned about my patients and their histories, the easier it was for me to figure out how to help them.

Balancing the Hormones with Herbs and Homeopathic Remedies

Chemicals in the environment create hormonal imbalances in the body which then stimulate cancer development. This makes chemical clean-up around the home and workplace important. Hormonal imbalances are a stumbling block to healing from cancer.

The medical community knows that a large number of cancers are hormonally-influenced, but I don't like the hormone-blocking drugs that are commonly prescribed to people with these types of cancer; aromatase-inhibitors, and others, like Tamoxifen, because the science behind them isn't very good. One of the most effective estrogen-blocking herbs is called puerarin, which is from Thailand. It's sometimes jokingly referred to as HRT (Herbal Remedy from Thailand). It blocks natural estrogenic activity, and is three times more powerful than soy isoflavones. Breast cancer is unknown in the region of Thailand where puerarin grows, and studies from universities all around the world have demonstrated the powerful estrogenic properties of this herb. It functions by attaching to estrogen receptors on cancer cells, so that these receptors are blocked from receiving natural estrogen, but it doesn't have estrogenic effects upon the body. This herb has more solid science behind it than any other that I know of and can be used in lieu of hormone-blocking drugs in people with hormonally-influenced cancers.

One of the problems that men with prostate cancer face is estrogen excess. As part of men's aging process, testosterone gets increasingly metabolized into dihydrotestosterone (DHT), which isn't actually testosterone, but a type of estrogen, the effects of which can be blocked with puerarin. I know men who take this herb as a prophylaxis to block the effects of male estrogen in their bodies.

Looking at and addressing other hormone imbalances in the body with homeopathic and other remedies is likewise important. There's a strong association between thyroid insufficiency and cancer. Thyroid insufficiency impacts the immune system, and I would prescribe supplements, such as homeopathic thyroid extracts, which stimulate the thyroid gland, to my patients with this condition.

Similarly, people with cancer also suffer from adrenal exhaustion, which also impacts the immune system. Their adrenal glands can't cope with stress, but these glands play an important role in healing the body from cancer, so restoring them is important. I found homeopathic remedies such as phosphoric acid, argentum nitricum, and gelsemium, (just to name a few) to be useful for supporting weak adrenals.

Finally, pancreatic shock ranks high on the list of triggering factors for any disease, including cancer, so I would commonly prescribe my patients homeopathic pancreatic formulas for this problem, as well. I would also attempt to discover what disease processes were impacting their pancreases. Sometimes I would find old diseases, such as scarlet fever, that were still exerting an influence, like a shadow, over their organs. I would then prescribe them homeopathic remedies to remove that influence.

Treatment Outcomes

People used to come to my clinic because I had a reputation for being a successful nutrition and food allergy doctor, but people with cancer also came to see me because they heard about the good results that I had with others who had cancer. Many people's cancers would halt when I gave them the right nutritional substances. Some would survive for years, even decades, as a result of my treatments. Their tumors wouldn't always shrink, but they would live for years, without getting worse. Others would see their tumor markers decrease. I produced many cancer arrests in my patients, even in those with late stage cancers, just by addressing their nutrition and food allergies alone. Many with stage three and four cancers lived for many years past their initial diagnoses as a result of what I did for them.

While I saw many people with cancer, I never analyzed specifically what percentage of my overall practice consisted of cancer patients, because I didn't gather statistics based on the types of disease that my patients had. I did, however, keep statistics based on the results of different treatments, and those were remarkably consistent. About 50 percent of the people that I saw were cured and able to stop their treatments, including my cancer patients. Another 25 percent were much better off as a result of their treatments. Only for a remaining 25 percent did none of my treatments seem to greatly impact their symptoms.

Considerations When Searching for a Cancer Doctor

People with cancer should seek out doctors who understand the power of nutrition, and who give it its proper place at the top of the list in importance for treating cancer. They should also look for qualified physicians who can administer nutritional IVs, because IVs are a faster and more direct way to deliver nutrition to the body. When taken orally, nutrients are notorious for not being effectively absorbed by the body and the problem of absorption is eliminated with an IV. Also, finding a practitioner who understands homeopathy is a good idea, because homeopathy is a whole different philosophy about disease which really works. It's not just another alternative practice. Those that really understand homeopathy know how to drive disease out of the body. Cancer isn't an alien entity that drops into people from outer space; it's a part of them that has "gone wrong," and if they nurture and treat it properly, it will go back into being a "friendly" part of them. This approach is better than treating cancer as if it were the enemy, and blasting it to death with substances.

Ultimately, people need to decide for themselves what treatments they need. They shouldn't be terrorized into a choice. In general, I think it's wise to avoid chemotherapy. Ample evidence demonstrates that the results of chemotherapy aren't as good as what people are led to believe. There are safer alternatives now, anyway. I recommend that people give those a chance, even though some oncologists would prefer to scare their patients, and say things like, "You have to do this (therapy) now, or you will die!"—which isn't true. If they follow an alternative treatment course, it will give them time to think through their options, because at the very least, natural treatments will slow down the progression of their diseases. I always advise people with cancer to make their own decisions, but if they were to say to me, "I want you to tell me what you think is best," I would always tell them to go the alternative route, even if they are in the later stages of cancer. I can't tell you the number of people that I know of who have practically come back from the grave by using only natural treatments. It's not true that the more aggressive and serious the cancer, the more heroic the solution needs to be. I used to get patients who were at death's door, and often, just one homeopathic remedy would turn their situations around. Just because people have dangerous, severe, stage four cancers, doesn't mean that their cures won't be simple and straightforward. Often, the gentler the treatment, the better it is. Doctors need to be gentle with really sick patients if those patients are to heal.

Low-Cost Cancer Treatments

If you, the patient, entrust your life to a doctor, you should do what that doctor says. If you can't afford good help, don't take a fatalistic view about your disease. Instead, do something at home to treat it, starting with your diet. But if you do find reliable help, follow that doctor's advice to the letter. People who don't have much money to see doctors can do many important things on their own which will help them to heal. Following a good diet costs very little. Anyone can afford a twenty-dollar book on diet. There's a book on the Gerson approach that costs less than that. Nobody needs to die from cancer just because they don't have enough money to treat it. People can make juices and fresh food, and they can get rid of the chemicals in their homes. Even being able to cry on a friend's shoulder can make a difference. Homeopathy is cheap; the remedies cost three to five dollars.

Although lack of money shouldn't be a reason for people to not effectively treat their cancers, some people don't know which therapy is best for them, and will agonize over treatment decisions. It isn't possible to try every treatment. That's why, in my practice, I established three treatment pillars, because I considered these to be the most important aspects of cancer treatment. Outside of these pillars, I would leave it up to my patients to decide, through their feelings, intuition, or research, what types of treatments they most needed.

Ineffective Cancer Treatments

I don't like laetrile, which is also known as amygdalin and Vitamin B-17. This is a substance found naturally in some fruits and vegetables, particularly apricot pits and bitter almonds. The active anti-cancer ingredient in laetrile is cyanide, but I don't accept the evidence for its effectiveness. I think people are fooling themselves with this remedy.

One of the problems with alternative medicine is that people go on a program that has many components, along with laetrile, and they think that it's the laetrile that worked for them, when they really don't know. I want to ask those who boast of its benefits whether they have ever taken it by itself. Most likely, they did a bunch of other treatments too, and it was probably their diet and other therapies which helped them more than the laetrile. The clinical trials on it just didn't produce great results. No researcher has done a good enough trial on laetrile to convince me of its effectiveness.

Patient/Practitioner Challenges to Healing

The greatest challenge of treating cancer in the United States is the legal hassles that doctors face in this country. They can go to jail for practicing natural medicine. In Europe, doctors don't have to deal with this nonsense. For me, the single biggest challenge that I faced in treating cancer patients in the UK was family and friends interfering with my patients' choice of treatment. People would often come to my office, motivated and with sincere intentions to follow a protocol, but they wouldn't have any emotional support from their families. For instance, a wife might have refused to cook new, healthier foods which her husband needed to overcome his cancer. This lack of support was the single most important barrier to my patients' healing. If everyone in the family is on the "same page," and is emotionally supportive of the person with cancer, that person's cancer often becomes very treatable.

How Friends and Family Can Support Their Loved Ones with Cancer

Friends and family can best support their loved ones with cancer by keeping their emotions to themselves. When they constantly wring their hands and weep, this doesn't help the sick person. Also, joining in on some of the treatment protocols is one of the best things that they can do. Sometimes, couples go through a similar type of emotional cathartic healing when they do this; when they get on the same diet program as the person with cancer, for example. It's the best kind of sympathy and support that they could offer them.

New Developments in Conventional Medicine

Conventional therapy is getting better and smarter. Developments are being made with "smart bomb" cancer treatments. These are cancer drugs which selectively burrow into tumors and detonate lethal doses of anti-cancer toxins, while leaving healthy cells unscathed. These drugs work for some types of cancer. Ultraviolet light is another type of anti-cancer treatment that has recently been developed, which involves shining UV light directly upon the tumor. The light serves to activate the chemotherapy treatments inside the tumor. Yet another method uses nano-particle balls that heat up and shine infrared heat upon the tumor. There are many clever tricks like this which conventional medicine is developing, but so far, there are only four or five types of cancers for which the survival rate has increased dramatically as a result of their use.

Increasingly, conventional medicine is coming up with strategies that target the chemotherapy to the tumor, and which don't damage other cells in the body as much. There's also a prostate cancer vaccine that it has had good results with. This vaccine creates antibodies to a specific cancer antigen, so it attacks only the antigen, and consequently, only the tumor itself. This is exciting. Any treatment that works via the immune system is harnessing nature's own healing processes. I support such treatments and am pleased that conventional medicine is developing them.

Still, there are many cancers that conventional medicine hasn't been able to improve the statistics for, such as colon and breast cancer. Furthermore, in medicine, there's a lot of "statistics massaging" to get people to believe that the success rate of conventional treatments is higher than what it is really is. And the truth is that, overall, the story still isn't improving for many kinds of cancers.

Final Words

Cancer is a wake-up call but it's not a death knell. It's a message to people: "Your health is in ruins, so you must change some things in your life, but you don't have to die." It's a signal for them to change, which they must pay attention to. If they do this, they can obtain favorable outcomes with their healing. I have had patients who have made positive changes in their lives. They have pulled themselves out of a rut, and ended up in a wonderful place. So in this regard, cancer can be a blessing.

While I'm no longer actively practicing medicine, I do consultations, and can coach people about the treatments and doctors that they should see. Such consultations can be done through the following website: www.alternative-doctor.com/consult.

Contact Information
Keith Scott-Mumby, MD, MB, ChB, PhD

www.alternative-doctor.com
www.cancerconfidential.com
E-mail: keith.scottmumby@gmail.com

•CHAPTER 14•

Chad Aschtgen, ND, FABNO
SEATTLE, WA

Biography

Chad Aschtgen, ND, FABNO, is Board Certified in naturopathic oncology and specializes in integrative cancer care. He received his Doctorate of Naturopathic Medicine from Bastyr University in Seattle, Washington in 2005, and subsequently completed a two-year, hospital-based naturopathic medical residency at the Cancer Treatment Centers of America (CTCA), near Chicago, Illinois. Dr. Aschtgen returned to the Pacific Northwest in 2008 and has been providing integrative oncology services since then at the Institute of Complementary Medicine in Seattle and at Providence Western Washington Oncology in Olympia.

Dr. Aschtgen provides expert naturopathic care for people with cancer or to those who want to prevent cancer or who have a family history of cancer. His primary role is to provide supportive treatments to patients who are also receiving conventional oncology treatments, such as chemotherapy, radiation, and surgery. He utilizes nutrition and lifestyle counseling, herbal medicines, vitamin and mineral therapies, as well as other modalities to support optimal wellness in his patients before, during, and after they receive treatments with their oncologists. Whether newly diagnosed, undergoing conventional treatments, or long-term survivors of cancer, those facing the difficulties of cancer have a great resource in Dr. Aschtgen.

Dr. Aschtgen works closely with his patients to create unique, customized, integrative, and holistic treatment plans that take into consideration all aspects of their health and medical care. His patients receive safe and effective natural therapies that are specifically designed to improve overall health and well-being, decrease symptoms, and aid in fighting disease. Committed to patient-centered care, Dr. Aschtgen is available to communicate and coordinate treatments with other members of his patients' care team, including their families, medical and/or radiation oncologists, surgeons, cancer care managers, and other practitioners.

Dr. Aschtgen is an active member of numerous professional organizations, including the American Association of Naturopathic Physicians (AANP), American Society of Clinical Oncology (ASCO), Oncology Association of Naturopathic Physicians (OncANP), Society for Integrative Oncology (SIO), and the Washington Association of Naturopathic Physicians (WANP).

The Benefits of Integrative Medicine

Conventional oncology focuses on eradicating the body's tumor burden. Surgery is very successful at removing gross disease, while radiation and chemotherapy are variably effective at destroying and/or controlling macro and microscopic disease. However, none of these modalities focus on changing the underlying factors that caused the cancer to develop in the first place, nor do they discourage ongoing tumor cell activity.

Integrative cancer care, which may involve naturopathic, complementary, allopathic, and other types of medicine, focuses upon altering the underlying processes that lead to cancer development and progression. There are some people, such as those with inherited genetic mutations, for whom some of these underlying processes can't be altered. Fortunately, only a minority of patients fall into this category. The majority of people within the scientific and medical community contend that most cancer is caused by environmental factors, or exposures that are external to the body, and will therefore respond to treatments.

What Is FABNO?

FABNO is an acronym for Fellow of the American Board of Naturopathic Oncology. Naturopathic physicians who have successfully completed advanced post-graduate training with an accredited integrative oncology residency program, and have passed a rigorous evaluation, are eligible for board certification in Naturopathic Oncology. According to the Oncology Association of Naturopathic Physicians, "These physicians meet the highest standard of the profession as specialists in naturopathic oncology... and have demonstrated competence in both naturopathic and conventional medical oncology." Furthermore, the organization states, "Naturopathic oncology is the application of the art and science of naturopathic medicine to the field of cancer care and treatment. Naturopathic oncologists work both in hospital oncology settings and in private practices, bringing their wisdom, perspective and experience to aid oncology treatment teams that seek the best positive outcomes for their patients." Board certified naturopaths take into account the best current medical evidence when making decisions about how to optimally care for their patients. This is a complex balancing act in which they must consider the scientific research literature, established practice guidelines, their clinical experience, and individual patient needs and desires when establishing a treatment protocol.

How My Training Has Affected How I Treat Cancer

Because of my training, I have both a deeper understanding of and greater appreciation for the conventional medical approach to cancer care than if I had been a non-residency trained naturopathic doctor. During my two years of post-graduate training, not only did

I use my naturopathic tools of care to support patients, but day in and day out, I worked alongside numerous physicians: medical, radiation, and naturopathic oncologists; gastroenterologists and surgeons, and witnessed their work firsthand. Occasionally, I assisted with major surgical procedures, radiation planning, chemotherapy infusions and managing complex, sometimes emergency medical situations. In my first year of residency alone, I had the opportunity to meet, track, interact, and have case discussions about more than 2,000 cancer patients, so my training has been greatly augmented by my direct clinical experience with these patients.

I am grateful for this experience, and believe that I have a higher level of competency in treating patients because of my training and experience. I'm able to complement my patients' conventional treatments more effectively because I understand and appreciate them. I'm also able to better assess the compatibility between my treatments and those of the oncologist, and ensure that potential adverse interactions between them are minimized. In fact, combining oncology treatments with naturopathic treatments can be inappropriate at times, because there may be potential interactions between, for example, herbs or nutrients, and chemotherapy. Because of my understanding of oncology treatments, in certain situations, I am more conservative with treatments than some of my colleagues who aren't residency-trained. Conversely, in other situations, I am more aggressive with certain treatments than my colleagues who aren't Board Certified (FABNO) or residency-trained.

Unfortunately, not all naturopathic physicians have the opportunity to do post-graduate residency training, nor do most state licensing boards require naturopathic doctors to undergo this type of training. Although I suspected it was valuable, I now believe that it's crucial for naturopathic doctors to have extensive, advanced training in an oncology environment if they wish to competently support their cancer patients while they are undergoing conventional treatments.

There is evidence that conventional medicine helps many people with cancer, which is why I collaborate with oncologists in my work. But we (medical professionals) also know that other types of therapies such as nutrition, physical activity, sleep and stress management; herbal medicines, and vitamin and mineral therapies, can help patients. I use treatments that have the best track record for effectiveness, based on the following: clinical evidence, the known mechanisms of action behind the treatment, the patient's biochemistry, and my past experience of treating patients. While some of my decision-making is based upon the results of placebo-controlled clinical trials, this type of evidence isn't available for all of the treatment interventions I might consider. Furthermore, these trials don't allow me to effectively evaluate the entire body and all of its systems, which is what we do in naturopathic medicine.

In summary, as a physician of integrative medicine, my goal is to support my patients' health as they go through chemotherapy and radiation, while providing them with additional therapies that may have anti-cancer benefits. As well, I try to provide treatments that will prevent their cancers from recurring and which will increase their long-term survival.

What Cancer Is and What Causes It

I tell my patients that cancer occurs when a person's cells no longer perform optimally, and stop following the directions provided by the body's DNA instruction manual. Of course, this is an over-simplification of the process because the body is a complex organism. Cancer-causing processes are occurring all the time in everyone as a result of numerous factors. These include: DNA damage from radiation (both natural and man-made), pollution (or other toxic environmental substances, such as industrial solvents), normal oxidative stress, and ordinary mistakes in DNA replication during cell division (typically corrected by normal cellular processes). These factors sometimes allow or even cause cells to thrive unchecked, and to continue to grow and divide inappropriately.

Local and systemic inflammation, infection, and an excess of insulin or estrogen may also stimulate ongoing and unwarranted cell growth and division, which can then initiate other processes that may cause mutations of the DNA code. For example, in a healthy person, estrogen stimulates breast tissue growth, which is one of estrogen's normal functions. But when a person has breast tissue cells that have been injured and transformed into diseased or pre-cancerous cells, both naturally-occurring and foreign sources of estrogen can cause excessive cell growth and division, further damage cells, and lead to increased DNA mutations and eventually, tumor cell activity.

A healthy body is typically able to correct many of these processes through its own DNA repair and pre-programmed cell death (apoptosis) processes and the immune system's surveillance strategies, which allow it to identify and destroy abnormal cells, but the body has a limited ability to sustain ongoing injury. When the immune system is under stress from any of the aforementioned factors (e.g., excessive insulin or estrogen, inflammation, and infections) it may not be able to prevent the development of cancer.

Environmental factors such as exposure to industrial carcinogens, radiation from the sun, environmental pollutants, contaminated foods, and changing lifestyle patterns are thought to cause as many as 90 percent of all cancers. The foods that we eat and our daily activities have changed significantly over the past 100 years. For example, as a society, we consume less natural food than our ancestors and are also more sedentary. Both of these factors have increased our risk for developing cancer, among other chronic diseases, including heart disease, diabetes, and autoimmune conditions.

As previously mentioned, infections also play a role in cancer development. For example, the human papilloma virus (HPV) is known to increase the risk for developing squamous cell tissue cancers, especially of the uterine cervix, but it's not a straightforward relationship, because not everyone who has this virus will get cervical cancer, nor does everyone with cervical cancer have the HPV virus. Similar correlations have been found among other types of cancer and infections.

Treatment Approach

My overall treatment approach is to provide optimal integrative cancer care that supports the whole person through a customized and dynamic treatment program.

As mentioned in my biography, I typically work with patients that are either currently undergoing conventional treatment, or who have received it in the past. Many of my patients, as well as their referring physicians, view me as the physician team member who uses natural therapies to support patients while they are being treated and/or monitored for cancer by their oncologists. However, my services are more than just "complementary"; they are an integral part of each patient's care. I don't provide "alternative" cancer care. My experience is that people diagnosed with cancer are best served by utilizing every tool available to treat not only their cancers, but also their overall health.

I also work with patients who have been told by their medical doctors that they have cancer but don't need active treatment yet. They are instead undergoing active surveillance; a process some-times referred to as "watchful waiting" to see how their cancers develop. This includes patients who have slow-growing cancers, such as early-stage prostate cancer, or indolent follicular lympho-ma. My goal for such people is to provide health-promoting and disease-preventing techniques that will keep their cancers from progressing.

I categorize my treatment goals into four broad categories, which include: safely preventing and minimizing the adverse effects of anti-neoplastic therapies, managing symptoms, improving the body's terrain, and supporting patients' overall health. While the conventional approach to medicine essentially focuses on treating the organ or system where the disease is located, the naturopathic approach takes into account the entire body. In the following sections, I describe some of the therapies that I use to accomplish these goals.

Preventing and Minimizing the Adverse Effects of Anti-Neoplastic Therapies

How many and what types of adverse reactions or side effects patients suffer from depends upon their specific treatments. It's important for me to know every patient's oncology treatment plan in advance so that I know what to expect in each case, because, for example, the side effects of adjuvant radiation to the breast are much different than the effects of radiation to the brain. Radiation to the breast in a typical adjuvant setting (in which a tangential beam is targeted specifically at the residual breast tissue) avoids exposing internal organs to the potentially damaging effects of radiation. On the other hand, whole brain radiation is targeted at the central nervous system, and often more adversely affects the patient's quality of life. Women who undergo breast radiation treatments may experience short-term changes to their quality of life, including minor fatigue and mild skin changes, whereas patients who receive brain radiation can suffer from balance, memory, cognitive and central nervous system problems; profound fatigue and hearing loss. Of course, this doesn't always happen, and some people seem to tolerate brain radiation well. Nonetheless, it's important that doctors understand the potential side effects of different treatments so that they know how to best prevent and/or treat them.

Also, there are multiple types of therapeutic radiation methods, and each has different effects—and side effects—upon the body. For instance, proton therapy is different from electron therapy, and the effects of both differ from the more commonly used photon-based radiation. Radiation seed implant is a type of radiation that is frequently used for prostate cancer, which has its own unique side effects. Systemic radioisotope therapies, which are given for thyroid cancer or certain lymphomas, present an additional level of complexity when choosing the right treatments to minimize adverse effects. Since many of my patients are also treated by radiation oncologists, I must understand the differences among all types of radiation therapy, in order to provide them with safe and effective treatments.

We see a similar, often more complex scenario, with multi-drug chemotherapy regimens, especially because drugs can interact with herbs and nutrients. Interpreting the symptoms that result from treatments can be complex and complicated, given that there are hundreds of different chemotherapy agents and supportive medications, and patients all have different needs.

It would take days to mention all of the treatments that I use to treat the different side effects of chemotherapy and radiation. Over the course of three years, including during my clinical residency program, I created a clinical handbook which describes many of these treatments. This handbook is now being used in all of the residency programs for this specialty at the many Cancer Treatment Centers of America.

Managing Symptoms

Insomnia

Many people with cancer, whether or not they are undergoing treatment, have difficulty sleeping—for many reasons. I typically treat this symptom by first addressing my patients' sleep hygiene, because many simply don't spend a sufficient amount of time in bed to get the recommended seven to nine hours of sleep. Also, many don't sleep in a cool, dark, quiet environment, without dogs, cats and other disruptive factors. No amount of sleep medication will help patients to sleep better if they don't address these underlying sleep hygiene issues, which is why I start by teaching them about sleep management. Then I might prescribe them a sleep remedy to address the specific nature of their insomnia, which may be due to anxiety, pain, Restless Leg Syndrome, frequent nighttime urination, or using steroid drugs (such as dexamethasone or prednisone, which are often given to patients to help them tolerate chemotherapy drugs). One remedy that I often recommend is chamomile tea, but it must be covered and steeped for five to ten minutes; otherwise, its sedative properties evaporate up and out of the drink. Other remedies that I recommend include: magnesium, valerian, melatonin, or glycine. If the cause of insomnia is complex, I may refer my patients to an expert in sleep medicine, who can do a sleep study on them and recommend additional treatments.

Peripheral Neuropathy

Peripheral neuropathy, which is typically caused by damage to nerves of the peripheral nervous system, is a common side effect of chemotherapy and sometimes, radiation. Taxol and Taxotere are chemotherapy drugs that commonly cause tingling, pain, or numbness in the hands and feet, and it's difficult to make these symptoms go away; more difficult than to prevent in the first place.

For this condition, I often prescribe my patients ten grams of L-glutamine, three times daily, which is typically a safe and effective remedy. Although the medical literature indicates that L-glutamine is only moderately effective for treating neuropathy, I find that it works very well for many people.

Local cold therapy is also helpful for preventing neuropathy caused by taxane-based drugs. It's common for women who are going through adjuvant chemotherapy for breast cancer to undergo a twelve-week course of Taxol treatment. During their chemotherapy infusions, which typically last 60-90 minutes, I give them a stainless steel water bottle filled with cold water and a couple of ice cubes to hold in their hands. This cools their hands and reduces the blood flow to their fingers, thereby decreasing the leakage of chemotherapy into their peripheral tissues, where it has no benefit and damages nerve cells. Local cold therapy is remarkable for preventing peripheral neuropathy in both the hands and feet, and it's a free, simple, and effective treatment. As with many treatment interventions, however, local cold therapy isn't appropriate for everyone. For example, another chemotherapy drug called oxaliplatin, which is frequently used to treat colorectal and sometimes pancreatic or gastric cancers, causes neuropathy but also cold sensitivity, so I wouldn't recommend local cold therapy to patients who are receiving this drug. Other substances that I commonly use to treat peripheral neuropathy include Vitamin E and alpha-lipoic acid, which I prescribe at moderate to high doses, except during active chemotherapy or radiation, due to the potential for these substances to interact with the medications. Vitamin B-6 can also be helpful, and there are other substances that I use, as well.

Fatigue

For fatigue that's attributable to cardiovascular problems, I may prescribe Coenzyme Q10, which is necessary for energy production at the mitochondrial or cellular level. Many patients with cancer take statin drugs, which are intended to lower their cholesterol levels; however, they also inhibit the body's production of CoQ10, which is why it may be important to give such people CoQ10.

Nutrient deficiencies and other nutritional problems also contribute to fatigue. Patients with nausea, diarrhea, constipation, taste changes, and other symptoms may have difficulty getting enough calories into their bodies, and/or may struggle to maintain a well-rounded diet. Also, patients who have undergone surgeries that affect the digestive tract may have problems absorbing their nutrients and will often experience fatigue and other symptoms.

Depending upon the circumstances, I may recommend protein supplements to help my patients get adequate nutrition. Other substances that I prescribe for fatigue, depending upon the cause, include B vitamins, Ayurvedic formulas consisting of multiple herbs, and acetyl-L-carnitine. The latter is an amino acid that can cross the blood-brain barrier and also relieve symptoms of "chemo brain" or post-chemotherapy cognitive impairment, problems with memory recall, concentration and mental focus that may occur as a result of chemotherapy. I have found, through research and clinical experience, that higher, more beneficial concentrations of L-carnitine are best achieved when dosed in a powdered formulation.

If patients have diarrhea and fatigue, simply increasing their fluid intake can improve their energy levels. Ultimately, I don't have a simple algorithm that I use when prescribing therapies. I make recommendations based upon my patients' specific circumstances, their biochemistry (which is assessed through laboratory tests), and what's causing their symptoms.

Changing the Body's Internal Terrain

Changing the body's internal terrain to make it less hospitable or supportive of cancer cells is another one of my treatment goals. Doing this involves addressing all of the following in my patients: poor immune system function, nutrient deficiencies, inflammation, oxidative stress, insulin and glucose balance, hypercoagulation, and stress. Lab test results help to guide my clinical decision making in these areas.

Treating Inflammation

Erythrocyte sedimentation rate (ESR) and C-reactive protein (CRP) are two common markers (tests) that I commonly use to evaluate my patients for systemic inflammation. ESR is generally used to measure inflammation in people who have arthritis and some autoimmune diseases, while CRP is primarily used to measure inflammation that specifically affects the cardiovascular system. Elevated CRP may be suggestive of cardiovascular disease, but not always. These tests are also useful for indicating to what degree people with cancer have systemic inflammation. This is important to know because high levels of inflammation are sometimes associated with poor long-term treatment outcomes. A half-dozen other tests can reveal the presence of inflammation, but I rarely run the full panel of those tests on all of my patients.

I treat inflammation using various anti-inflammatory substances, which range from non-steroidal anti-inflammatory drugs to dietary supplements and herbal medications that are well-known for their anti-inflammatory properties. Such supplements include omega-3 fatty acids, curcumin, boswellia, and bromelain, among others.

Addressing Nutrient Deficiencies

Reviewing my patients' dietary habits can give me an idea of what their nutrient deficiencies are, although I may also order laboratory tests to help determine this. Vitamin D and omega-3 fatty acids are two common deficiencies that I find, so I frequently recommend supplementation with fish oil, flax seed oil, or other foods containing essential fatty acids. However, people with cancer must understand that no amount of a capsule product can make up for a terrible diet. It's difficult for me to justify prescribing a highly concentrated omega-3 fish oil product to my patients if they have a diet that consists entirely of fast and processed foods. Most patients reap greater benefits from changing their dietary and lifestyle habits than from taking multiple vitamin and mineral supplements.

Eliminating Oxidative Stress and Increasing the Body's Antioxidant Capacity

Some of the tests that I do to determine the body's levels of oxidative stress and its antioxidant capacity include: a lipid peroxide profile, oxidized LDL (low-density lipids), gamma-glutamyl transferase (a liver enzyme), ferritin, and blood levels of Coenzyme Q10. If my patients' test results are abnormal, I may prescribe them supplemental antioxidants such as Vitamin E or resveratrol, or work to increase their glutathione activity by providing them with glutathione precursors. There's much debate and disagreement among practitioners about whether antioxidants are safe to use during chemotherapy, but the answer isn't as simple as saying that all antioxidants interfere with chemotherapy or that all antioxidants are safe to use in combination with anti-cancer treatments. Neither is entirely correct because the issue is complex, so I evaluate my patients on an individual basis and then treat them accordingly.

Balancing Insulin and Glucose

I may also test my patients' fasting glucose, insulin, hemoglobin A1c and insulin-like growth factor levels, as well as others. Whenever any of these are abnormal, I recommend that they eat foods that will prevent them from having frequent blood sugar spikes after they eat. Unfortunately, blood sugar spikes (in which the body's blood sugar rapidly rises, causing it to release an excessive amount of insulin) are common in people who follow a standard American diet (SAD). Many of my patients need to change their eating habits, but they are often pleasantly surprised when they learn that I don't recommend that they follow a strict diet of "twigs and seeds." I also don't advocate that they follow any specific fad diet. Rather, I try to get them to maintain a well-balanced, whole-foods based diet that's mostly comprised of plants and small portions of animal products (primarily meat and eggs).

Treating Hypercoagulation

Many cancers increase the risk of developing blood clots. These need to be prevented and/or aggressively managed because the processes that lead to clotting, as well as some of the results of clotting, such as blood vessel injury, can cause cell signaling within the body that prompts tumor cell growth. I often test my patients' fibrinogen, homocysteine, D-dimer, and even vascular endothelial growth factor (VEGF) levels to determine whether hypercoagulation is present. Treatments for hypercoagulation include green tea, Nattokinase, and Coenzyme Q10, among others. High VEGF, which promotes new blood vessel growth, is treated with drugs like Avastin (bevacizumab).

Improving Immune Function

Some of the tests that we do to determine our patients' immune system status include natural killer cell (NK) activity, as well as white blood cell and absolute neutrophil counts. As well, we measure their Vitamin D levels. These are all important indicators of immune function. Interventions range from protein supplementation to the use of short-term, high-dose Vitamin D or medicinal mushroom extracts, such as coriolus, reishi, maitake, and agaricus.

Minimizing the processes that encourage cancer cell survival, growth and division, such as hypoxia (oxygen deprivation), cancer cell signaling and mitochondrial dysfunction, is also an important component of my treatment plan. Many clinicians and medical scientists are spending an increasing amount of time and financial resources studying each of these areas in a quest to improve cancer treatments and prevention strategies.

Physical Therapies

Physical therapy can benefit patients in their healing and help them to feel better. Treatments that I often recommend to my patients include simple forms of hydrotherapy, Epsom salt baths for muscle aches and pains, massage, acupuncture, and local cold treatments during chemotherapy infusions to prevent or minimize peripheral neuropathy. I don't do acupuncture myself, but I have a network of practitioners that I refer my patients to, who have extensive training and experience in working with people with cancer. Acupuncture is useful for alleviating symptoms, but I'm not aware of any data which suggests that it does anything to mitigate the underlying causes of cancer.

Dietary Recommendations

My dietary recommendations are based upon a whole foods diet. Although there are many good diets that can help people to improve their eating habits and general health, such as Dr. D'Adamo's Blood Type diet, the Mediterranean diet and the Paleolithic diet, I try to make good nutrition as simple as possible for my patients. I encourage them to consume whole foods, and to minimize/eliminate processed and fast food. Author Michael Pollan has some great ideas about healthy eating in his books, so I regularly recommend these to my patients.

I often emphasize many of the basic concepts upon which the US Department of Agriculture's Food Pyramid was founded. The Food Pyramid encourages the consumption of a wide variety of fruits (two to three pieces or cups/day), vegetables (three to four cups/day) and whole grains (two cups of cooked whole grains) per day.

People with cancer should avoid foods that are processed: anything in a box, bag, bottle, jar, or can should be considered as processed unless their ingredients labels show convincing evidence to the contrary. There are some exceptions to this guideline, as frozen fruits and vegetables are often considered 'whole foods,' even though they usually come packaged in bags. People with cancer should also minimize their consumption of animal products, including dairy. Meat and dairy should be hormone and antibiotic-free and primarily consumed as 'condiments.' It's also okay for people with cancer to freely consume wild-caught fish but they should avoid farmed fish entirely, because these fish have a higher incidence of disease, are genetically modified and often given antibiotics. Also, they are fed a non-native diet, and have potentially decreased omega-3 fatty acid content and increased contamination from polychlorinated bi-phenyls and other environmental pollutants, among other problems. Tropical fish, such as tuna and swordfish, should only be eaten in moderation. I also recommend high amounts of vegetables and fruits, green drinks, and omega-3 fatty acids (as mentioned above).

In America, it seems as though people have to be "alternative" or "counter-culture" to maintain a healthy lifestyle. Of course, this shouldn't be an earth-shattering revelation, as many studies have found that the average American is terribly deficient in essential nutrients, due to their consumption of poor quality foods.

Detoxification

I recommend that my patients eliminate as many toxic exposures as possible from their lives. This includes tobacco, alcohol, recreational and unnecessary prescription drugs, as well as toxic chemicals in the workplace and in the home. Such chemicals include solvents, paints, lubricants, petrochemicals, harsh cleaners, and typical anti-microbial agents (including bleach). There are many healthy, non-toxic alternatives out there, but many people don't take the time to learn about these products and their benefits.

I also recommend that my patients maximize their innate detoxification processes by consuming at least 64 ounces of clean, filtered water daily. Green leafy, cruciferous and root vegetables are also important, as are culinary herbs and spices, lots of garlic and onions, and mild teas that support liver and kidney function.

I don't advocate aggressive detoxification regimens involving colonic irrigation, fasting, frequent constitutional hydrotherapy and/or sauna therapy, while patients are undergoing active chemotherapy, radiation, and/or immediately before or after surgery. These types of detoxification procedures can deplete the body and are therefore contraindicated during active anti-neoplastic treatments. While they may be effective for removing toxins, they can also remove vital nutrients from the body that patients need in order to get through their oncology treatments. Furthermore, complex detoxification programs may compromise the effectiveness of chemotherapy or radiation.

I do, however, encourage gentle detoxification, because it's a critical component of healing, and detoxification is also a part of our body's normal physiological processes. So I try to support its inherent ways of doing that.

Some doctors prescribe heavy metal chelation to their cancer patients, but I find that metals are rarely my patients' principal concern. I don't do this type of treatment anyway when they are undergoing chemotherapy, because chelation involves drawing metals out of the tissues, which may increase the amount of metals that circulate throughout the body. This then creates neurological, cardiovascular, and digestive symptoms. I would be doing my patients a great disservice by exposing them to more mercury, because it would create too much of a toxic burden for their bodies.

I generally work with my patients to establish some type of detoxification protocol after they complete their chemotherapy, though as previously mentioned, it's usually a bad idea to do any type of aggressive detoxification protocol during chemotherapy, not just because of the excessive toxic burden that it could create for the body, but also because the goal of a detoxification protocol is to decrease some type of toxic substance in the body. Chemotherapy regimens are designed to deliver a certain amount of a toxic drug to the body over a period of time, and ideally, in a controlled environment. Detoxification would potentially decrease the amount of the active drug in the body, thereby limiting its effectiveness.

Therefore, my detoxification protocol during chemotherapy is basically geared towards maximizing the body's innate detoxification processes. We aren't "sweeping out the dust," but rather, helping the body to stimulate the removal of that dust. Fundamentally, I want to ensure that my patients receive adequate nutrition and fluids, and that they are physically active on a regular basis. I may also give them herbs such as milk thistle (in capsule, tea, or liquid form), or antioxidants that support their detoxification organs, especially the liver and kidneys.

Supporting the Hormones

It's important for me to address hormonal imbalances in my patients because, for example, high levels of insulin and estrogen can contribute to tumor cell activity, so any excess of these hormones needs to be treated. Hyperparathyroidism, which leads to excess serum calcium, is a rare condition, but can be exacerbated by cancer and conventional cancer treatments. It can lead to further calcium deregulation, so managing this condition is important, as well. If patients have other imbalances, such as hypothyroidism, I also evaluate and manage those.

Hypothyroidism is a common condition that develops as people age, especially in women. We don't know all of the causes behind it, but it seems to be somewhat related to declining health. It can also be caused by autoimmune disease. When patients suffer from an uncomplicated case of hypothyroidism related to aging, thyroid hormone supplementation may be appropriate. When it's related to autoimmune disease or cancer, treating the disease may be a better first step.

Sex hormones, like others, are complex in their biological function and should be respected as such. Many practitioners prescribe their patients estrogen, progesterone, and testosterone replacement therapies, without due regard for the potential long-term effects that these supplemental hormones may have upon the body. This isn't to say that patients can't benefit from this type of therapy, but it's a very complex area of medicine, so I don't focus much on estrogen or testosterone supplementation in my practice. However, I do test my patients' estrogen and testosterone levels, using blood and urine tests, whenever I suspect that these hormones might be affecting their cancers, and then balance them with herbs or medications.

Supporting the adrenal glands is also important for healing, although some practitioners believe that adrenal insufficiency doesn't even exist. The majority of naturopaths and many other doctors, including me, however, suspect that it does, and I believe that many people with cancer suffer from challenges to their overall adrenal function. I try to ensure that my patients have adequate nutrients to support their adrenals, such as Vitamin C and certain minerals. Many adaptogenic herbs are thought to support adrenal function, so I also use these frequently in my practice.

Finally, glucocorticoid steroid drugs, which are prescribed to many cancer patients, change the balance of the body's internal steroid hormones, especially cortisol. Corticosteroids can be difficult to assess and manage, and imbalances can negatively impact the body, especially with long-term use. Drugs like dexamethasone or prednisone, which are often given to help patients tolerate Taxol chemotherapy, can cause severe insomnia, anxiety, digestive problems, and even nausea and vomiting, so I treat these problems whenever they arise in my patients.

Hormone management is complex and complicated. I take a conservative approach to it, because hormones affect every tissue and organ system of the body. In general, I treat my patients' hormones depending upon their level of dysfunction and whether or not they are directly affecting their cancers. If patients have uncontrolled diabetes or other complex hormonal issues, though, they should be under the management of doctor skilled in insulin management, or an endocrinologist, not me. A naturopath in my practice focuses on this area, and I sometimes refer my patients to her, as well as to endocrinologists in Seattle or Olympia, Washington.

Lifestyle Recommendations for Healing

Adequate, appropriate nutrition, sleep, physical activity, and effective stress management are foundational for good health, so I address all of these areas in my patients. I may also recommend that they take dietary supplements to correct for any nutritional deficiencies and to support their overall health.

My exercise prescription depends upon my patients' circumstances, including their co-morbidities, or other health problems. Ideally, I recommend that they be physically active for at least 30-45 minutes per day, 4-5 days per week. The form and intensity of the exercise should be varied and tailored to their needs, and can include a combination of cardiovascular, stretching, and/or muscle strengthening techniques. I always recommend that they limit their physical activity if they experience increased fatigue and/or pain because of the activity. Their goals should be realistic, safe, and achievable.

I also generally recommend that they get seven to eight hours of sleep nightly, but these recommendations can vary widely. If they are taking corticosteroids, for instance, they may not be able to sleep for more than four to five hours at a time, anyway.

To help my patients with their mental health, I assess their stress levels and ability to manage that stress. I look at factors such as whether or not they have sleep disturbances and anxiety, whether they are interested in healthy life activities (work and/or social engagements), and whether they are supported by others in their healing process and lives.

How patients manage their stress doesn't matter, as long as the strategies that they use are effective for them. There are many ways to relieve stress, including psycho-social techniques such as counseling; physical strategies such as biofeedback, exercise, yoga, tai chi, etc.; social strategies, including support groups; spiritual strategies, such as meditation and religious activities, and, of course, symptom management, which I described earlier in this chapter.

I may also make recommendations for improving certain areas of their lives, in addition to prescribing remedies to alleviate the symptom-related aspects of their stress. For instance, I might encourage them to stop smoking or to avoid excessive alcohol consumption, especially during chemotherapy, and to lose weight if they are overweight or obese. They should consider cancer treatment as a full-time job, schedule other obligations and occupational responsibilities accordingly, and do additional activities only as they are able.

Treatment Considerations

Every patient is unique and requires an individualized treatment plan. I typically start off my patients' visits by asking them what their goals are in seeing me that day. This ensures that I am able to address the issues that are most important to them. I also learn a tremendous amount about them by doing this, which helps me to serve them beyond their initial goals and in ways that they may not have expected.

When determining a treatment regimen, I take into consideration their specific disease (including histological subtype, grade, stage, etc.), lab test results, and oncology treatment plan. I also consider their nutritional status and habits, their level of physical activity and/or ability to be productive, as well as any relevant physical limitations. Their food sensitivities, digestive problems, toxic environmental exposures and other major and minor health problems, are likewise important. Their finances and motivation to do treatments also play a role in my treatment recommendations, as do their lifestyle habits, including, for example, whether or not they smoke or drink excessive amounts of alcohol.

I also take into account family issues. It's common for me to see patients whose families are adamant about the supplements or dietary strategies that they think their loved ones should do. I try to serve as an expert reference for them and diffuse the stress that can arise between patients and spouses or other family members. I have at least one patient whose family member is a sales person for a multi-level or network marketing company that sells supplements, and this has created a difficult situation for the patient when she is trying to make treatment decisions, because the family member inadvertently pressures her into taking stuff that she doesn't want to take.

Additionally, I coordinate my patients' care with treatments that they receive from other providers. It's common for me to see patients on drugs that contraindicate other therapies, or patients who are continuing on prescription medicines that were initiated prior to their cancer diagnoses and which they no longer need. When this happens, I may contact their other doctors to find out whether they really need to be on those medications anymore. Or when they have co-morbid conditions, I may refer them to other practitioners for management of these conditions. For instance, sometimes patients' blood pressure is affected by chemotherapy, so I may need to refer them back to their family practitioners or to a cardiologist. Others may require the assistance of their primary care physicians or an endocrinologist to help them manage their anti-hyperglycemic or insulin medications. Basically, I work with a variety of other doctors, so my patients end up receiving the best care possible. I also routinely send a copy of their chart notes to their managing oncologists, to make sure that we are all on the same page, and to help them understand what my treatment recommendations are and why.

I try to be as helpful as possible to my patients without overwhelming them, because people with cancer are already overwhelmed as it is. For many, cancer treatment is a full time job and anything I can do to make those treatments easier and more efficient is usually appreciated. When I make a supplement recommendation, for instance, I tell them which brand and how much of that supplement to take, what time of day to take it, and where they can get it. I typically offer them three to four different options, so that they don't have to research the products themselves. Similarly, when recommending counselors and acupuncturists, I try to help them find providers who participate in their insurance plans and who have extensive experience in working with people with cancer. It's nice for patients to not have to do this research. We also help those who don't have financial resources for treatments to find organizations and/or people that provide this kind of support to those with cancer.

Treatment Outcomes

My treatments definitely provide my patients with a better quality of life than what they would have had if they had done conventional treatments alone. They are also effective for mitigating the side effects of chemotherapy and radiation. I would like to think that they extend their lifespan, and ensure them a disease-free life, as well, but this is difficult to ascertain without a prospective controlled study in which I could follow up with them long-term. Data on patient survival as a result of conventional oncology treatments are also lacking. Ultimately, I believe that people live better and survive longer because of my work.

Some people with terminal cancers who do integrative treatments live for years beyond their initial prognoses. But we also witness this in people who have presumably done just conventional treatments (the standard of care). Outcomes vary, based upon the stage and histological subtype of the disease, and patients' initial overall prognoses (which can be anywhere from a few months to several years or longer). My experience has been that people who utilize integrative treatments do far better than those who rely solely upon conventional treatments.

It's hard to track statistics for diseases like breast cancer, which is typically diagnosed earlier than other types of cancers. Outcomes for the early stages are favorable, and people tend to have fewer recurrences down the road. Many women who have breast cancer live for ten years without a recurrence, much less die from the disease, so it's something that takes decades to evaluate, compared to the more aggressive types of cancer.

I left CTCA three years ago and started my own practice here in Washington. Since that time, I have been treating a couple of patients with lung and metastatic pancreatic cancer, and so far, they are still alive. I don't know if their cases are unusual. We have statistics and data on certain treatments, which are relevant for a population, but not for individual people. This is because data is based on thousands of people that are all pooled together, and there are many individual factors which are not accounted for in these kinds of statistics.

I can make some well-educated guesses, and say that a person with advanced diabetes or who has a history of a stroke won't likely do as well as the person who doesn't have these types of health problems, and there is data which suggests that maintaining certain lifestyle habits matters. Studies have shown, for instance, that people with lung cancer who eat vegetables will survive longer than those who don't. Overweight women with breast cancer have a 30 percent increased likelihood of recurrence than those who are at a healthy body weight. People who don't drink alcohol do better with their treatments than those that do. People who exercise have fewer recurrences of aggressive breast cancer. We know that some of these individual factors matter, but part of the problem of trying to fit the naturopathic model into clinical research is that in most studies, only one factor is accounted for. And in my practice, I am usually changing ten different factors in my patients' day-to-day regimens, so it's hard to compare the absolute effectiveness of a single strategy from one patient to the next, much less do a large scale study with 400 patients where we change eight parameters of treatment, and then do another study where we alter a different set of parameters on 400 different patients, and then look at the data and say, "this is the outcome." It would be too expensive, time consuming, and logistically impossible. But taken independently, many of the tools that I utilize to treat my patients have proven to be beneficial, and their safety and effectiveness is supported by research data.

Roadblocks to Healing

Sometimes, my patients have really aggressive cancers and there's nothing that I, nor their oncologists, can do for them, so this is obviously a roadblock to healing. Social, financial, or motivational factors can also be roadblocks to healing: for instance, if patients don't follow a treatment protocol, refuse to change their diets, and/or keep smoking. While a lack of compliance can be a road-block to healing, I also firmly believe that it's difficult to be healthy in America. You have to be "counter-culture" to maintain a healthy diet. In cities like Boulder, Colorado where I did my undergraduate work, or Seattle, Washington, where I live now, it's easier to identify and obtain healthy food and more socially acceptable to eat healthy food. But outside of Seattle, in other parts of Washington, for instance, it's common for people to misunderstand what organic food is or not have easy access to that food. Also, our society values aggressive, unsustainable work habits, at the unfortunate cost of a person's health. We have to recognize this and take steps to recreate what it means to be healthy in the United States. I educate my patients on the value of things like a good diet, exercise, and sleep. Balance in all aspects of life is important.

What More Patients Should Understand When Researching Cancer Treatments

First, people with cancer should know that it's okay to get a second opinion when researching medical treatments. Every physician is a tool for helping them to heal. Also, it's important that they ask questions about their treatments: any and all that are meaningful to them. They should understand that the word 'cancer' includes many different diseases and when they hear or read things like, "Product X is good for cancer," know that the product may not be beneficial for their specific situation. Also, the quality of supplements that they take matters, often significantly.

People with cancer shouldn't wait until they have had a recurrence of cancer before they improve their dietary habits. They should begin working with a well-trained and experienced naturopathic physician or other integrative doctor as soon as possible. There's so much more available to cancer patients than just oncology treatments. From an outcomes perspective, I believe most people do much better if they incorporate naturopathic strategies into their lives sooner rather than later, along with a chemotherapy regimen. I don't think that a naturopath should be the only type of integrative provider that patients see, though. There are many other types of practitioners, such as integrative oncologists, who do the type of work that I do, in addition to conventional therapies, and who are good at what they do.

Resources for Low-Income Cancer Patients

Some hospitals and community organizations have financial assistance programs to help people who don't have the funds to pay for their treatments. For instance, I work with Providence St. Peter Hospital in Olympia, which has a foundation to help cancer patients. There's also a group here in Seattle called Cancer Lifeline. Their mission is to connect people with the resources that they need to heal from cancer, and this can include money for their treatments and living expenses. Thus, financial aid can come from places besides government and church organizations. Other resources exist, and I help my patients to find their way to those resources, whenever appropriate.

Fortunately, most of my patients' insurance plans pay for my services, because the state of Washington mandates insurance coverage for naturopathic physicians and many other types of health care providers, including medical doctors. Typically, insurance plans cover naturopathic care only in states that offer licensing in naturopathic medicine, although not all insurance companies pay for naturopathic care, regardless of the state. I also give a "time of service" discount to people who pay cash for their treatments, whenever they lack insurance benefits. This is considered to be industry standard. I believe that every practitioner should consider offering such discounts, so if people don't have insurance and need to pay for their treatments "out of pocket," they have an option to avoid paying the premium for services. I try to work with my patients to make cancer care affordable for them.

How Family and Friends Can Support Their Loved Ones with Cancer

Friends and family should listen to their loved ones with cancer, and learn to prioritize their needs over their own. They should also try to be patient, understanding, and forgiving.

Sometimes I have patients that come to me because they have been dragged here by family and friends. They don't necessarily have an interest in integrative or naturopathic care. They may be overwhelmed with other things. It's common for spouses to push nutrition on their husbands or wives with cancer, but their spouses might not be interested in good nutrition. Family members and caregivers want to be able to do something to help, and doing things like offering dietary suggestions gives them a sense of control and a way to help. Yet it's also important for them to listen to their loved ones, because trying to convince them to do something against their will can be a source of stress for them, which is the last thing they need while battling cancer.

I sometimes manage this stress relationship between family members, and end up becoming an authority that says to the patient, "If you want to have pizza tonight, that's okay. If you can't take 23 supplements today, that's okay. Let's back it up to just three capsules and next week, try to add in one or two more." Such suggestions can relieve the person with cancer, while also providing a sense of legitimacy to the spouse who is pushing for him or her to get on a better diet and take supplements. So I try to help friends and family to be as effective as possible in their roles as helpers. I am not a counselor but all health care practitioners provide some degree of counseling to their patients. Counseling is inherent in all practitioner-patient relationships.

Dangerous/Ineffective Cancer Treatments

The majority of medical interventions, whether conventional (standard of care) or otherwise, carry some degree of risk that needs to be weighed against the benefits in each patient's situation. Of course, all therapies have limitations, whether they involve conventional drugs, radiation, or natural medicine. It's important for patients to understand the potential benefits/risks that they might experience from different treatments, as well as the alternatives that are available.

Many ineffective and dangerous therapies are advertised on the Internet and described in seemingly authoritative books that are available at local markets. Ultimately, I recommend that people who are considering natural or complementary therapy consult with an expert before combining such therapies with their conventional oncology treatments.

Recommended Books/Websites

Following are books which contain more information on integrative cancer care, as well as on whole foods nutrition and recipes for those with cancer.

1. *Food Rules* or *In Defense of Food: An Eater's Manifesto* – Michael Pollen.

2. *Anti-Cancer: A New Way of Life* – David Servan-Schreiber, MD

3. *The Journey Through Cancer: An Oncologist's Seven-Level Program for Healing and Transforming the Whole Person* – Jeremy R. Geffen, MD

4. *Definitive Guide to Cancer: An Integrated Approach to Prevention, Treatment and Healing* – Lise N. Alschuler, ND & Karolyn A. Gazella

5. *Life Over Cancer: The Block Center Program for Integrative Cancer Treatment* – Keith I. Block, MD

6. *The Cancer Fighting Kitchen: Nourishing, Big-Flavor Recipes for Cancer Treatment and Recovery* – Rebecca Katz

7. *The Whole Life Nutrition Cookbook: Whole Foods Recipes for Personal and Planetary Health* – Alissa Segersten and Tom Malterre, MS

8. Also, see The Environmental Working Group website at www.EWG.org for additional information on organic versus conventionally-grown produce, as well as healthier home cleaning and personal care products.

9. Society of Integrative Oncology (SIO) - www.integrativeonc.org

10. Memorial Sloan Kettering Cancer Center: About Herbs, Botanicals and Other Products, www.mskcc.org/mskcc/html/11570.cfm

11. Oncologist-approved cancer information from the American Society of Clinical Oncology – www.cancer.net

Contact Information
Chad Aschtgen, ND

Institute of Complementary Medicine
1600 E. Jefferson, Suite 603
Seattle, WA 98122
Phone: (206) 726-0034
www.instituteofcomplementarymedicine.com

•CHAPTER 15•

Finn Skøtt Andersen, MD
HUMLEBÆK, DENMARK

Biography

Finn Skøtt Andersen, MD, has been the chief physician at Humle-gaarden cancer clinic since 1979. Founded in 1945, Humlegaarden is situated amidst idyllic surroundings in the small town of Hum-lebæk, just five miles south of Elsinore and approximately thirty miles north of Copenhagen, Denmark. Through his work with cancer patients, Dr. Andersen has become one of the most well-known and innovative cancer doctors in Scandinavia. He uses holistic methods for treating cancer, and has treated thousands of patients from all over the world during his thirty-two years at Humlegaarden. He has achieved exceptional results in his patients, especially in those with prostate cancer.

What Cancer Is and What Causes It

Describing cancer in just a few words is difficult, because cancer is actually many diseases, and several factors are implicated in their development. All human beings have small, dormant tumors in their bodies. These tumors are very little: perhaps no larger than a millimeter or two in size. Autopsies performed on the breasts of middle-aged women and the prostates of men (who died of other causes besides cancer) have revealed the presence of these dormant cancers. These little cancers are also commonly found in the thyroid gland. People can live with such small, dormant tumors for years without ever developing cancer.

The small dormant tumors can, however, start to produce growth factors such as platelet-derived growth factor (PDGF), vascular endothelial growth factor (VEGF), and fibroblast growth factor (FGF). These growth factors attach themselves to receptors on nearby blood vessel walls and induce biochemical processes that create new blood vessels, which then sprout out from the walls towards the dormant tumor. The sprouting vessels then grow into the tumor, thus enabling it to obtain oxygen and nutrients and grow at an accelerated rate. The production of new blood vessels from existing blood vessels is called angiogenesis.

What triggers a dormant tumor to start producing these growth factors at a certain point in time is an interesting question. Perhaps a dormant tumor may be triggered to start growing when all of the well-known cancer-promoting factors that we are exposed to in our lifetimes reach a "tipping point." However, our experience at Humlegaarden suggests that there is usually just one primary factor which finally triggers tumor development, which is different for everyone. If patients could discover this factor, and neutralize or eliminate it, their prognoses would be majorly impacted.

Emotional trauma may be the most relevant or important factor in the development of some cancers. Pancreatic and breast cancers are psychosomatic cancers, according to our experience, especially pancreatic cancer, which often occurs after an emotional shock. This shock can be a bankruptcy, a difficult divorce, or any traumatic event in a person's life. Some people have an "inner balance" which allows them to cope with even the most challenging life traumas, while others can't get them out of their systems. The energy of those traumas then accumulates in the solar plexus area of the body. Ancient Chinese doctors have said that cancers arise wherever a person has an accumulation, or overabundance, of Chi (energy) in a specific area of the body. Setting this excess energy into motion so that it leaves the body is important and necessary for treating psychosomatic cancers. Of course, environmental contamination also contributes to cancer, and there's no doubt that it has increased the incidence of cancer in recent years.

Cancer Treatments

Local Hyperthermia

Humlegaarden is known as a center of excellence for hyperthermia treatments. Since 1984, we have been the only clinic in Scandinavia that does these treatments on cancer patients, so we have obtained in-depth knowledge about how to treat cancer using this method.

We don't use a standard hyperthermia unit to do local hyperthermia treatments. Instead, we have been using an EHY-2000 OncoTherm machine for almost twenty years, which combines hyperthermia with electro-therapy. During this therapy, patients lie on a waterbed. A bolus electrode is positioned at the site where the patient is to be treated, and a counter electrode is positioned under the waterbed's mattress. A modulated electric field with a carrier frequency of 13.56 MHz is then generated by the two active electrodes, which each have a diameter of 17 cm.

Since malignant tissue has a higher electrical conductivity than healthy human tissue, the electric field flows predominantly through the malignant tumor tissue. The combination of deep layer heating and the electric field stimulates malignant tumor cells. This, in turn, triggers increased apoptosis activity in the tumor and cancer cell death. Compared with classic hyperthermia, which can burn the patient, a significantly lower temperature is used in oncothermia. Classic hyperthermia increases the body's temperature to 42 degrees Celsius (107.6 degrees Fahrenheit), but oncothermia achieves a greater effect in the body by only raising its temperature to 38 degrees Celsius (100.4 degrees).

Oncothermia selectively heats tumor tissue while leaving healthy tissue virtually untouched. For this reason, it's used primarily for treating localized solid tumors. It doesn't matter whether the tumors are located deep within the body or on its surface. Oncothermia also allows "mobile" areas of the body to be treated, such as the lungs or thermo-sensitive regions such as the brain. It's also effective in areas of the body where there is high blood flow, such as the liver, as well as in areas of high air circulation, such as the lungs.

In general, oncothermia can be used to treat all stages and types of cancer, although its principal use is for advanced solid tumors that are either barely operable or inoperable, or for recurrent tumors and metastases.

People can often be successfully treated with oncothermia whenever conventional therapy approaches such as surgery, chemotherapy, and radiation therapy have proven to be inadequate or are unlikely to be successful. It can be used on all of the following tumors, even if there are metastases in other organs of the body: astrocytomas and glioblastomas; bronchial, cervical, colorectal, hepotocellular, stomach, renal cell, esophageal, ovarian, pancreatic, head, breast, squamous epithelium, urethra, and throat carcinomas, as well as malignant melanomas.

Usually, we treat our patients using 13.56 MHz radio frequency waves, for an hour to an hour and a half, every other day. We recommend that they do ten treatments.

Whole Body Hyperthermia

A healthy body reacts to the threat of illness with regulated temperature increases. In acute cases of illness, these increases may progress, until the person has a high fever, which then triggers an enhanced immune response.

Body temperature plays a crucial role in immune system regulation. Fevers might be considered as a natural, temporary "special program" which the immune system is set up to follow at times. Accordingly, an artificially induced increase in body temperature can result in the sustained stimulation of otherwise inhibited powers of self-healing, even in cases of disease involving chronic or malignant processes.

Martin Heckel, MD, a German radiologist and doctor of internal medicine, has developed a cancer treatment method which involves irradiating the entire body in a heat-insulated treatment cabin with high intensity infrared rays, which are emitted from four 300-watt halogen wolfram lamps. The intensity of the treatment is adjusted individually for each patient, and for those who are able to tolerate it, a body temperature of more than 40° Celsius (104 degrees Fahrenheit) can be achieved.

Besides counteracting symptoms by stimulating the immune system, a controlled increase in body temperature can also influence faulty regulatory processes within the entire body, promote cell reparation and regeneration, and create sustained muscle relaxation, even in the deepest, most inaccessible muscle layers of the body. It enhances numerous immunological processes, especially lymphocyte migration to sites of inflammation and malignant processes, and increases the efficiency of various antibiotic and chemotherapeutic substances.

In 1996, we had a Norwegian patient with melanoma come into our clinic. He had suffered three recurrences of cancer to his lumbar and thoracic spine, as well as to his ribs and left hip (which had lesions). He had also had surgery, but within a year following his operation, bone metastases were found in his spine, ribs, femur, and pelvis. During the three weeks that he was at our clinic, he received weekly whole body hyperthermia treatments, in which we were able to raise his body temperature to 40-40.5° C (104-105.8 degrees Fahrenheit). He also received mistletoe injections. After he left our clinic, he continued with the mistletoe injections and returned to Humlegaarden on a yearly basis to receive whole body hyperthermia sessions. By 2002, we decided that he no longer needed treatments, but he continued to do mistletoe treatments on his own. Today, he is doing very well, and has never had a recurrence of cancer since his stay here.

Whole-body hyperthermia is a supportive therapy that can be combined synergistically with other therapies to treat cancer and other diseases.

HL (High Level) Whole Body Hyperthermia

We will soon be one of the first cancer facilities in Europe to use High Level Whole Body Hyperthermia, which is another efficient cancer treatment method whereby we raise the patient's body temperature to 43.5 - 44 °C (approximately 110-111.2 degrees Fahrenheit). Raising the body's temperature to this level kills cancer cells.

For the procedure, the patient is lowered into a 47 degree Celsius (116.6 degrees Fahrenheit) hot water bath, for just under an hour. This is done under the supervision of a team of doctors and nurses. Due to the very high temperature of the water, anesthesia is given to the patient prior to the treatment. After awhile, the patient's body temperature peaks to 43.4-44 degrees Celsuis (110-111.2 degrees Fahrenheit) for about six minutes, which is sufficient for adequately stimulating the immune system. High Level Whole Body Hyperthermia has been extensively tested, and clinical results show that patients don't suffer from any side effects from it, and neither have any resulting fatalities ever been reported. We are very encouraged about the results that other clinics have had so far with this new treatment, and are looking forward to implementing it here in Denmark in the near future. We will be the first clinic in Scandanavia to use it.

Low-Dose Metronomic Chemotherapy

Since 1970, global angiogenesis research has taken place at the Judah Folkman laboratories at the Dana-Farber Institute in Boston, MA, USA. A majority of the world's top angiogenesis researchers have been working here or in close connection with Judah Folkman, the medical doctor who first discovered that all cancer tumors are angiogenesis-dependent. (Angiogenesis is the creation of new blood vessels from existing blood vessels. These blood vessels are the most important way that cancer cells obtain their nutrition.) Dr. Folkman surmised that if a tumor could be stopped from growing its own blood supply, it would wither and die. Unfortunately, he died of a heart attack in January 2008 at Denver International Airport. He was 75 years old. Because of his untimely death, he didn't win the Nobel Prize in medicine, which he really deserved.

At Humlegaarden, we have acquired extensive knowledge about metronomic chemotherapy, a non-damaging chemotherapy treatment which cuts off the tumor's blood supply rather than destroying the tumor itself. It does this by destroying endothelial cells within the blood vessels that feed the cancer. While full-dose chemotherapy also destroys the endothelial cells which are in the small blood vessels, in the usual two to three week break that is given in-between chemotherapy sessions, these cells have time to grow and reestablish themselves, so that the blood vessels are able to reach into the cancer again.

Metronomic chemotherapy, which is given daily or every other day, doesn't allow blood vessels to get reestablished. It doesn't matter what type of cancer cells are involved or if those cells have become resistant to full-dose chemotherapy and/or other treatments, because doctors don't attack cancer cells with metronomic therapy; they attack the blood vessels that feed the cancer.

On February 23, 2008 at the 28th annual German Cancer Congress, the American cancer researcher D. McDonald, MD, from San Francisco, presented an interesting lecture at a symposium entitled: "Anti-angiogenesis Therapy for Solid Tumors." At this lecture, he showed pictures from his research, which illustrated that as soon as a day after treatment with an anti-angiogenesis remedy is stopped, the endothelial cells (the cancer's blood vessel wall cells) start sprouting and sending out growth processes from the basal membrane. Within just a week of stopping anti-angiogenesis treatment, the blood vessels and the blood supply to the cancer tumor are able to fully reestablish themselves, which is why metronomic chemotherapy is given daily or every other day.

Over the long run, endothelial cells can become resistant to treatments just like cancer cells, but they take much longer than cancer cells to develop this resistance. When a patient who is doing metronomic chemotherapy has a shrunken tumor that ceases to remain stable and starts to grow again, this indicates that endothelial resistance has occurred. The period of stability which patients experience with metronomic therapy can last for years, but at some point, as blood vessels become resistant to angiogenesis treatments, the cancer can start to grow again. At that point, patients should change to a different treatment agent or combination of metronomic substances.

Because of its extreme usefulness in stopping angiogenesis, we give metronomic chemotherapy to our patients whenever needed. It represents one of the greatest medical advances in the entire history of cancer treatment.

For patients, this newer way of treating cancer is beneficial because it has practically no side effects. Many different substances can be used in metronomic chemotherapy, most of which are prescribed in tablet form. Research has shown their effects upon cancer to be comparable to what patients would experience from regular, full-dose chemotherapy. The only difference is that with full-dose chemotherapy, high-dose drugs are given every second or third week, and they tend to produce serious side effects.

One hundred tablets of cyclophosphamide, a natural substance that's sometimes used in metronomic chemotherapy, costs approximately 30 US dollars: enough for 3.5 months of treatment, so cancer patients who don't have a lot of money can use this as part of a formidable treatment plan.

CHAPTER 15: Finn Skøtt Andersen, MD

Mistletoe

One of the main therapies that we utilize at Humlegaarden is mistletoe injections. The mistletoe that we use comes from different trees: most commonly, spruce, apple and pine trees. The first person to suggest mistletoe for cancer treatment was Rudolph Steiner, an Austrian-Swiss philosopher who founded the Anthroposophical Society in 1912. Mistletoe injections have been used in Europe to treat cancer for almost 100 years, since 1917. Since that time, millions of patients have been treated with it. A recent survey revealed that 60 percent of cancer patients in Germany use mistletoe as part of their treatment protocols. It's also popular in Switzerland, France, and Austria.

Mistletoe affects cancer in several ways. First, it kills cancer cells directly, without harming healthy cells. It does this through the actions of lectins and viscotoxins, which are proteins produced by the plant's leaves and stems. These proteins are toxic to cancer cells and cause necrosis (premature cell death), and apoptosis (programmed cell death, in which the cancer cell self-destructs). They also stimulate the immune system. Lectins are considered to be the most important substances in mistletoe. In addition to killing cancer cells, mistletoe increases endorphins, and has many other positive effects upon the body. More than 200 studies have been done on this incredible plant.

People with cancer who receive mistletoe injections have a better quality of life and higher tolerance for chemotherapy, as well as increased longevity, or survival from cancer.

We start our patients on a small dose of mistletoe and slowly increase it, as we look for local skin reactions which are often present at the beginning of treatment. Fortunately, these reactions typically resolve after a few injections, and if not, we are usually able to find a different dose or preparation which patients can tolerate. Iscador or Helixor are the two most common mistletoe products in Europe, and we have very good results with these. Sometimes, the results are absolutely astounding.

Mistletoe therapy is mostly prescribed by medical doctors, and we have thousands of well-documented case stories of cancer patients who have done mistletoe injections for up to fifteen or twenty years.

I once had a patient from Norway who had a tumor that measured 25 cm (approximately 9.8 inches) by 12-14 cm (4.7-5.5 inches) on the left side of his liver, along with metastases on the right side. He was told that he had a month or two to live. If you had seen him, you wouldn't have believed your eyes. He was 77 years old and his liver was huge! He came to my clinic for three weeks. I gave him Helixor (a mistletoe compound), at a dosage of 100 mg, three times per week, along with hyperthermia treatments. Three years later, I spoke with him and discovered that his quality of life was good; he was fishing every day, and going out to enjoy the hills of Norway every Sunday. He lived for seven years following his treatment at my clinic, until he was 84 years old. His case is an example of how mistletoe, even when used alone, can produce excellent results and significantly improve and extend one's life.

Mistletoe can be used as a standalone treatment, but it can also be combined with chemotherapy and other therapies. There are rules for its use, though. For instance, it shouldn't be given if patients have a fever above 37.7 Celsius (99.86 degrees Fahrenheit), or on the same day that they receive intravenous treatments of any kind, including chemotherapy. It can, however, be given on the day before or the day after such treatments. In fact, mistletoe enables patients to tolerate chemotherapy and radiation treatments better. A Danish architect that I know did mistletoe injections while undergoing chemotherapy. He was the only one in the cancer ward at his local hospital who was taking mistletoe. Doctors couldn't understand why his white blood cell counts stayed so high during chemotherapy. Many studies have shown that people tolerate conventional treatments better when they take mistletoe, because it keeps their immune parameters high.

Low-Dose Naltrexone

Low-dose naltrexone (LDN) is another excellent cancer treatment remedy that we have been giving our patients for over ten years. Many Internet websites describe the benefits of low-dose naltrexone for treating cancer, so its use in treating cancer is becoming well-known. It's also beneficial for treating autoimmune diseases. Patients that take this drug feel dramatically better within days because it releases endorphins, kills cancer cells via apoptosis, and reduces inflammation.

The first person to take this medication for cancer was a woman from France, who had four brain metastases from melanoma. This is a very aggressive cancer, and there was nothing that conventional oncologists could do for her. She had heard about Dr. Bernard Bihari, the medical doctor who discovered the clinical effects of LDN, and went to hear him speak in Paris. She asked him for some LDN, which he gave her. She began to take it, in a dose of three milligrams daily. Seven months later, her brain metastases disappeared! She took LDN for twelve years, but after twelve years, she stopped, as every time she took a pill, she was reminded of the fact that she had cancer. About seven months later, she began to have multiple metastases on her lungs and on the skin of her arms. She called Dr. Bihari, and resumed taking LDN for another seven months, during which time her lung and skin metastases disappeared. She was forty-two years old at the time, and I don't know what has happened to her since then. Now, LDN is given to many cancer patients. It's completely non-toxic and is very effective for treating some cancers, especially when given in conjunction with alpha-lipoic acid.

Prostate Cancer Treatment

There are many effective treatment options for prostate cancer, but there is a trade-off between treatment efficacy and the patient's ability to be sexually active. Understanding patients' attitudes and preferences is important when choosing what treatments to give them, especially when they are first diagnosed. Fortunately, all three of the following types of patients can be efficiently treated:

1. Those who want to do the most promising and effective treatments available, even if it means they will run the risk of impotence and incontinence as a result.
2. Those who don't want to risk being permanently impotent. Medical castration (using drugs to impair or block the release of male hormones, which feed cancer) only causes temporary impotence.
3. Those who won't accept impotency for any period of time.

There is currently extensive knowledge and research about prostate cancer within the medical community, and countless divergent opinions about what people should do when they get prostate cancer. Every newly diagnosed prostate cancer patient feels a deep need to obtain further information about his disease and we at Humlegaarden try to meet this need. We offer a week-long training course for prostate cancer patients every month, whereby we share the most current knowledge about prostate cancer and treatment principles. Following is some information about the latest discoveries on effective prostate cancer treatments.

First, androgens, or steroid hormones that are responsible for the development of male characteristics in humans, are also able to stimulate cancer growth later in life in prostate cancer patients. Therefore, treatments which suppress or block the production or function of male sex hormones are an important part of prostate cancer therapy. Men who have started these treatments should know that a paradigm shift has taken place on this issue after the February 2011 Genitourinary Cancers Symposium, which was arranged by the American Society of Clinical Oncology in Orlando, Florida. Intermittent, rather than ongoing, androgen-suppressing treatments are now recommended as the new standard of care for most patients who have cancer recurrences after having received aggressive anti-cancer therapies. This means that androgen-suppressing treatments should be given to patients for only eight months, and should be restarted only if their prostate-specific antigen (PSA) values increase to levels greater than 10ng/ml. Multiple clinical trials have proven that giving patients these treatments for only eight months provides equally beneficial results as treating them with androgen suppression for longer periods—even years. What's more, the costs and side effects of treatment are minimized by doing therapy intermittently.

What can doctors do for their patients when their PSA levels rise, despite the fact that they have undergone surgical castration,[2] or been given anti-hormone substances to suppress the production of male hormones that feed their cancers?

The first thing that doctors should do is make sure that their patients are actually "sufficiently castrated."[3] For example, that their blood testosterone levels are preferably below 20 nanograms/dl (= <0.69 mmol/l). Earlier guidelines recommended 50 nanograms/ dl, but today it's recommended that doctors bring their patients' testosterone levels to below 20 nanograms/dl.

We know that 37.5 percent of medically castrated patients[4] don't have levels of testosterone under 20ng/dl, and that 12.5 percent don't have levels that are less than 50ng/dl.

Medical castration removes one of the body's sources of testosterone, which is important because testosterone feeds cancer cells. But testosterone isn't just produced in the testicles; it's also produced in the adrenal glands and in cancer cells themselves. Ninety percent of the testosterone which circulates in the blood is bound to a protein substance called sex hormone-binding globulin (SHBG), while the other ten percent of testosterone enters prostate cancer cells and is

---

[2] "Surgical castration" refers to surgical removal of the testicles.
[3] "Sufficiently castrated" means that the body's androgen, or male hormone, levels have been sufficiently reduced.
[4] "Medical castration," otherwise known as chemical castration, involves giving patients hormones that either prevent the body from making androgens or which block their effects upon the body.

irreversibly converted to dihydrotestosterone (DHT) by the enzyme 5-alpha reductase.

DHT has a much greater affinity for androgen receptors on cancer cells (its binding capacity is two to five times greater than testosterone). It also has at least a fifty-fold greater affinity for androgen receptors than known anti-androgen medications such as Casodex (bicalutamide), as well as a tenfold greater ability to stimulate androgen receptor signalling to the cell's nucleus, which in turn stimulates cancer cell growth.

Interestingly, though, if doctors measure the DHT levels of their medically castrated male patients, they often find that these levels are within the normal range (30–80 ng/dl), despite the fact that the men's testosterone has been successfully lowered by castration.

Men that have persistently high DHT levels must be treated with a medication which inhibits the transformation of testosterone to DHT. This medication is called Avodart (dutasteride), and when given in dosages of 0.5 mg per day in tablet form, it reduces the amount of DHT to four percent of the amount that would have otherwise been present. We measure our patients' testosterone as well as dihydrotestosterone (DHT) levels so that we can identify whether they need dutasteride (Avodart).

We try to inhibit prostate cancer growth in three different ways, using androgen deprivation therapy (ADT), which includes all of the following:

1. Gonadotropin releasing hormone (GnRH) agonists like Zoladex (which nearly eliminates the production of testosterone in the testicles)
2. An androgen receptor blocker like Casodex
3. Dutasteride (Avodart)

Often, androgen receptors develop hypersensitivity to even very small amounts of DHT and testosterone. Whenever this happens, cancer cells may grow rapidly, even when the serum (blood) levels of testosterone in the body are 1/10 to 1/1000 of normal. Fortunately, a number of studies have shown that the anti-androgen medication Casodex, when given in daily dosages of 150 mg – 250 mg, can inhibit the growth of such hyper-sensitive cancer cells.

Because castration affects only testosterone production in the testicles, but not that which comes from the adrenal glands and the cancer cells themselves, we often add the anti-fungal remedy Ketoconazole (200 mg x 3), and 10 mg of the corticosteroid drug prednisone daily, to the ADT-3 treatment to reduce the adrenal glands' production of androgens.

Because of all the aforementioned factors, it can be difficult to provide a 100 percent effective treatment to patients who have hormone-sensitive cancers such as prostate cancer, so the medical community must appreciate and be open to new ways of treating this cancer besides using the treatments that are commonly known in oncology.

In our opinion, one of the most promising therapies for "castrate-resistant"[5] prostate cancer is low-dose metronomic chemotherapy. As previously mentioned, high-dose conventional chemotherapy attacks cancer cells and low-dose metronomic chemotherapy blocks angiogenesis (the formation of new cancer cell blood vessels).

Up until now, we have only done two studies which show the effects of conventional chemotherapy upon prostate cancer patients. Both studies were done in 2004 and involved giving castrate-resistant patients Taxotere, which increased their median survival from 15-16 months, to 17-18 months, thereby giving them only two more months of life.

By comparison, metronomic chemotherapy has yielded very interesting, and more beneficial, results. In one study, for example,

---

[5] "castrate-resistant" cancer refers to cancer that is resistant to both medical and surgical castration, because neither approach is, or has been, effective for stopping cancer growth.

responders had a median survival of five years, even when the therapy was given after patients had taken Taxotere.

One very interesting metronomic chemotherapy protocol is called KEES, which originated from Sahlgrenska University hospital in Sweden. It involves the use of cyclophosphamide (an alkylating antineoplastic agent), ketoconazole, prednisone, etoposide (a chemotherapy agent) and Estramustine (another chemotherapy agent), which are all given in low doses. Many other protocols are in use today. Whenever doctors give their patients metronomic chemotherapy, the cancer cell's sensitivity to hormones becomes irrelevant.

Other effective prostate cancer treatments include: pomegranate, resveratrol, Cool Cayenne (a chili product), artemisinin (Chinese wormwood), lycopene (a phytochemical from tomatoes), noscapine (a well known cough remedy), Vitamin D-3, transdermal estrogen, Sandostatin (a growth hormone inhibitor), milk thistle (which slows cancer cell growth), mistletoe compounds like Iscador and Helixor, as well as many others. Their mechanism of action upon the cancer varies, depending upon the substance, but all either have anti-neoplastic or immune-stimulating properties.

When prostate cancer becomes really resistant, other options, such as vaccines, may also work well for treatment. Soon, a more universal testosterone-inhibiting medication called Abiraterone will be out on the market. It is expected to be approved in most countries within the next year.

Many of the above methods are not used by conventional urologists, but many prostate cancer discussion groups on the Internet eagerly debate and comment on their effectiveness.

The Art of Combining and Switching Cancer Therapies

Today, the integrative medical community has a large group of different treatment modalities at its disposal. Cancer treatment options can be compared to a person who is traveling from one town to another. To get to the next town, he can travel by car, bus, train, or even airplane, and can choose many alternate routes to reach his final destination. Monotherapy, or using a single treatment modality, can be compared to traveling along just one of these routes, using a single mode of transportation. If the therapy (or transportation) is effective, the cancer's growth will be blocked for awhile, but sooner or later, it will attempt to use an alternate route. The best approach is to combine multiple therapies that block most of the cancer's survival routes and hope that it dies from a lack of nutrition before it finds a new route. Combining multiple therapies at the beginning of treatment is also important.

Because there are a multitude of routes, or strategies, that cancer can use for its survival, it often recurs despite a multi-faceted treatment approach. Good integrative physicians, however, have a multitude of therapies to choose from, and can often succeed at blocking the new route that the cancer has taken with a different treatment approach.

Fortunately, cancer treatments can also be synergistic with one another. When two compatible therapies are given together, they can sometimes provide better results than if two non-synergistic therapies are given together. One example of an effective combination strategy would be using different androgen deprivation therapies together, each of which functions to disable the prostate cancer in a different way. For example, doctors might first treat their patients with a GnRH agonist like Zoladex to stop or reduce the body's testosterone production. Next, they might add Avodart to their patients' regimens, to inhibit the transformation of testosterone to dihydrotestosterone. Finally, they might block the cancer cell's androgen receptors with an anti-androgen agent such as Casodex. In this way, they can simultaneously block three hormonal strategies that the cancer uses for its proliferation, which is clearly better than just blocking one of them.

There is no reason for people with cancer to despair if their cancers recur. Their doctors just have to block another route that the cancer has taken for its survival, which can be accomplished by effectively combining different treatments.

Tumor Markers and CTCs (or Circulating Tumor Cell) Tests

Over the past fifteen to twenty years, we have used tumor marker measurements extensively to evaluate our patients' progress on their treatment regimens. Our frequent use of these markers is due partly to the fact that we have an excellent tumor marker department at the Danish Serum Institute in Copenhagen.

A tumor marker is a substance in the blood, urine or tissues that is found in higher amounts in people with cancer because it is produced by cancer cells. Many different tumor markers exist, because almost every cancer produces its own unique markers.

Tumor markers can be used to monitor the effectiveness of a given treatment, and in many cases, to detect whether the histology (microscopic anatomy) of the tumor tissue and the tumor marker match. Often they don't, and the pathologist has to change the initial diagnosis. Tumor marker counts also provide information about the aggressiveness of a particular cancer.

The most frequent tumor markers that we use are: PSA (prostate specific antigen) for prostate cancer, CA-125 (cancer antigen 125, for ovarian cancer and sometimes adenocarcinomas); CA-19-9 for pancreatic, bile duct, and sometimes, colon and stomach cancers; CA-15-3 for breast cancer; S-100 for malignant melanomas; NSE and chromogranin A for neuro-endocrine cancers; CEA for colon cancer (and often also breast cancers); HCG for testicular cancers; alpha-phoetoprotein for primary liver cancer (and testicular cancer); and ferritin, which is a non-specific marker.

The most recent tumor marker that we have been using is called Circulating Tumor Cells (CTC). This diagnostic test collects and identifies CTCs, which are live tumor cells that have separated from solid tumors and are circulating in the blood. It then identifies and counts the exact number of circulating tumor cells within an ordinary 7.5 ml blood sample. The cut-off limit for a positive prognosis is five, so if patients have less than five cancer cells within a given blood sample, their prognoses are far better than if more than five CTCs are found in their blood samples. For patients that have a cell count above five, the goal of treatment would be to get their CTC counts to below five, in order to substantially improve their prognoses. For patients whose CTC numbers are less than five, we can use milder and less toxic treatments, and thus save them from having to endure the severe side effects of more aggressive therapies.

With the CTC test, it's possible to determine whether a given treatment works as early as three weeks into treatment. If it doesn't, we can stop it immediately and replace it with another type of treatment. This saves patients valuable time because they can avoid unnecessary harsh treatments, which often have many side effects. Also, the CTC test is able to predict patients' prognoses much more accurately than previously.

Dietary Recommendations

It's important for people with cancer to establish good nutritional habits. Fatigue is the single most important symptom that doctors must address in their cancer patients, because energy is vital for recovery. For that reason, we recommend foods that will increase the body's energy. This is an integral part of our nutritional protocols. Such foods are fresh; they are not frozen or canned, and are ideally organic and mostly vegetarian. Consuming lots of fresh organic vegetables is especially important!

We also recommend that people with cancer avoid sugar. Cancer cells have twenty times more glucose (sugar) receptors on the surface of their membranes than normal cells, which means that they proliferate when fed sugar. Ideally, cancer patients should follow a diet similar to that of diabetics, and avoid all sugars. Instead, they should use natural sweeteners like Stevia. They can also have a little honey but not much, as it's important for them to keep their blood sugar low.

We sometimes give our patients Metformin, which is the most commonly prescribed diabetes drug in the world, because it reduces the body's blood sugar levels, and inhibits a hormone called insulin-like growth factor-1 (IGF-1) which plays a crucial role in cancer growth. In June 2010, I met a researcher at the American Society of Clinical Oncology conference in Chicago, who gives her cancer patients three tablets of Metformin, in doses of 500 mg per day, and seemingly without complications. However, I think this dose is a bit high for people who don't have diabetes, so at our clinic, we prescribe our patients just two tablets per day, which should be taken only with meals, and have seen some excellent clinical results at this dosing.

It's important for sugar addicts to understand this message, because most of the sugar that people consume feeds cancer cells. For every glucose molecule that enters a cancer cell, two molecules of ATP (the energy currency of the cells' mitochondria) are produced in the cancer cell. If the same molecule of glucose is burned in a normal cell, it produces 36 molecules of ATP. This means that eighteen times more energy is produced in a normal cell from a single glucose molecule than what would be produced in a cancer cell from a single glucose molecule. Since cancer cells require copious amounts of glucose to function, they steal all that they can from the body so that little is left over for the normal cells. This is the main reason why cancer patients are tired, lose weight, and suffer from other symptoms.

People with cancer should get their energy from the sugar that comes from complex carbohydrates, including grains and vegetables, as well as some fruits. I don't believe that they necessarily need to be vegetarians, although studies have shown vegetarian diets to be the most ideal for people with cancer. In a major study that was done in Heidelberg in 1992, researchers tracked 2000 vegetarians for ten years, and found that they had 50 percent less cancer and cardiac conditions than the general population. In another study that was done in Britain in 1998, researchers tracked 11,000 vegetarians, and found that they had a 40 percent lower mortality rate from cancer than the general population. In yet another study, 7,500 Seventh-day Adventists, (who don't eat pork and who generally eat less meat than most people), had dramatically lower levels of cancer than the general population.

Lifestyle Strategies for Healing

Cancer patients should do three things to improve their chances for recovery. First, they should seek to attain a good quality of life that has purpose and meaning. Secondly, they should adhere to a cancer-fighting diet (as described in the previous section), and thirdly, they should exercise.

People with cancer should pursue activities that they can look forward to doing every day, and have things that they feel good about in their daily lives. It's also important for them to have hobbies that they really enjoy. We have witnessed, time and again, beneficial results in cancer patients who pursue hobbies. In 1984, we had a fourteen-year old female patient with brain cancer whose tumor had grown into her brain stem. Her doctors told her that she had between one and two months to live. In the meantime, she developed a hobby out of collecting key rings, which turned out to be a very important, purposeful activity for her. She didn't die, and when she came back to visit our clinic in 1996, she told me that she had compiled around 2,200 key rings. She came back again in 2007, and by that time, had 8,400 key rings. She was proud of her collection of key rings; it gave her a sense of purpose, and she is still alive today, 26 years after being given a terminal cancer diagnosis.

Another patient of mine had lung metastases from kidney cancer. She came to our clinic in 1981, at the age of 56. The oncologists in the hospitals couldn't help her, so she came to see us and we gave her mistletoe injections as part of her therapy. Every time I saw her at the clinic while she was doing treatments, she was writing poems and festive songs. After three weeks of therapy here, her metastases were gone completely and she's still alive and well today. At 86 years of age, she still writes. I cite these examples to illustrate how important it is for cancer patients to partake in and focus on meaningful activities.

Exercise

Several studies on cancer and exercise have proven that exercise is of utmost importance when fighting cancer. At Humlegaarden, we have always emphasized this to our patients. The exercise program that they do must be tailored to their health and overall condition; it's not necessary that they run a marathon! What matters most is continuity, whether they walk, jog, lift weights, play soccer, or do any other type of physical activity. We witness over and over again that patients who exercise have a far better quality of life, more energy, and better results from their treatments.

Exercise is the most important therapy for cancer, in my opinion. Cancer patients don't die from cancer or from the size of their tumors. If all of a patient's tumor tissue were placed on a table, it would weigh perhaps only a kilogram (2.2 pounds) or less, and might amount to the size of a fist. So how is it possible for a person to die from something so small? The answer is: because cancer is an energy vampire! It steals energy from people, so that they become increasingly tired, and finally end up bedridden. They die from fatigue, which is the most common cancer symptom.

A nurse with ovarian cancer, who was born in 1938, did chemotherapy for four or five years prior to coming to our clinic in 2001. When we saw her, her tumor marker (CA-125) levels were around 3,800 (A healthy person would have a tumor marker level of less than 30). Her situation was dire, and conventional doctors could do nothing to help her, so I gave her mistletoe injections. She also began to run two miles or ride her bicycle every other day. That was ten years ago, and I sincerely believe that her daily exercise regimen is the single most important reason why she's still doing well today. Her last CA-125 was 7. Over the last ten years, she has maintained a healthy lifestyle, and continued with her daily exercise regimen.

If patients walk, run, swim, or bike the same distance every day, they can control their energy levels better, even if the distance that they run or walk isn't significant. But the activity that they do has to be measurable and consistent. That's the secret to success. For instance, if they are going to run, then it should be the same distance daily, and it should be done at regular intervals. Of course, not everyone with cancer is able to walk or run two miles daily. Maybe they can only walk for ten minutes. That's okay, as long as they are consistent with the exercise.

Also, exercise is the most important tumor marker there is. By evaluating their energy levels daily, people with cancer can obtain feedback from their bodies, which will let them know whether or not they are doing okay with their treatments. That is one reason why exercise is so important.

The other reason why exercise is so important is because it stimulates the immune system, and is even directly cytotoxic to cancer cells. Much research on the effects of exercise in people with cancer has demonstrated it to be the most important, non-specific cancer treatment that there is.

In 1978, a German cancer patient went into surgery, but was found to be inoperable, because his cancer was so advanced. After the operation, he was sent home to die by conventional oncologists. He bought an exercise bike, and started biking. Seventeen years later, I read a story in a German newspaper that stated he had just biked across the USA!

In 1975, I met the famous German sports and cancer physician, Ernst van Aaken, who wrote several books about cancer and exercise. He believed that all people with cancer should aim to increase their heart rate through aerobic exercise to at least 132 beats per minute, for 30 minutes daily. Today, doctors and researchers at all of the major cancer conferences around the world present studies demonstrating the beneficial effects that exercise has upon cancer.

In one study, a researcher in Berlin sent ten or fifteen breast cancer patients to southern France to do a 7-800 km walk. The results of the study proved that the walk had demonstrable, positive effects upon the patients' cancers. Other studies on cancer and exercise can be found by doing a Google search on the Internet.

Most cancer patients, however, find many excuses not to exercise, out of pure ignorance of the important positive biochemical processes that happen in the body while doing it.

Even if people with cancer only walk 25 meters (or 82 feet) every day, I believe that this can make a difference. It's the discipline to do it every day that matters. If people don't make excuses for why they can't exercise, and just do it, it's the best thing that they can do to heal themselves.

The Importance of Treating Infections and Toxicity in the Mouth

Infections in the sinuses, mouth and tonsils can cause immune problems and compromise recovery from cancer, and should therefore be treated. In 1978, I attended a three-day conference in Munich with doctors and dentists who were studying the phenomenon of foci, or localized areas of infection in the body, which weaken the immune system and create toxins that get sent out into the bloodstream. These infections are most commonly found in the teeth, and especially, in root canals. Root canals create cavitations and obstructions in the mouth, and bacteria reside and produce toxins there. Subsequently, these infections and toxins spread to the rest of the body.

Also, if people with cancer have dental amalgams, they must get them removed for the best chance at recovery, or if they want to remain healthy once their cancers are in remission. These fillings contain high amounts of toxic mercury which poison the body. A dentist from Colorado once came to Denmark and presented a lecture which demonstrated the detrimental effects of amalgams upon white blood cell counts in cancer patients. Three patients with leukemia and dental amalgams initially had white blood cell counts between 60,000-70,000, but when they had their amalgams taken out, their lab values normalized.

In summary, focal infections in the tonsils, teeth, or sinuses must be treated, and root canals must be removed. People with cancer may also need to have their tonsils taken out, if they are severely infected. Treating these issues is one of the most important things that people with cancer can do to assist with their recovery.

Final Words

You (the cancer patient) must always nourish hope in your heart, even if you are given very bad news from your oncologist. Many patients have survived with cancer for many years, even after having been given a death sentence.

Contact Information
Finn Skøtt Andersen, MD

Humlebæk Strandvej 11
DK - 3050 Humlebæk
Tel.: (+45) 49 13 24 65
Fax: (+45) 49 13 44 98
Website: www.humlegaarden.com
Email: info@humlegaarden.com

About Author Connie Strasheim

Connie Strasheim is a medical researcher and writer who has experienced the hardships of chronic illness firsthand through her seven-year battle with Lyme disease and Chronic Fatigue Syndrome. She is the author of three other books, including:

The Lyme Disease Survival Guide: Physical, Lifestyle and Emotional Strategies for Healing (available from www.LymeInsights.com or www.LymeBook.com)

Insights Into Lyme Disease Treatment: Thirteen Lyme-Literate Health Care Practitioners Share Their Healing Strategies (available from www.LymeInsights.com or www.LymeBook.com)

Healing Chronic Illness: By His Spirit, Through His Resources (available from www.HealingChronicIllness.org)

Ms. Strasheim's second Lyme disease book, *Insights Into Lyme Disease Treatment*, has been a bestseller within the Lyme disease community since its release in September, 2009.

In addition to writing books on medicine and spiritual healing, Connie maintains a blog on chronic illness and Lyme disease, which can be accessed here: www.Lymebytes.Blogspot.com. She also leads a bi-monthly prayer conference call group for the chronically ill across the United States.

Prior to becoming a medical researcher, she was a medical interpreter for Spanish-speaking patients, as well as Spanish instructor, novelist and flight attendant for United Airlines. Her travels to over fifty countries on six continents have provided her with broad and unique perspectives on healing, and life.

Press inquiries can be made to the publisher, BioMed Publishing Group, in South Lake Tahoe, CA, by calling (530) 573-0190 or by emailing us at: bmpublish@gmail.com.

BioMed Publishing Group
Product Catalog

Books and DVDs on Cancer & Related Topics

To order online: www.cancerbooksource.com/store
To order by phone: (530) 573-0190

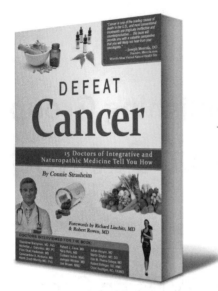

Book • $39.95

Defeat Cancer: 15 Doctors of Integrative & Naturopathic Medicine Tell You How

By Connie Strasheim
Foreword by Richard Linchitz, M.D. & Robert Rowen, M.D.

If you traveled the world for appointments with fifteen cancer doctors, you would discover many of the cutting-edge treatments used to heal the body from cancer. You would also spend thousands of dollars on hotels, plane tickets, and medical appointment fees—not to mention the time that it would take to embark on such a journey. Even if you had the time and money to travel, would the physicians have enough time to answer all of your questions? Would you even know which questions to ask?

In this long-awaited book, health care journalist Connie Strasheim has done all the work for you. She conducted intensive interviews with fifteen highly regarded doctors who specialize in cancer treatment, asking them thoughtful, important questions, and then spent months compiling their information into organized, user-friendly chapters that contain the core principles upon which they base their approach to healing cancer. The practitioners interviewed are medical, osteopathic and naturopathic doctors, trained in a variety of integrative approaches to cancer treatment. **Meet the physician interviewees, representing 5 countries:**

- Colleen Huber, NMD
- Juergen Winkler, MD
- Joe Brown, NMD
- Julian Kenyon, MD
- Martin Dayton, MD, DO
- Elio M. Rivera-Celaya, MD
- Robert Eslinger, DO, HMD
- Chad Aschtgen, ND, FABNO

- Stanislaw Burzynski, MD, PhD
- Nicholas J. Gonzalez, MD, PC
- Finn Skøtt Andersen, MD
- Constantine A. Kotsanis, MD
- Keith Scott-Mumby MD, PhD
- Robert J. Zieve, MD
- Nina Reis, MD
- *Physicians from 5 countries!*

All aspects of treatment are covered, from anti-neoplastic (anti-cancer) remedies and immune system support, to dietary and lifestyle choices that result in the best outcomes for patients.

The book also offers unique insights into healing, such as the pros and cons of different treatments and how to intelligently use chemotherapy. Finally, it offers helpful insights to the friends and families of those coping with cancer. Cancer treatment is complex and controversial, and this book puts the treatment information you need in the palm of your hand.

> "… a valuable perspective you will likely not hear from your oncologists."
>
> **- Joseph Mercola, DO**

Paperback book, 7 x 10", 435 pages, $39.95

Cancer is Curable Now!

DVD documentary, produced by Marcus & Sabrina Freudenmann

With 31 leading global cancer experts, scientists, doctors and authors, "Cancer is Curable Now" is the most comprehensive and conclusive DVD documentary about cancer and holistic cancer treatments ever made. In addition to a multitude of physical and dietary treatments, this groundbreaking documentary uncovers the various problems, physical and emotional, that promote and cause cancer.

The information given in the movie transforms your life and provides you with all the tools you need to take charge of your own health. We have avoided hype, false claims and marketing strategies that are only designed to make you pull out your purse. The information provided is useful and scientifically based.

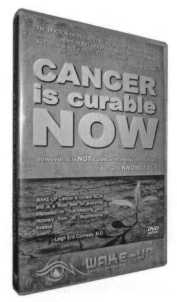

DVD • $34.95 • 115 Minutes

The movie is divided into 7 sections, for a total of 115 minutes. Following is a list of sections, as well as the sub-sections within each section of the film:

- Chapter 1: A FAULTY SYSTEM. Greed, fear, pressure, obedience, blind faith.
- Chapter 2: THE CAUSE OF CANCER. Household toxins, food toxins, plastics, vaccination, environmental toxins, emotional toxins, "overwhelmed by life," the real cause of cancer, dealing with the cause.
- Chapter 3: THE JOURNEY TO HEALTH. Self-responsibility, the pain of change, victory is a decision, cancer is a wake-up call, finding good support, common sense, self confidence, a new way of healing, healing is possible, your body heals itself.
- Chapter 4: MANDATORY CANCER TREATMENT. Exercise, oxygen, sunshine/Vitamin D3, cancer diet, alkalize, detox diet, Gerson therapy, detoxification, supplements, Vitamin C, enzymes, immune boosting.
- Chapter 5: MEDICAL CANCER TREATMENT. Whole body hyperthermia, local hyperthermia, prostate treatment, ozone treatment, dental cavitations, root canal fillings, antineoplastons, hormone harmonizers, nature has no side effects, low dose insulin potentiation, metronomic low dose.
- Chapter 6: MENTAL CANCER TREATMENT. People are waking up, healthy habits, motivation, mental detox, meditation.
- Chapter 7: BLESSINGS FROM CANCER. Secondary gains, blessing for all involved, we vote with our shopping cart, it's time to change ...and much more!

> "*Cancer is Curable Now* is the best video on the subject we have seen. ("We" includes myself, and my wife, Terri Su, MD). It was very broad, covering all aspects of healing, many of which are costless."
>
> **- Robert Rowen, M.D.**

Do not miss this cancer DVD, which is a perfect companion resource to the book *Defeat Cancer* (opposing page).

DVD, 115 Minutes, $34.95

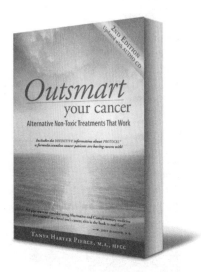

Book and Audio CD • $26.95

Outsmart Your Cancer: Alternative Non-Toxic Treatments That Work, by Tanya Harter Pierce

Why BLUDGEON cancer to death with common conventional treatments that can be toxic and harmful to your entire body?

When you OUTSMART your cancer, only the cancer cells die — NOT your healthy cells! *OUTSMART YOUR CANCER: Alternative Non-Toxic Treatments That Work* is an easy guide to successful non-toxic treatments for cancer that you can obtain right now! In it, you will read real-life stories of people who have completely recovered from their advanced or late-stage lung cancer, breast cancer, prostate cancer, kidney cancer, brain cancer, childhood leukemia, and other types of cancer using effective non-toxic approaches.

Plus, *OUTSMART YOUR CANCER* is one of the few books in print today that gives a complete description of the amazing formula called "Protocel," which has produced incredible cancer recoveries over the past 20 years. **A supporting audio CD is included! New 2nd Edition!**

Paperback book, 6 x 9", 506 pages, with audio CD, $26.95

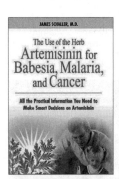

Book • $32.95

The Use of the Herb Artemisinin for Babesia, Malaria and Cancer

By James Schaller, M.D.

This book is the only patient book written in English offering practical, clear, and carefully researched help on Artemisinin medications. Artemisinin herbals are powerful treatments for infections like Malaria and Babesia, as well as cancer.

Artemisinin can be used as an alternative to pharmaceutical treatments for Babesia and similar infections—or it can be used synergistically with prescription drugs. This book is a must-have for all patients and physicians seeking an artemisinin education.

One of the benefits of artemisinin is that it is available over the counter, and it is an affordable herb. However, the quality of various retail substances can vary, and you should only use this herb (as well as any other treatment) under the care of a physician.

Paperback book, 7x10", 160 pages, $32.95

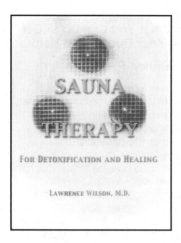

Book • $22.95

Sauna Therapy for Detoxification and Healing

By Lawrence Wilson, MD

This book provides a thorough yet articulate education on sauna therapy. It includes construction plans for a low-cost electric light sauna. The book is well referenced with an extensive bibliography.

Sauna therapy, especially with an electric light sauna, is one of the most powerful, safe and cost-effective methods of natural healing. It is especially important today due to extensive exposure to toxic metals and chemicals.

Fifteen chapters cover sauna benefits, physiological effects, protocols, cautions, healing reactions, and many other aspects of sauna therapy.

Dr. Wilson is an instructor of Biochemistry, Hair Mineral Analysis, Sauna Therapy and Jurisprudence at various colleges and universities including Yamuni Institute of the Healing Arts (Maurice, LA), University of Natural Medicine (Santa Fe, NM), Natural Healers Academy (Morristown, NJ), and Westbrook University (West Virginia). His books are used as textbooks at East-West School of Herbology and Ohio College of Health. Go to www.CancerBookSource.com for free book excerpts!

Paperback book, 8.5 x 11", 167 pages, $22.95

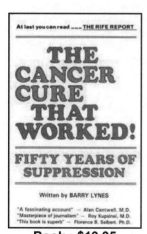

Book • $19.95

Over 50,000 Copies Sold!

The Cancer Cure That Worked: Fifty Years of Suppression At Last You Can Read... The Rife Report

By Barry Lynes

Investigative journalism at its best. Barry Lynes takes readers on an exciting journey into the life work of Royal Rife. In 2011, we became the official publisher of this book. Call or visit us online for wholesale terms.

"A fascinating account..."
-Alan Cantwell, M.D.

"This book is superb."
-Florence B. Seibert, PhD

"Barry Lynes is one of the greatest health reporters in our country. With the assistance of John Crane, longtime friend and associate of Roy Rife, Barry has produced a masterpiece..." -Roy Kupsinel, M.D., editor of *Health Consciousness Journal*

Paperback book, 5 x 8", 169 pages, $19.95

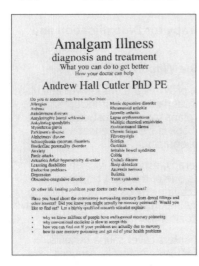

Book • $35

Amalgam Illness, Diagnosis and Treatment: What You Can Do to Get Better, How Your Doctor Can Help

By Andrew Cutler, PhD

This book was written by a chemical engineer who himself got mercury poisoning from his amalgam dental fillings. He found that there was no suitable educational material for either the patient or the physician. Knowing how much people can suffer from this condition, he wrote this book to help them get well. With a PhD in chemistry from Princeton University and extensive study in biochemistry and medicine, Andrew Cutler uses layman's terms to explain how people become mercury poisoned and what to do about it. The author's research shows that mercury poisoning can easily be cured at home with over-the-counter oral chelators – this book explains how.

In the book you will find practical guidance on how to tell if you really have chronic mercury poisoning or some other problem. Proper diagnostic procedures are provided so that sick people can decide what is wrong rather than trying random treatments. If mercury poisoning is your problem, the book tells you how to get the mercury out of your body, and how to feel good while you do that. The treatment section gives step-by-step directions to figure out exactly what mercury is doing to you and how to fix it.

"Dr. Cutler uses his background in chemistry to explain the safest approach to treat mercury poisoning. I am a physician and am personally using his protocol on myself."

- Melissa Myers, M.D.

Sections also explain how the scientific literature shows many people must be getting poisoned by their amalgam fillings, why such a regulatory blunder occurred, and how the debate between "mainstream" and "alternative" medicine makes it more difficult for you to get the medical help you need.

This down-to-earth book lets patients take care of themselves. It also lets doctors who are not familiar with chronic mercury intoxication treat it. The book is a practical guide to getting well. Sections from the book include:

- Why worry about mercury poisoning?
- What mercury does to you – symptoms, laboratory test irregularities, diagnostic checklist.
- How to treat mercury poisoning easily with oral chelators.
- Dealing with other metals including copper, arsenic, lead, cadmium.
- Dietary and supplement guidelines.
- Balancing hormones during the recovery process.
- How to feel good while you are chelating the metals out.
- How heavy metals cause infections to thrive in the body.
- Politics and mercury.

This is the world's most authoritative, accurate book on mercury poisoning.

Paperback book, 8.5 x 11", 226 pages, $35

Hair Test Interpretation: Finding Hidden Toxicities

By Andrew Cutler, PhD

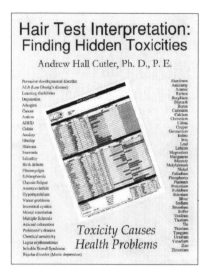

Hair tests are worth doing because a surprising number of people diagnosed with incurable chronic health conditions actually turn out to have a heavy metal problem; quite often, mercury poisoning. Heavy metal problems can be corrected. Hair testing allows the underlying problem to be identified – and the chronic health condition often disappears with proper detoxification.

Hair Test Interpretation: Finding Hidden Toxicities is a practical book that explains how to interpret **Doctor's Data, Inc.** and **Great Plains Laboratory** hair tests. A step-by-step discussion is provided, with figures to illustrate the process and make it easy. The book gives examples using actual hair test results from real people.

Book • $35

One of the problems with hair testing is that both conventional and alternative health care providers do not know how to interpret these tests. Interpretation is not as simple as looking at the results and assuming that any mineral out of the reference range is a problem mineral.

Interpretation is complicated because heavy metal toxicity, especially mercury poisoning, interferes with mineral transport throughout the body. Ironically, if someone is mercury poisoned, hair test mercury is often low and other minerals may be elevated or take on unusual values. For example, mercury often causes retention of arsenic, antimony, tin, titanium, zirconium, and aluminum. An inexperienced health care provider may wrongfully assume that one of these other minerals is the culprit, when in reality mercury is the true toxicity.

"This new book of Andrew's is the definitive guide in the confusing world of heavy metal poisoning diagnosis and treatment. I'm a practicing physician, 20 years now, specializing in detoxification programs for treatment of resistant conditions. It was fairly difficult to diagnose these heavy metal conditions before I met Andrew Cutler and developed a close relationship with him while reading his books. In this book I found his usual painful attention to detail gave a solid framework for understanding the complexity of mercury toxicity as well as the less common exposures. You really couldn't ask for a better reference book on a subject most researchers and physicians are still fumbling in the dark about."
- Dr. Rick Marschall

So, as you can see, getting a hair test is only the first step. The second step is figuring out what the hair test means. Andrew Cutler, PhD, is a registered professional chemical engineer with years of experience in biochemical and healthcare research. This clear and concise book makes hair test interpretation easy, so that you know which toxicities are causing your health problems.

Paperback book, 8.5 x 11", 298 pages, $35

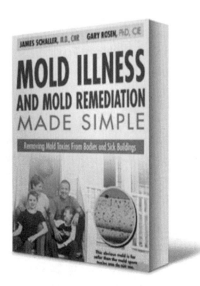

Book • $32.95

Mold Illness and Mold Remediation Made Simple: Removing Mold Toxins from Bodies and Sick Buildings

By James Schaller, M.D. and Gary Rosen, Ph.D.

Indoor mold toxins are much more dangerous and prevalent than most people realize. Visible mold in and around your house is far less dangerous than the mold you cannot see. Indoor mold toxicity, in addition to causing its own unique set of health problems and symptoms, also greatly contributes to the severity of most chronic illnesses.

In this book, a top physician and experienced contractor team up to help you quickly recover from indoor mold exposure. This book is easy to read with many color photographs and illustrations.

Dr. Schaller is a practicing physician in Florida who has written more than 15 books. He is one of the few physicians in the United States successfully treating mold toxin illness in children and adults.

Dr. Rosen is a biochemist with training under a Nobel Prize winning researcher at UCLA. He has written several books and is an expert in the mold remediation of homes. Dr. Rosen and his family are sensitive to mold toxins so he writes not only from professional experience, but also from personal experience.

Together, the two authors have certification in mold testing, mold remediation, and indoor environmental health. This book is one of the most complete on the subject, and includes discussion of the following topics:

- Potential mold problems encountered in new homes, schools, and jobs.
- Diagnosing mold illness.
- Mold as it relates to dryness and humidity.
- Mold toxins and cancer treatment.
- Mold toxins and relationships.
- Crawlspaces, basements, attics, home cleaning techniques, and vacuums.
- Training your eyes to discern indoor mold.
- Leptin and obesity.
- Appropriate/inappropriate air filters and cleaners.
- How to handle old, musty products, materials and books, and how to safely sterilize them.
- A description of various types of molds, images of them, and their relative toxicity.
- Blood testing and how to use it to find hidden health problems.
- The book is written in a friendly, casual tone that allows easy comprehension and information retention.

> "A concise, practical guide on dealing with mold toxins and their effects."
>
> **- Bryan Rosner**

Many people are affected by mold toxins. Are you? If you can find a smarter or clearer book on this subject, buy it!

Paperback book, 8.5 x 11", 140 pages, $32.95

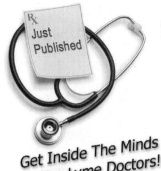

Just Published

13 Lyme Doctors Share Treatment Strategies!

In this new book, not one, but thirteen Lyme-literate healthcare practitioners describe the tools they use in their practices to heal patients from chronic Lyme disease. Never before available in book format!

Get Inside The Minds Of Top Lyme Doctors!

Insights Into Lyme Disease Treatment: 13 Lyme Literate Health Care Practitioners Share Their Healing Strategies

By Connie Strasheim

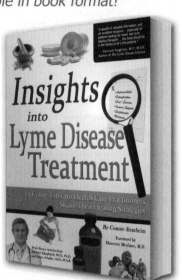

If you traveled the country for appointments with 13 Lyme-literate health care practitioners, you would discover many cutting-edge therapies used to combat chronic Lyme disease. You would also spend thousands of dollars on hotels, plane tickets, and medical appointment fees—not to mention the time it would take to embark on such a journey.

Even if you had the time and money to travel, would the physicians have enough time to answer all of your questions? Would you even know which questions to ask?

In this long-awaited book, health care journalist and Lyme patient Connie Strasheim

Paperback • 443 Pages • $39.95

has done all the work for you. She conducted intensive interviews with 13 of the world's most competent Lyme disease healers, asking them thoughtful, important questions, and then spent months compiling their information into 13 organized, user-friendly chapters that contain the core principles upon which they base their medical treatment of chronic Lyme disease. The practitioners' backgrounds span a variety of disciplines, including allopathic, naturopathic, complementary, chiropractic, homeopathic, and energy medicine. All aspects of treatment are covered, from anti-microbial remedies and immune system support, to hormonal restoration, detoxification, and dietary/lifestyle choices. **PHYSICIANS INTERVIEWED:**

- Steven Bock, M.D.
- Ginger Savely, DNP
- Ronald Whitmont, M.D.
- Nicola McFadzean, N.D.
- Jeffrey Morrison, M.D.
- Steven J. Harris, M.D.
- Peter J. Muran, M.D., M.B.A.

- Ingo D. E. Woitzel, M.D.
- Susan L. Marra, M.S., N.D.
- W. Lee Cowden, M.D., M.D. (H)
- Deborah Metzger, Ph.D., M.D.
- Marlene Kunold, "Heilpraktiker"
- Elizabeth Hesse-Sheehan, DC, CCN
- Visit our website to read a <u>FREE CHAPTER</u>!

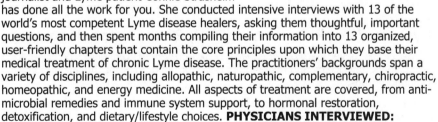

Paperback book, 7 x 10", 443 pages, $39.95
For all of our Lyme-related products, see: LymeBook.com

Dietrich Klinghardt, MD, PhD
"5 Levels of Healing"
5-DVD Set

15% off! Now only $125

Dietrich Klinghardt, MD, PhD, is legendary and known in almost all health circles for his innovative strategies for healing chronic disease, heavy metal toxicity, autism, cancer, and numerous other health conditions. This set includes his "Fundamental Teachings" series, with 5 DVDs:

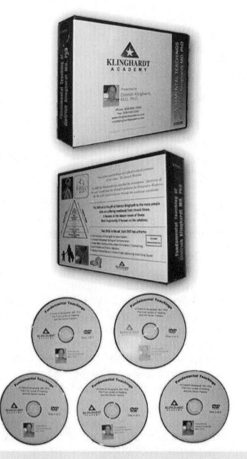

  • DISC 1: The Five Levels of Healing and the Seven Factors

  • DISC 2: Autonomic Response Testing and Demonstration

  • DISC 3: Heavy Metal Toxicity and Neurotoxin Elimination / Electrosmog

  • DISC 4: Lyme disease and Chronic Illness

  • DISC 5: Psycho-Emotional Issues in Chronic Illness & Addressing Underlying Causes

All 5 discs are included with your order.

5-DVD Set, $125 (15% off Suggested Retail Price)

Physicians' Desk Reference (PDR) Books (opposing page)

Most people have heard of *Physicians' Desk Reference* (PDR) books because, for over 60 years, physicians and researchers have turned to PDR for the latest word on prescription drugs.

You may not know that Thomson Healthcare, publisher of PDR, offers PDR reference books not only for drugs, but also for herbal and nutritional supplements. No available books come even close to the amount of information provided in these PDRs.

THOMSON™

We carry all three PDRs. For the supplements, herbs, and drugs included in the books, you will find the following information: Pharmacology, description and method of action, available trade names and brands, indications and usage, research summaries, dosage options, history of use, pharmacokinetics, and much more! See opposing page for information about each of the three PDRs.

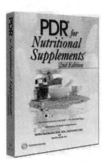

PDR for Nutritional Supplements *2ⁿᵈ Edition!*

This PDR focuses on the following types of supplements:

- Vitamins
- Minerals
- Amino acids
- Hormones
- Lipids
- Glyconutrients
- Probiotics
- Proteins
- Many more!

"In a part of the health field not known for its devotion to rigorous science, [this book] brings to the practitioner and the curious patient a wealth of hard facts."

- Roger Guillemin, M.D., Ph.D., Nobel Laureate in Physiology and Medicine

Book • $69.50

The book also suggests supplements that can help reduce prescription drug side effects, has full-color photographs of various popular commercial formulations (and contact information for the associated suppliers), and so much more! Become educated instead of guessing which supplements to take.

Hardcover book, 11 x 9.3", 800 pages, $69.50

PDR for Herbal Medicines *4ᵗʰ Edition!*

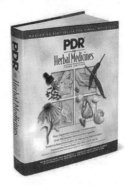

PDR for Herbal Medicines is very well organized and presents information on hundreds of common and uncommon herbs and herbal preparations. Indications and usage are examined with regard to homeopathy, Indian and Chinese medicine, and unproven (yet popular) applications.

In an area of healthcare so unstudied and vulnerable to hearsay and hype, this scientifically referenced book allows you to find out the real story behind the herbs lining the walls of your local health food store.

Use this reference before spending money on herbal products!

Book • $69.50

Hardcover book, 11 x 9.3", 1300 pages, $69.50

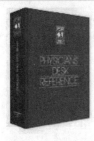

PDR for Prescription Drugs   *Current Year's Edition!*

With more than 3,000 pages, this is the most comprehensive and respected book in the world on over 4,000 drugs. Drugs are indexed by both brand and generic name (in the same convenient index) and also by manufacturer and product category. This PDR provides usage information and warnings, drug interactions, plus a detailed, full-color directory with descriptions and cross references for the drugs. A new format allows dramatically improved readability and easier access to the information you need now.

Book • $99.50

Hardcover book, 12.5 x 9.5", 3533 pages, $99.50

Renegade Patient: The No-Nonsense, Practical Guide to Getting the Health Care You Need
By Tedde Rinker, D.O.

Stop! Before you pick up the phone to make an appointment with your local cancer doctor, take a few deep breaths, and ask yourself: "Am I an empowered patient who knows what I need from my physician and how to get it? Am I in control of my health care, and if not, who is?"

Dr. Rinker, an experienced osteopathic physician practicing medicine in Redwood City, California, believes that all patients should become empowered and responsible, equipped with the necessary education and knowledge to navigate the maze of modern medical services. This book includes tools for dealing with all aspects of the medical industry, from insurance companies and physicians' offices to requesting your medical chart and monitoring treatment progress. **This is a hands-on workbook with document templates and forms that you can actually use.**

Book • $22.95

Above: Paperback book, 6x9", 245 pages, $22.95
Below: Hardcover book, 8.5x11", 730 pages, $99.95

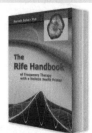

The Rife Handbook of Frequency Therapy, With a Holistic Health Primer, New Revised Edition!
By Nenah Sylver, PhD

This is the most complete, authoritative Rife technology handbook in the world. A hardcover book, it weighs over 2 lbs. and has more than 730 pages. A broad range of practical, hands-on topics are covered. This is the book to get if you want to learn as much as possible about Rife therapy in one place.

Book • $99.95

Easy Ordering: Toll Free (866) 476-7637
www.CancerBookSource.com/Store

Our website does not offer all of the products you see here in the catalog. If the product you want is missing from our website, call us to place your order. We offer wholesale pricing to bookstores, health food stores, and cancer support groups. We can also send you free product flyers or additional catalogs.

Do you have a book inside you? Submit your book proposal to:
bmpublish@gmail.com

Sign up for our newsletter at: www.cancerbooksource.com/newsletter

DISCLAIMER: Our materials are for informational and educational purposes only. They are not intended to prevent, diagnose, treat, or cure disease. These products are not intended to substitute for professional medical advice.

INDEX

F

P

X

Y

Z

W